a LANGE medical book

BASIC RADIOLOGY

2ND EDITION

Editors

Michael Y. M. Chen, MD
Associate Professor of Radiology
Department of Radiology
Wake Forest University School of Medicine
Winston-Salem, North Carolina

Thomas L. Pope, MD
Professor of Radiology
Department of Radiology and Radiologic Science
Medical University of South Carolina
Charleston, South Carolina

David J. Ott, MD
Professor of Radiology
Department of Radiology
Wake Forest University School of Medicine
Winston-Salem, North Carolina

D1710634

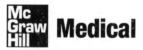
McGraw Hill **Medical**

New York   Chicago   San Francisco   Lisbon   London   Madrid   Mexico City
Milan   New Delhi   San Juan   Seoul   Singapore   Sydney   Toronto

Basic Radiology, Second Edition

1 2 3 4 5 6 7 8 9 0 DOC/DOC 14 13 12 11 10

ISBN 978-0-07-162708-5
MHID 0-07-162708-1

Notice

Medicine is an ever-changing science. As new research and clinical experience broaden our knowledge, changes in treatment and drug therapy are required. The authors and the publisher of this work have checked with sources believed to be reliable in their efforts to provide information that is complete and generally in accord with the standards accepted at the time of publication. However, in view of the possibility of human error or changes in medical sciences, neither the authors nor the publisher nor any other party who has been involved in the preparation or publication of this work warrants that the information contained herein is in every respect accurate or complete, and they disclaim all responsibility for any errors or omissions or for the results obtained from use of the information contained in this work. Readers are encouraged to confirm the information contained herein with other sources. For example and in particular, readers are advised to check the product information sheet included in the package of each drug they plan to administer to be certain that the information contained in this work is accurate and that changes have not been made in the recommended dose or in the contraindications for administration. This recommendation is of particular importance in connection with new or infrequently used drugs.

This book was set in Minion by Aptara, Inc.
The editors were Michael Weitz and Karen G. Edmonson.
The production supervisor was Phil Galea.
Project management was provided by Sandhya Joshi Aptara, Inc.
The designer was Alan Barnett.
The cover art director was Anthony Landi.
Cover images: *Left*, kidney (coronal reformat and volume rendered CT by terarecon technique; see Figure 9-7). *Middle*, brain (PASL, perfusion technique; see also Figure 12-5). *Right*, lower extremity (PET/CT; see Figure 6-36B).
RR Donnelley was printer and binder.

This book is printed on acid-free paper.

Library of Congress Cataloging-in-Publication Data

Basic radiology / editors, Michael Y.M. Chen, Thomas L. Pope, David J. Ott.—2nd ed.
    p. ; cm.
  Includes bibliographical references and index.
  ISBN-13: 978-0-07-162708-5 (alk. paper)
  ISBN-10: 0-07-162708-1 (alk. paper)
  1. Radiography, Medical.   2. Diagnostic imaging.   I. Chen, Michael Y. M.
  II. Pope, Thomas Lee.   III. Ott, David J. (David James), 1946-
  [DNLM:1. Diagnostic Imaging—methods.   WN 180 B311 2010]
  RC78.B34 2010
  616.07′54—dc22
                                              2010011952

To the memory of my mother
M.Y.M.C.
To Susan, Stephen, and the memory of my parents and father-in-law
D.J.O

Contents

Contributors

Joseph S. Ayoub, MD
Fellow, Department of Radiology, Baylor College of Medicine, Houston, Texas

Robert E. Bechtold, MD
Professor, Department of Radiology, Wake Forest University School of Medicine, Winston-Salem, North Carolina

Michelle S. Bradbury, MD, PhD
Assistant Attending Radiologist, Molecular Imaging & Neuroradiology Sections Department of Radiology, Memorial Sloan Kettering Cancer Center
Assistant Professor of Radiology, Weill Medical College of Cornell University, New York, New York

Melanie P. Caserta, MD
Assistant Professor, Department of Radiology, Wake Forest University School of Medicine, Winston-Salem, North Carolina

Fakhra Chaudhry, MD
Mecklenburg Radiology Associates, Charlotte, North Carolina

Michael Y. M. Chen, MD
Associate Professor, Department of Radiology, Wake Forest University School of Medicine, Winston-Salem, North Carolina

Caroline Chiles, MD
Professor, Department of Radiology, Wake Forest University School of Medicine, Winston-Salem, North Carolina

Robert L. Dixon, PhD
Professor, Department of Radiology, Wake Forest University School of Medicine, Winston-Salem, North Carolina

Rita I. Freimanis, MD
Associate Professor, Department of Radiology, Wake Forest University School of Medicine, Winston-Salem, North Carolina

Jud R. Gash, MD
Professor, Department of Radiology, University of Tennessee at Knoxville, Knoxville, Tennessee

Lawrence E. Ginsberg, MD
Professor of Radiology and Head and Neck Surgery, Department of Radiology, University of Texas, M. D. Anderson Cancer Center—Houston, Texas

Nandita Guha-Thakurta, MD
Assistant Professor, Diagnostic Radiology, Department of Radiology University of Texas, M. D. Anderson Cancer Center, Houston, Texas

Shannon M. Gulla, MD
Mid-South Imaging and Therapeutics, Memphis, Tennessee

Tamara Miner Haygood, MD, PhD
Assistant Professor, Department of Diagnostic Radiology, University of Texas, M. D. Anderson Cancer Center, Houston, Texas

Jacob Noe, MD
Chief Resident, Department of Radiology, University of Tennessee at Knoxville, Knoxville, Tennessee

David J. Ott, MD
Professor, Department of Radiology, Wake Forest University School of Medicine, Winston-Salem, North Carolina

Thomas L. Pope, MD
Professor, Department of Radiology and Radiologic Science, Medical University of South Carolina, Charleston, South Carolina

James G. Ravenel, MD
Professor, Chief of Thoracic Imaging, Department of Radiology and Radiologic Science, Medical University of South Carolina, Charleston, South Carolina

Mohamed M. H. Sayyouh, MD
Assistant Lecturer, Department of Radiology, National Cancer Institute, Cairo University, Egypt

Paul L. Wasserman, DO
Assistant Professor, Department of Radiology, Wake Forest University School of Medicine, Winston-Salem, North Carolina

Christopher T. Whitlow, MD, PhD
Fellow, Department of Radiology, Wake Forest University School of Medicine, Winston-Salem, North Carolina

Daniel W. Williams III, MD
Professor, Department of Radiology, Wake Forest University School of Medicine, Winston-Salem, North Carolina

Michael E. Zapadka, DO
Assistant Professor, Department of Radiology, Wake Forest University School of Medicine, Winston-Salem, North Carolina

Preface

The primary goal of this book was to create a concise text on current radiologic imaging for medical students and residents not specializing in radiology. After the first two introductory chapters, subsequent chapters employ an organ-system approach. Imaging techniques pertinent to the organ system, including their appropriate indications and use, are presented. Question-oriented exercises highlight the most commonly encountered diseases for each organ system.

The first chapter describes the various diagnostic imaging techniques that are available: conventional radiography, nuclear medicine, ultrasonography, computed tomography (CT), and magnetic resonance (MR) imaging. In recent years, many new techniques, such as CT angiography, CT colonography, MR angiography, MR cholangiopancreatography, and positron emission tomography (PET)/CT have emerged with new generations of CT and MR equipment. The second chapter gives an overview of the physics of radiation and its related biological effects, ultrasound, and magnetic resonance imaging. The remaining chapters focus on the individual organ systems of the heart, lungs, breast, bones, joints, abdomen, urinary tract, gastrointestinal tract, liver, biliary system, pancreas, brain, and spine. The chapters have a similar format to provide a consistent presentation. Each chapter briefly describes recent developments in the radiologic imaging of these organ systems. This is followed by a description of the normal anatomy and a discussion of the most appropriate and rational imaging techniques for evaluating each organ system. Each chapter stresses the proper selection of each imaging examination based on clinical presentation, need for patient preparation, and potential conflicts between techniques. Finally, all chapters end with questions and imaging exercises to enhance and reinforce the principles of each chapter. All exercises include numerous images and specific questions focusing on common diseases or symptoms. One question per case is used in all exercises, and the case and question numbers are matched for clarity. A short list of suggested readings and general references is included at the end of each chapter.

We hope that this book will help medical students and residents not specializing in radiology to better comprehend the basics of each imaging technique. Ideally, this book will also aid them in selecting and requesting the most appropriate imaging modality for each patient's presenting symptoms. Our further hope is that the interactive exercises presented will familiarize readers with the more common diseases that current radiologic imaging can best evaluate.

We wish to thank Allen D. Elster, MD, Director of the Division of Radiologic Sciences and Professor and Chairman of the Department of Radiology of the Wake Forest University School of Medicine, and C. Douglas Maynard, MD, now retired former Director of Division of Radiologic Sciences and Professor and Chairman of the Department of Radiology of the Wake Forest University School of Medicine, who have provided us with the supportive environment needed to complete this endeavor. This book would not have been possible without the able support of Michael Weitz, Karen Edmonson, Laura Libretti, and their fine associates at Lange Medical Books/McGraw-Hill.

Scope of Diagnostic Imaging

Michael Y. M. Chen, MD
Christopher T. Whitlow, MD, PhD

Conventional Radiography
  Contrast Studies
  Computed Tomography

Ultrasonography
Magnetic Resonance Imaging
Nuclear Medicine

For almost half a century following the discovery of x-rays by Roentgen in 1895, radiologic imaging was mainly based on plain and contrast-enhanced radiography. Those images were created by exposing film to an x-ray beam attenuated after penetrating the body. The production of x-rays and radiographic images is described in the next chapter. In the recent half century, diagnostic radiology has undergone dramatic changes and developments. Conventional angiography, nuclear medicine, ultrasonography, and computed tomography (CT) were developed between 1950 and 1970. Magnetic resonance (MR) imaging, interventional radiology, and positron emission tomography (PET) were developed later. Conventional radiology, including contrast-enhanced radiography and CT, uses ionizing radiation created from x-ray equipment. Nuclear medicine uses ionizing radiation that is emitted from injected or ingested radioactive pharmaceuticals in various parts of the body. Ultrasonography and MR imaging modalities use sound waves and magnetism, respectively, rather than ionizing radiation.

Radiologic subspecialties have been developed based on organ systems, modalities, and specific fields. Organ-oriented subspecialties of radiology include musculoskeletal, breast, neurologic, abdominal, thoracic, cardiac, gastrointestinal, and genitourinary imaging. Modality-oriented subspecialties comprise nuclear medicine, interventional, ultrasonography, and MR imaging. Specific field subspecialties include pediatric and women's imaging. Functional and metabolic imaging methods are now being used clinically, with genetic and molecular marker imaging expected in the future.

This chapter is intended to provide an overview of a variety of modalities in diagnostic radiology and basic knowledge regarding radiologic image-based diagnosis. Specific modality settings in each field and diagnostic interpretation for the use of these modalities in evaluating various organ systems are described in subsequent chapters.

CONVENTIONAL RADIOGRAPHY

Conventional radiography refers to plain radiographs that are generated when x-ray film is exposed to ionizing radiation and developed by photochemical process. During development, the metallic silver on the x-ray film is precipitated, rendering the latent image black. The amount of blackening on the film is proportional to the amount of x-ray radiation exposure. Plain radiography relies on natural and physical contrast based on the density of material through which the x-ray radiation must pass. Thus, gas, fat, soft tissue, and bone produce black, gray-black, gray, and white radiographic images, respectively, on film (Figure 1-1).

Although other image modalities such as CT, ultrasonography, and MR imaging are being used with increasing frequency to replace plain radiographs, conventional radiography remains a major modality in the evaluation of chest, breast, bone, and abdominal diseases.

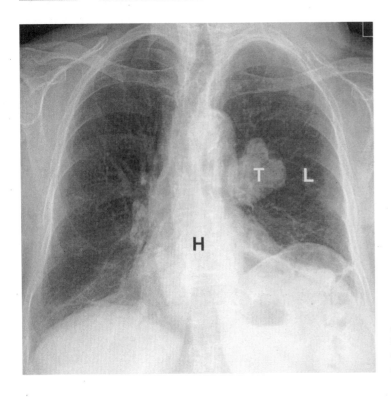

▲ **Figure 1-1.** Standard posteroanterior chest radiograph demonstrated the striking contrast between the heart (H) and lungs (L). A tumor (T) is seen at the left hilum.

Computed radiography (CR) or digital radiography is presently replacing conventional screen-film combination techniques. The most common CR technique, photostimulable phosphor computed radiography (PPCR), uses a phosphor-coated plate to replace the film-screen combination. When a cassette containing the phosphor-coated plate is exposed to x-rays, the phosphor stores the absorbed x-ray energy. The exposed cassette is then placed in a PPCR reader that uses a laser to stimulate release of electrons, resulting in the emission of short-wavelength blue light. The brightness of the blue light is dependent on the amount of absorbed x-ray photon energy. This luminescence generates an electrical signal that is reconstructed into a gray-scale image, which may be displayed on a monitor or printed as a hard copy. Digital images generated from PPCR are capable of being transmitted through a picture archiving and communications system (PACS), similar to other digital images acquired from CT or MR facilities. PPCR is better than plain radiography in linear response to a wide range of x-ray exposure. However, PPCR provides less spatial resolution than plain radiography. Another CR technique that is being developed uses an amorphous selenium-coated plate, which directly converts x-ray photons into electrical charges.

Fluoroscopy uses a fluorescent screen instead of radiographic film to view real-time images generated when an x-ray beam penetrates through a certain part of the body. An image intensifier absorbs x-ray photons and produces a quantity of light on the monitor. The brightness of the image is proportional to the number of incident photons received. Fluoroscopy is a major modality used to examine the gastrointestinal tract. For example, fluoroscopy can be used to follow the course of contrast materials through the gastrointestinal tract, allowing the evaluation of both structure and function. Spot filming or video recording may be used synchronously with fluoroscopy to optimally demonstrate pathology. Fluoroscopy is also used to monitor catheter placement during angiography and to guide interventional procedures. In recent years, digital detectors (such as charge-coupled devices, CCDs) have begun to replace video cameras on fluoroscopy units.

Conventional tomography produces an image of one intended area by blurring structures superimposed on both sides of a focus plane. This technique, however, has been largely replaced by CT.

Mammography uses a film-screen combination technique to evaluate breast lesions for the early detection of breast carcinoma. A mammographic unit is installed with a special x-ray tube and a plastic breast-compression device. A standard mammogram obtains views in two projections, producing craniocaudal (CC) and mediolateral oblique (MLO) images of the breast. Additional images of the breast in other projections, such as mediolateral (ML) views, and using diagnostic techniques such as magnification and/or spot compression views may also be obtained to further characterize potential pathologic findings. Ultrasonography (US) is also used in breast imaging as a complementary modality to further characterize breast pathology. Several image-guided breast interventional procedures, such as preoperative needle placement for lesion localization and core needle biopsy using stereotactic ultrasound or MR guidance, are widely available.

▶ Contrast Studies

Contrast materials are used to examine organs that do not have natural inherent contrast with surrounding tissues. Contrast media are commonly used to evaluate the gastrointestinal tract, the urinary tract, the vascular system, and solid organs. Contrast media used in MR imaging are described in the MR modality section.

Barium suspension is still used daily in the examination of the gastrointestinal tract. Barium suspension is a safe contrast media that provides high imaging density on upper gastrointestinal (UGI) series, small-bowel studies, and evaluation of the colon. Both single-contrast and double-contrast techniques may be used to evaluate the gastrointestinal tract (Figure 1-2). In the single-contrast study, barium suspension is administered alone. In the double-contrast study, both barium and air are introduced to delineate the details of the mucosal surface, which facilitates the identification of superficial lesions in the bowel lumen. In the UGI double-contrast study, air is introduced into the bowel lumen by administering oral effervescent agents. For double-contrast evaluation of the lower GI tract with barium enema, air is introduced into the bowel lumen via direct inflation with a small pump through a rectal catheter. Small-bowel contrast studies include peroral, enteroclysis, and retrograde techniques. The peroral small-bowel study is performed by feeding barium suspension to the patient and recording the progress of contrast through the small bowel. Enteroclysis is performed by placing a catheter in the proximal jejunum and infusing barium suspension through the catheter. Enteroclysis is preferred for evaluating focal small-bowel lesions or the cause of small-bowel obstructions. Retrograde small-bowel examination is performed by retrograde reflux of barium suspension into the small bowel during barium enema or via direct injection through an ileostomy.

Water-soluble contrast media are commonly used for angiography, interventional procedures, intravenous urography, and enhancement of CT. All water-soluble contrast media are iodinated agents that are classified as high or low osmolar, ionic or nonionic, and monomeric or dimeric in chemical nature. The iodine atoms in contrast medium absorb x-rays in proportion to the concentration in the body when radiographed. The most common water-soluble contrast

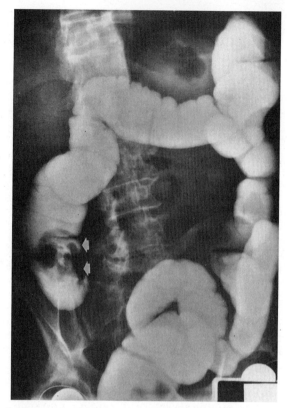

▲ **Figure 1-2.** A single-contrast retrograde colonic enema in the left posterior oblique view demonstrates an annular lesion representing a cecal carcinoma (arrows). Bilateral hip prostheses are an incidental observation.

media are the high osmolar ionic contrast agents (diatrizoate and its derivatives). Low osmolar contrast media include ionic (meglumine ioxaglate) and nonionic (iohexol, iopamidol, ioversol, iopromide) monomers, as well as nonionic dimers (iodixanol). Low osmolar contrast media have an overall lower incidence of adverse reactions, including nephrotoxicity and mortality, than high osmolar ionic agents; however, lower osmolar agents are also three to five times more expensive.

The occurrence and severity of adverse reactions after administration of iodinated contrast material are unpredictable. These reactions are categorized as mild, moderate, or severe based on degree of symptoms. Mild adverse reactions include nausea, vomiting, and urticaria that do not require treatment. The incidence of mild adverse reactions may be less if using a lower osmolality contrast agent. Moderate reactions include symptomatic urticaria, vasovagal events, mild bronchospasm, and/or tachycardia that requires treatment. Severe and life-threatening reactions, such as severe bronchospasm, laryngeal edema, seizure, severe hypotension, and/or cardiac arrest, are unpredictable and require prompt recognition and immediate treatment.

Contrast-induced nephropathy (CIN) is characterized by renal dysfunction after intravenous administration of iodinated contrast material. There is no standard definition of CIN. Findings with CIN include percent increasing serum creatinine from baseline (such as 20% to 50%) or increasing absolute serum creatinine above baseline (such as 0.5 to 2.0 mg/d) within 24 to 48 hours (or in 3 to 5 days). The incidence of CIN is variable. Patients with renal failure or underlying renal diseases are several times more likely to develop CIN than those with normal renal function following the administration of iodinated contrast material.

Water-soluble contrast agents are used in the gastrointestinal tract when barium suspension is contraindicated, when perforation is suspected, when surgery is likely to follow imaging, when confirmation of percutaneous catheter location is necessary, and when gastrointestinal opacification is required during abdominal CT evaluation. Unlike barium suspension, water-soluble contrast agents are readily absorbed by the peritoneum if extraluminal extravasation occurs, but provide less image density. High osmolar water-soluble contrast agents may cause severe pulmonary edema if aspirated. High osmolar contrast agents may also cause fluid to shift from the intravascular compartment into the bowel lumen, resulting in hypovolemia and hypotension, which is less likely to occur with low osmolar water-soluble contrast media.

Intravenous urography (IVU) uses ionic or nonionic water-soluble contrast agents to evaluate the urinary tract. Renal excretion/concentration of intravenously administered iodinated contrast material opacifies the kidneys, ureters, and bladder approximately 10 minutes postinjection. Intravenous urography has been largely replaced over the past decade by unenhanced helical CT evaluation. IVU, however, remains useful for the evaluation of subtle uroepithelial neoplasms and other diseases of the renal collecting system, and it can provide additional information that complements data from cross-sectional image modalities. Additional contrast-enhanced imaging examinations of the genitourinary system include cystography, voiding cystourethrography, and retrograde urethrography to evaluate the bladder and urethra.

Hysterosalpingography is primarily used to evaluate the patency of fallopian tubes and uterine abnormalities in patients with infertility. Hysterosalpingography is also used for postsurgical evaluation and to define anatomy for reanastomosis procedures.

Hysterosalpingography is performed by inserting a catheter into the uterus and subsequently injecting water-soluble contrast medium (some institutions prefer oil-based iodine contrast) to delineate the uterine cavity and the patency of the fallopian tubes. A fluoroscopic spot image is taken once contrast medium fills the uterus and fallopian tubes, but before spillage into the peritoneum. A second image is taken

after fallopian tube spillage appears. A transcervical recanalization of obstructed fallopian tube has been introduced to improve the fertility rate.

Angiography is the study of blood vessels following intra-arterial or intravenous injection of water-soluble contrast agents. A series of rapid exposures is made to follow the course of the contrast medium through the examined blood vessels. Angiographic images are recorded by standard or digital imaging, and/or stored digitally.

Thoracic aortography is performed when there is suspicion of traumatic aortic injury, dissection (Figure 1-3), or atherosclerotic aneurysm, and to evaluate cerebral and upper extremity vascular disease. Multidetector CT has largely replaced conventional aortography as the initial modality to evaluate aortic trauma (Figure 1-4). Conventional aortography, however, remains important in specific settings, such as planning endovascular stent graft therapy and assessing small branch vessel injuries in stable patients. Abdominal aortography is used to evaluate vessel origins in vascular occlusive disease or prior to selective catheterization. Abdominal aortography is also used for vascular mapping prior to aneurysm repair or other intra-abdominal surgery. Coronary angiography is most commonly performed to evaluate coronary occlusion. Pulmonary angiography is used in patients who are suspected of having pulmonary embolus, especially in the setting of equivocal results on ventilation-perfusion imaging. Inferior venacavography is performed to evaluate for caval occlusion from venous thrombosis, obstruction or compression by retroperitoneal lymphadenopathy, or fibrosis. Inferior venacavography is also performed to evaluate the configuration of the inferior vena cava before filter placement. In recent years, conventional angiography has been replaced by CT angiography and MR angiography.

Less commonly used contrast studies include myelography (evaluating disk herniation and spinal cord compression), fistulography (sinus tracts for abscesses and cavities), sialography (evaluating the salivary glands for ductal obstruction or tumor), galactography (assessing the breast ductal system), and oral cholecystography, cholangiography (evaluating the biliary tree), and lymphangiography (assessing lymph nodes and lymph channels for malignancies).

▶ Computed Tomography

Computed tomography, an axial tomographic technique, produces source images that are perpendicular to the long axis of the body (Figure 1-5). Attenuation values generated by CT reflect the density and atomic number of various tissues and are usually expressed as relative attenuation coefficients, or Hounsfield units (HUs). By definition, the HUs of water and air are zero and −1,000, respectively. The HUs of soft tissues range from 10 to 50, with fat demonstrating negative HU. Bone is at least 1,000 HU. The contrast resolution of vascular structures, organs, and pathology, such as

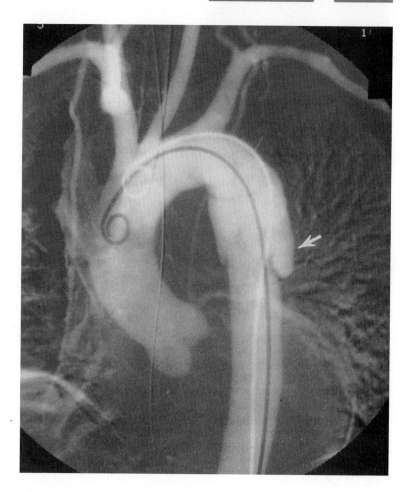

▲ **Figure 1-3.** An aortogram demonstrated transection (arrow) of the aortic arch at the aortic isthmus extending about 4 cm below.

hypervascular neoplasms, can be enhanced following intravenous infusion of water-soluble contrast media. The type, volume, and rate of administration as well as the scan delay time vary with specific study indication and protocol. Additionally, oral contrast material, namely, water-soluble agents or barium suspensions, can be administered for improved bowel visualization. Artifacts may be produced by patient motion or high-density foreign bodies, such as surgical clips.

Variety Scanners

Conventional CT scanners have traditionally operated in a step-and-shoot mode, defined by data acquisition and patient positioning phases. During the data acquisition phase, the x-ray tube rotates around the patient, who is maintained in a stationary position. A complete set of projections are acquired at a prescribed scanning location prior to the patient positioning phase. During this latter phase, the patient is transported to the next prescribed scanning location.

The first helical (spiral) CT scanner was introduced for clinical applications in the early 1990s. Helical CT is characterized by continuous patient transport through the gantry while a series of x-ray tube rotations simultaneously acquire volumetric data. These dynamic acquisitions are typically obtained during a single breath hold of about 20 to 30 seconds. Higher spatial resolution can be achieved with narrower collimations. The advantages of helical CT technology include reduced scan times, improved speeds at which the volume of interest can be adequately imaged, and increased ability to detect small lesions that may otherwise change position in non-breath-hold studies. In addition, gains in scan speed permit less contrast material to be administered for the same degree of vessel opacification.

The evolution of multidetector CT (MDCT) scanners has resulted from the combination of helical scanning with multi-slice data acquisition. In this CT system, a multiple-row detector array is employed. Current state-of-the-art models are capable of acquiring 64, 128, or 256 channels of helical data

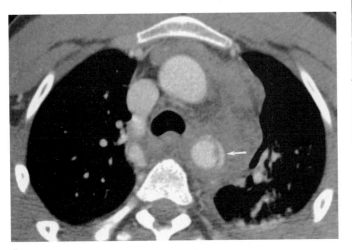
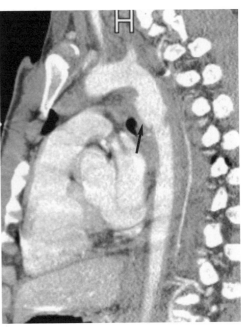

A   **B**

▲ **Figure 1-4.** Axial (**A**) and sagittal (**B**) view of CT angiography (CTA) on a patient with a motor vehicle accident showing aortic transection (arrow) at the level of the ductus arteriosus with a surrounding mediastinal hematoma that extends superiorly along the aorta.

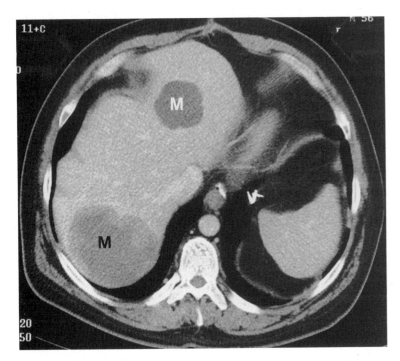

▲ **Figure 1-5.** Contrast-enhanced CT image of the upper abdomen demonstrated two low-attenuation areas (M) confirmed as multiple hepatic metastases from a gastrointestinal stromal tumor.

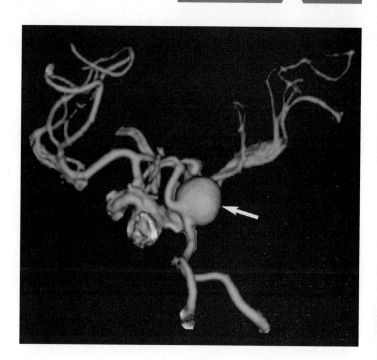

▲ Figure 1-6. 3D reformatted image from CT angiography of brain shows a 16-mm aneurysm (arrow) arising from the left lateral aspect of the mid basilar artery.

simultaneously. For a given length of anatomic coverage, multidetector CT can reduce scan time, permit imaging with thinner collimation, or both. The use of thinner collimation (0.4 mm to 2 mm) in conjunction with high-resolution reconstruction algorithms yields images of higher spatial resolution (high-resolution CT), a technique commonly used for evaluation of diffuse interstitial lung disease or the detection of pulmonary nodules. Multidetector CT offers additional advantages of decreased contrast load, reduced respiratory and cardiac motion artifact, and enhanced multiplanar reconstruction capabilities. These innovations have had a significant impact on the development of CT angiography (CTA). Multidetector CT has replaced conventional angiography as a primary modality in patients with acute aortic injuries.

CT Angiography

CT angiography protocols combine high-resolution volumetric helical CT acquisitions with intravenous bolus administration of iodinated contrast material. Using an MDCT scanner, images are acquired during a single breath hold, ensuring that data acquisition will commence during times of peak vascular opacification. This has permitted successful imaging of entire vascular distributions, in addition to minimizing motion artifact and increasing longitudinal spatial resolution, thus potentially lowering administered contrast doses. The time between the start of contrast injection and the commencement of scanning can be tailored in response to a particular clinical question, permitting image acquisition

during the arterial, venous, and/or equilibrium phases. Exquisite anatomic detail of both intraluminal and extraluminal structures is revealed using this technique, including detection of intimal calcification and mural thrombosis. CT angiography has become an important tool for assessment of the abdominal and iliac arteries and their branches, the thoracic aorta, pulmonary arteries, and intracranial and extracranial carotid circulation (Figure 1-6).

CT Colonography

CT colonography (virtual colonoscopy), introduced in 1994, is a relatively new noninvasive method of imaging the colon in which thin-section helical CT data are used to generate two-dimensional or three-dimensional images of the colon. This technology has been used primarily in the detection and characterization of colonic polyps, rivaling the traditional colonoscopic approach and conventional barium enema examinations. These images display the mucosal surface of the colon and internal density of the detected lesions, as well as directly demonstrating the bowel wall and extracolonic abdominal/pelvic structures.

ULTRASONOGRAPHY

Diagnostic ultrasound is a noninvasive imaging technique that uses high-frequency sound waves greater than 20 kilohertz (kHz). A device known as a *transducer* is used to emit and to receive sound waves from various tissues in the body.

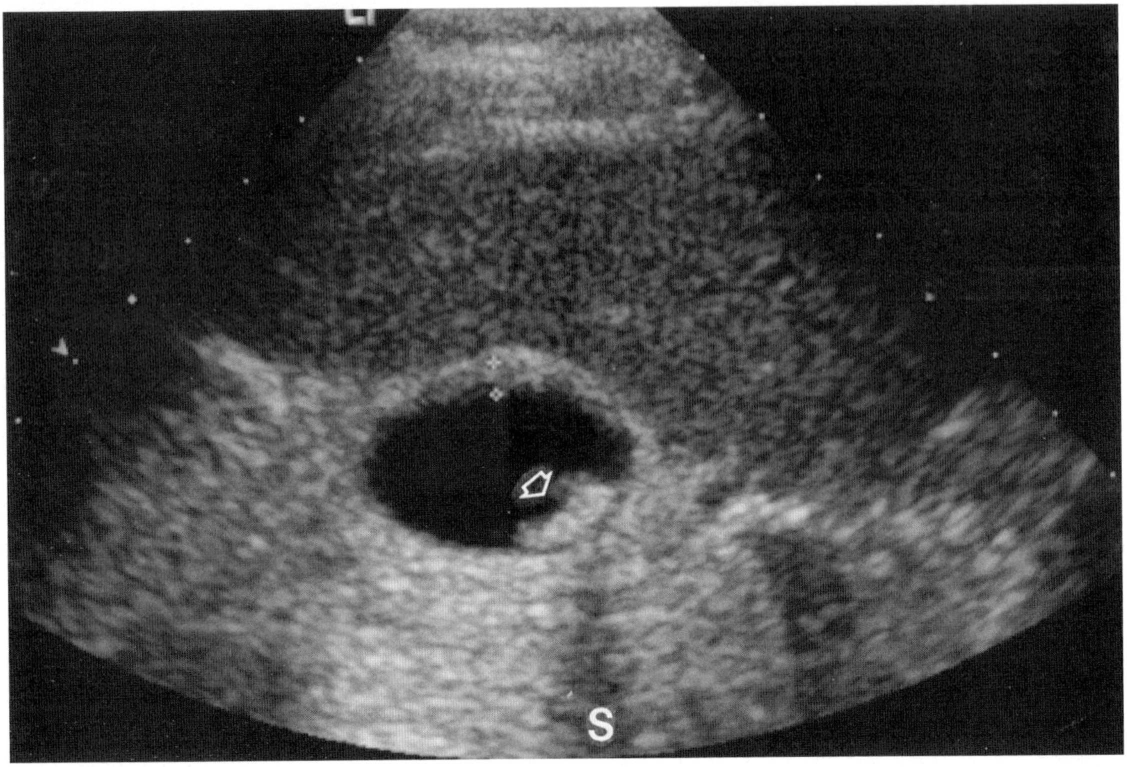

▲ **Figure 1-7.** A transverse ultrasound image of the gallbladder demonstrates a gallstone (arrow) with the characteristic distal acoustic shadowing (S) because sound waves cannot penetrate the gallstone.

The transducer is placed against the patient's skin with a thin layer of coupling gel. This gel displaces the air that would otherwise reflect virtually the entire incident ultrasound beam. As sound travels into the patient, wave fronts spread out, diminishing the overall beam intensity. Beam attenuation also occurs secondary to partial tissue absorption with associated heat conversion. At tissue interfaces, the beam is partially reflected and transmitted. The reflected sound waves, or echoes, travel back to the transducer and are converted into electric signals and amplified. The amplitude of the returning wave partially depends on the degree of beam absorption. A shade of gray is then assigned to each amplitude, with strong echoes being typically assigned a shade near the white end of the spectrum, and weak echoes assigned a shade near the black end of the spectrum. In addition, the depth of the reflecting tissue can be calculated from the known total beam travel time and the average sound velocity in human tissue (1,540 m/s). Limitations of this modality are primarily operator-dependent in nature. Additional limitations include variable visualization of midline abdominal organs (pancreas) and vasculature when obscured by overlying bowel gas, as well as inability of sound waves to penetrate gas or bone.

There are many common applications of ultrasonography, including imaging of the abdomen (liver, gallbladder, pancreas, kidneys) (Figure 1-7), pelvis (female reproductive organs), fetus (routine fetal surveys for detection of anomalies), vascular system (aneurysms, arterial-venous communications, deep venous thrombosis), testicles (tumor, torsion, infection), breasts, pediatric brain (hemorrhage, congenital malformations), and chest (size and location of pleural fluid collections). In addition, ultrasound-guided interventions are routinely used to facilitate lesion biopsy, abscess drainage, and radiofrequency ablation.

Doppler ultrasound is used primarily to evaluate vascular flow by detecting frequency shifts in the reflected beam, utilizing a principle termed the *Doppler effect*. This effect occurs when a sound emitter or reflector is moving relative to the stationary receiver of sound. Objects moving toward the detector appear to have a higher frequency and shorter wavelength, whereas objects moving away from the detector appear to have a lower frequency and longer wavelength. If the ultrasound beam strikes a reflector moving toward it, the reflected sound will have a higher frequency than the original beam. Alternatively, if the ultrasound beam strikes a reflector moving away from it, the reflected sound will have a lower frequency than the original beam. The Doppler shift is the frequency difference between the original beam frequency and the reflected beam frequency. Frequency differences are used to calculate the corresponding flow velocities, from which a Doppler waveform, or tracing, can be generated. This tracing depicts the relationship between velocity and time and is unique to the flow pattern within the vessel. Color flow Doppler assigns colors (blue and red) to structures according to their motion toward or away from transducers. This information can be superimposed on a gray-scale image. Endoluminal sonography uses a high-frequency catheter-based transducer (9 to 20 megahertz [MHz]) to image structures beyond the lumen of the hollow viscus. It is accurate in local staging of cancer and in detecting small lesions that may not be visualized with other imaging modalities. Limitations for optimal evaluation include inability to precisely position the transducer within an area of interest that may restrict full entry.

Diverse applications of ultrasonography are presented as follows. Gastrointestinal (GI) applications of endoluminal sonography include quantification of the size and wall thickness of esophageal carcinoma or to detect and characterize esophageal varices. Transrectal ultrasound is performed to evaluate the prostate gland. Transesophageal echocardiography is used for evaluating cardiovascular abnormalities. Genitourinary (GU) applications include guidance of collagen injections, examination of the severity and length of ureteral strictures, diagnosis of upper-tract neoplasms and urethral diverticula, identification of submucosal calculi, and visualization of crossing vessels prior to endopyelotomy. Evaluation of the uterus, adnexa, and fetus can be conducted using a transvaginal probe in the presence of an empty bladder. Sonohysterography, an ultrasound-guided procedure, requires instillation of a sterile saline solution into the uterine cavity following cannulation for evaluation of endometrial masses or other abnormalities. More recently, intravascular application of sonography has been promising for quantitating the degree of arterial stenosis, and for monitoring the therapeutic effects of angioplasty in both peripheral and coronary arteries. Intravascular ultrasound (IVUS) has been applied to modeling plaque morphology, blood flow, and the geometry of the vessel lumen. Three-dimensional ultrasound (3D-US) has been developed with advancements in computer processing power and has rapidly achieved widespread use for some clinical applications, including the evaluation of normal embryonic and/or fetal development, as well as cardiac morphology in specific congenital anomalies.

MAGNETIC RESONANCE IMAGING

In 1952, Felix Bloch and Edward Purcell were awarded the Nobel Prize for their independent discovery of the magnetic resonance phenomenon in 1946. Between 1950 and 1970, nuclear magnetic resonance (NMR) was developed and used for chemical and physical molecular analysis. In 1971, Raymond Damadian demonstrated that NMR had utility in cancer diagnosis, based on prolonged relaxation times in pathologic tissue. The first 2D proton NMR image of a water sample was generated in 1972 by Paul Lauterbur using a back-projection technique, similar to that used in CT. In 1975, Richard Ernst used phase and frequency encoding, as well as Fourier transform analysis, to form the basis of current magnetic resonance imaging (MRI) techniques. All of these experiments used defined, nonuniform magnetic fields or linear variations in field strength along all coordinate axes. The application of these nonuniform fields (magnetic field gradients) permitted discrimination of various signals from different spatial locations. In MR imaging, a pulsed radiofrequency (rf) beam is used in the presence of a strong main magnetic field to generate high-quality images of the body. These images can be acquired in virtually any plane, although sagittal, coronal, and axial images are commonly obtained.

Although a detailed explanation is beyond the scope of this chapter, substances (eg, fluid) that have a long Tl will appear dark on Tl-weighted images, whereas those with short Tl (fat) will display high signal intensity. On T2-weighted images, a long-T2 substance (fluid) will appear bright. Advantages of MR imaging include superb contrast resolution, high spatial resolution, and lack of ionizing radiation.

The most commonly used clinically approved contrast agents for MR imaging are gadolinium-based compounds that produce T1 shortening. Tissue relaxation results from interactions between the unpaired electron of gadolinium and tissue hydrogen protons, which significantly decrease the T1 of the blood relative to the surrounding tissues. Adverse reactions to this agent are far less frequent than those seen with iodinated compounds, with common reactions including nausea, vomiting, headache, paresthesias, or dizziness.

Hydrogen nuclei are favored for MR imaging. On placement of a patient in an MR scanner, the randomly oriented hydrogen nuclei align with the static magnetic field. In order to detect a signal, a perturbing rf pulse is transiently applied to the patient, resulting in a net change in alignment of these nuclei. When the rf pulse is turned off, the spins return to their equilibrium state by dissipating energy to the surrounding molecules. The rate of energy loss is mediated by the intrinsic relaxation properties of the tissue, designated as the longitudinal (T1) and transverse (T2) relaxation times. T1 represents the restoration of the longitudinal magnetization along the axis of the main magnetic field, whereas T2 represents the decay time of the magnetization in the transverse plane.

Technical advances in gradient hardware have resulted in faster and stronger gradients that permit subsecond image scan times. Newer pulse sequences have been developed that currently augment conventional MR pulse sequences (spin echo and gradient echo), increasing the sensitivity of clinical studies to disease detection. These rapid imaging techniques offer major advantages over conventional MR imaging, including decreased image acquisition times, minimized patient discomfort, and increased ability to image physiologic processes in the body. In addition, single-breath-hold scanning can be performed, reducing respiratory artifact.

Fast spin echo, fast gradient echo, diffusion imaging, perfusion imaging, and echo planar imaging (EPI) are examples of fast imaging techniques that can be performed on clinical scanners. Diffusion-weighted imaging is exquisitely sensitive to the microscopic molecular motion of water, demonstrating areas of limited (restricted) intracellular diffusion following an acute ischemic event. This sequence is utilized routinely in clinical neuroimaging protocols but is somewhat nonspecific for pathology, as diffusion changes that are characteristic of acute ischemia can be observed with infection and some tumors. Perfusion-weighted MRI, a less frequently used technique, provides information about the blood supply to a particular area of the brain following rapid bolus injection of gadolinium-based contrast agent. Echo planar imaging allows the collection of all data required for image reconstruction in a fraction of a second, after a single rf pulse. This technology has resulted in significant clinical and scientific advances, such as in stroke evaluation and functional brain imaging, respectively. Functional MRI studies of the human brain using EPI techniques have allowed physiological investigations of the functional organization of the brain.

MR angiography includes contrast-enhanced MR angiography and non-contrast-enhanced MR angiography. Three-dimensional contrast-enhanced magnetic resonance angiography (MRA) is used for noninvasive assessment of many vascular abnormalities, including aneurysms, dissection, vessel anomalies, and coarctation. It has evolved from the use of fast scanning techniques on high-gradient-strength units, in combination with contrast. Using this technique, volumetric acquisitions can be performed in a single breath hold. Improvements in contrast resolution are achieved, regardless of the plane of acquisition. This has allowed reductions in the number of image sections needed to display a large vascular territory, as well as overall imaging acquisition times. Multiphase dynamic imaging is usually performed after intravenous gadolinium administration, with the arteries best seen during the early phase and veins during the later phases. Noncontrast MRA methods, such as 3D time-of-flight (TOF) MR, is used to evaluate intracranial arterial (Figure 1-8) and carotid arteries. In addition, 2D TOF MR imaging is used to evaluate peripheral vascular diseases.

Clinical Applications

MRI has traditionally been used for neurologic indications, including brain tumors (Figure 1-9), acute ischemia, infection, and congenital abnormalities. MRI has been used for a number of nonneurologic indications, namely, spine, musculoskeletal (MSK), cardiac, hepatic, biliary, pancreatic, adrenal, renal, breast, and female pelvic imaging. Spine MR studies are useful for evaluating degenerative changes, disk herniation, infection, metastatic disease, and congenital abnormalities. Common MSK applications involve imaging of

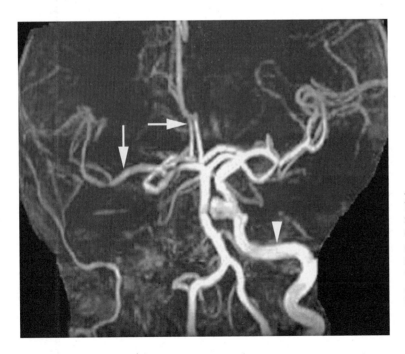

▲ **Figure 1-8.** 3D reformatted image from noncontrast MR angiography shows absent signal in the right internal carotid artery (ICA), indicating complete occlusion of the right ICA or a high-grade stenosis with extremely slow blood flow. Flow in the right anterior and middle cerebral arteries (arrows) is supplied by a small anterior or posterior communicating artery. (Arrowhead: left internal carotid artery.)

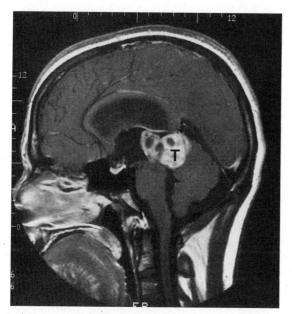

▲ **Figure 1-9.** A midline sagittal T1-weighted contrast-enhanced MR image depicts a large tumor (T) in the region of the pineal gland.

large joints, such as knee, shoulder, and hip. The primary common indication for MRI of the knee is the assessment of menisci and ligaments following internal derangement. Rotator cuff tear is a typical shoulder indication. Cardiac studies are performed to identify complex malformations, cardiac function, myocardiac viability, valvular disease, myocardial perfusion, and congenital heart disease. In the abdomen, hepatic MRI studies are often used to diagnose atypical presentations of liver lesions, metastatic disease, and hepatocellular carcinoma. Adrenal studies are performed primarily to distinguish adrenal adenomas from metastatic disease. Atypical renal masses, found incidentally on US or CT, can often be better characterized on MRI. In addition, renal MRI is used to establish the presence and extent of tumor thrombus in cases of renal-cell carcinoma for tumor staging purposes. Breast MRI is utilized to stage cancer, to screen patients at high risk, to look for unknown primary cancer in patients with positive axillary nodes, for delineation of residual cancer after chemotherapy, and sometimes for patients with equivocal mammographic and/or US findings. Finally, oncologic applications in the female pelvis include the diagnosis and characterization of cervical and endometrial carcinomas, as well as adnexal lesions. MR enterography is used in the evaluation of small-bowel disease (Figure 1-10).

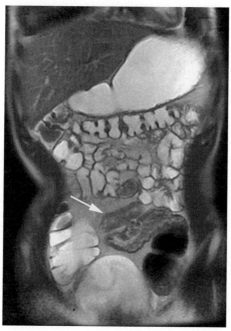

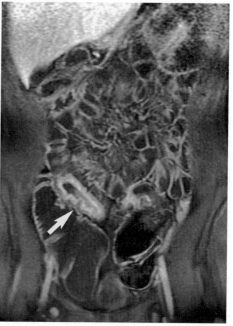

A   **B**

▲ **Figure 1-10.** MR enterography on a patient with Crohn disease. **A.** Coronal T2-weighted image shows wall thickening and stenotic ileum (arrow). **B.** Coronal gadolinium-enhanced fat suppressed T1-weighted image shows increased contrast enhancement of one thickened segment of ileum (arrow).

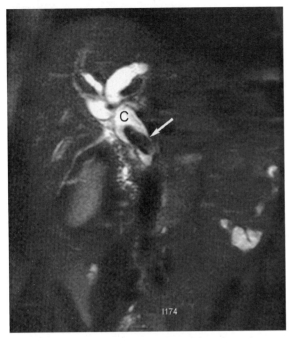

▲ **Figure 1-11.** An unenhanced MRI of the upper abdomen consisting of MRCP sequences showing the dilated common bile duct (C). Within the common bile duct, there is an ovoid filling defect (arrow) measuring 3.8 × 1.7 cm in the coronal plane, indicating a biliary calculus. The intrahepatic and extrahepatic biliary ducts are markedly dilated.

Magnetic Resonance Cholangiopancreatography

Magnetic resonance cholangiopancreatography (MRCP) is used to evaluate choledocholithiasis, retained gallstones, pancreatobiliary neoplasms, strictures, primary sclerosing cholangitis, and chronic pancreatitis (Figure 1-11). This noncontrast technique relies on the relatively stationary nature of bile (compared with blood) to depict the predominantly fluid-filled pancreatic ducts and biliary tree. Rapid heavily T2-weighted breath-hold sequences are utilized, resulting in visualization of high signal-intensity ductal structures. In patients who have failed endoscopic retrograde cholangiopancreatography (ERCP), or who are unable to tolerate this procedure, MRCP has become a suitable alternative. MRCP is particularly useful in postoperative patients, patients with biliary system anomalies, and as a screening tool in patients with an otherwise low probability of a biliary abnormality. ERCP is generally reserved for therapeutic purposes, such as stent placement, stone extraction, or stricture dilatation.

Nephrogenic Systemic Fibrosis

Since 2006, it has been reported that the administration of gadolinium-based contrast agents for MR imaging is associated with the development of nephrogenic systemic fibrosis (NSF) in some patients with renal insufficiency. Although NSF was first reported in 1997, the exact cause of development of NSF remains unknown. The dissociation of gadolinium ion from the chelating ligand recently has been proposed as an etiologic factor in the development of NSF. The incident of NSF ranges from 0.003% to 0.039% depending on the report cited. The incidence of NSF may increase to 1% to 7% in patients with severe chronic kidney disease following exposure to gadolinium-based contrast media. All patients in published case reports developed NSF within 6 months following administration of gadolinium-based contrast agent. The majority of patients with renal insufficiency in these published reports, however, did not develop NSF following administration of gadolinium chelates. The development of NSF following the administration of a gadolinium chelate contrast has been reported to be particularly associated with patients who have acute or chronic renal disease with a glomerular filtration rate (GFR) lower than 30 mL/min/1.73 m^2, and in those with acute renal insufficiency. The estimated GFR was calculated by using the patient's age, weight, and race and serum creatinine level. Some risk factors, such as concurrent proinflammatory conditions, metabolic conditions including acidosis and high calcium-phosphate products, or concurrent tissue injury, surgery, and ischemia, are associated with the development of NSF in patients who underwent gadolinium-based contrast MR imaging.

In 2007, the US Food and Drug Administration (FDA) requested that a warning be added to all five FDA-approved gadolinium-based contrast agents regarding the potential risk of NSF in patients with renal failure. These five FDA-approved products include gadodiamide (Omniscan, GE Healthcare, Oslo, Norway), gadopentetate dimeglumine (Magnevist, Bayer Healthcare, Wayne, NJ), gadobenate dimeglumine (MultiHance, Bracco Diagnostics, Princeton, NJ), gadoteridol (ProHance, Bracco Diagnostics, Princeton, NJ), and gadoversetamide (OptiMARK, Tyco-Mallinckrodt, St Louis, MO). One recent recommendation aimed at decreasing the risk of NSF has been to use 0.1 mmol/kg of gadolinium contrast for patients with GFR lower than 30 mL/min. If a patient is in a dialysis program, some experts believe that it may be prudent to dialyze after administration of gadolinium-based contrast agent. Alternative imaging examinations, such as arterial spin-labeling perfusion MRI, may replace administration of gadolinium for some.

MR imaging is contraindicated for patients with metal implants or foreign bodies, such as intracranial aneurysm clips, intraorbital metallic foci, cardiac pacemakers, or specific types of cardiac valves. In these instances, these objects may be dislodged or damaged by the magnetic field. MR imaging may also be contraindicated for claustrophobic or uncooperative patients who may not respond to conscious sedation protocols.

NUCLEAR MEDICINE

Nuclear medicine studies, in general, are very sensitive, but relatively nonspecific in the detection of pathology. It is very important, therefore, to correlate nuclear medicine examinations with pertinent history, physical findings, laboratory data, and other diagnostic imaging studies in order to optimize the diagnostic utility of these studies. Nuclear medicine imaging examinations are performed by administering various radiopharmaceuticals to the patient and subsequently recording in vivo distribution. Radiopharmaceuticals consist of two main components: (1) the main component that is distributed to various organs via a number of different mechanisms, and (2) the radionuclide that is tagged to the main component, which emits gamma rays, permitting detection of the compound in the body.

Most nuclear medicine studies are performed with gamma cameras, which provide planar (2D) images. Single photon emission computed tomography (SPECT) is a special technique that creates tomographic images using a rotating gamma camera system. Positron emission tomography (PET) is another unique technique that creates tomographic images by detecting gamma rays produced when positrons interact with electrons.

Some common nuclear medicine procedures include (1) cardiac studies to evaluate myocardial perfusion and/or ventricular function; (2) skeletal studies to evaluate for early bony metastases (Figure 1-12), skeletal trauma, osteomyelitis, and primary bone neoplasms; (3) renograms and renal scans to evaluate kidney function and morphology; (4) ventilation-perfusion studies to evaluate for suspected pulmonary emboli; and (5) PET studies to diagnose or stage tumors (eg, lung, lymphoma, melanoma, colorectal, breast), evaluate dementia, monitor for brain tumor recurrence, track post-therapy changes, and evaluate myocardial viability.

Less common nuclear medicine studies include (1) thyroid evaluation of nodules and therapy for hyperthyroidism and thyroid cancer; (2) hepatobiliary studies to evaluate for acute cholecystitis and bile duct patency; (3) brain imaging to evaluate dementia and brain death; (4) white blood cell studies to detect infection and inflammation; (5) gastrointestinal bleeding studies to detect and localize small gastrointestinal bleeds; (6) lymphoscintigraphy to identify sentinel lymph nodes for surgery; and (7) parathyroid studies to identify adenomas and hyperplasia.

Positron Emission Tomography/CT (PET/CT)

Positron emission tomography (PET) with fluorine (^{18}F) fluorodeoxyglucose (FDG) is a functional imaging method that plays an important role in the diagnosis and staging of malignancy, as well as in treatment monitoring. CT is an anatomic imaging modality that provides excellent spatial localization of pathology. The first combined PET/CT scanner was in operation in 2001. Combined PET/CT

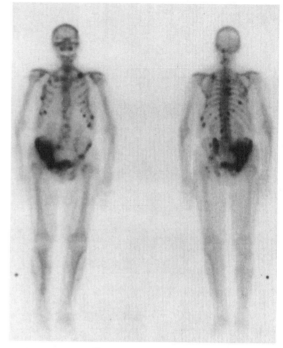

▲ **Figure 1-12.** A ^{99m}Tc-MDP bone scan in the anterior and posterior projections demonstrates multiple foci of increased radiopharmaceutical accumulation (spine, ribs, pelvis, and left clavicle) with the typical appearance of bone metastases.

scanners have separate individual imaging components that reside in the same unit. In general, a CT scan is performed first and the PET scan follows. Output from PET/CT imaging includes separate CT and PET images, as well as the coregistered fused images that overlay the anatomic CT and metabolic data. The combined anatomic and functional images can be acquired in a single examination. The use of CT images for attenuation correction of the PET emission data also significantly reduce PET scan time. The combined PET/CT is more sensitive and specific for detecting otherwise occult malignancy, tumor staging, and detecting disease recurrence and/or metastasis. PET/CT has also proven useful for following post-therapy changes, such as squamous-cell carcinoma of the head and neck. Fused PET/CT images consistently outperform separately collected CT and PET images for the detection of pathology, even when the separate nonfused imagines are viewed simultaneously.

Acknowledgments *Special thanks to my colleagues, Drs. John Leyendecker, MC, and Caroline Chiles, MD, for providing me with the CT and MR images used in this chapter.*

SUGGESTED READING

1. McAdams HP, Samei E, Dobbins J III, Tourassi GD, Ravin CE. Recent advances in chest radiography. *Radiology*. 2006;241: 663-683.

2. Rubesin SE, Levine MS, Laufer I. Double-contrast upper gastrointestinal radiograph: a pattern approach for diseases of the stomach. *Radiology*. 2008;246:33-48.

3. Steenburg SD, Ravenel JG. Acute traumatic thoracic aortic injuries: experience with 64-MDCT. *AJR Am J Roentgenol*. 2008; 191:1564-1569.

4. Nandalur KR, Hussain HK, Weadock WJ, et al. Possible biliary disease: diagnostic performance of high-spatial resolution isotropic 3D T2-weighted MRCP. *Radiology*. 2008;249:883-890.

5. Maccioni F, Bruni A, Viscido A, et al. MR imaging in patients with Crohn disease: value of T2- versus T1-weighted gadolinium-enhanced MR sequences with use of an oral superparamagnetic contrast agents. *Radiology*. 2006;238:517-530.

6. Prince MR, Zhang H, Morris M, et al. Incidence of nephrogenic systemic fibrosis at two large medical centers. *Radiology*. 2008; 248:807-816.

7. von Schulthess GK, Steinert HC, Hany TF. Integrated PET/CT: current applications and future directions. *Radiology*. 2006;238: 405-422.

8. Miyazaki M, Lee VS. Nonenhanced MR angiography. *Radiology*. 2008;248:20-43.

9. American College of Radiology. *Manual on Contrast Media*. 6th ed. Reston, Va: American College of Radiology; 2008:23-37.

The Physical Basis of Diagnostic Imaging

Robert L. Dixon, PhD
Christopher T. Whitlow, MD, PhD

IMAGING WITH X-RAYS

What Is an X-ray?

An x-ray is a discrete bundle of electromagnetic energy called a photon. In that regard, it is similar to other forms of electromagnetic energy such as light, infrared, ultraviolet, radio waves, or gamma rays. The associated electromagnetic energy can be thought of as oscillating electric and magnetic fields propagating through space at the speed of light. The various forms of electromagnetic energy differ only in frequency (or wavelength). However, because the energy carried by each photon is proportional to the frequency (the proportionality constant is called Planck's constant), the higher frequency x-ray or gamma ray photons are much more energetic than, for example, light photons and can readily ionize the atoms in materials on which they impinge. The energy of a light photon is of the order of one electron-volt (eV), whereas the average energy of an x-ray photon in a diagnostic x-ray beam is on the order of 30 kiloelectron volts (keV) and its wavelength is smaller than the diameter of an atom (10^{-8} cm).

In summary, an x-ray beam can be thought of as a swarm of photons traveling at the speed of light, each photon representing a bundle of electromagnetic energy.

Production of X-rays

Electromagnetic radiation may be produced in a variety of ways. One method is the acceleration or deceleration of electrons. For example, a radio transmitter is merely a source of high-frequency alternating current that causes electrons in an antenna wire to which it is connected to oscillate (accelerate and decelerate), thereby producing radio waves (photons) at the transmitter frequency. In an x-ray tube, electrons boiled off from a hot filament (Figure 2-1) are accelerated toward a tungsten anode by a high voltage on the order of 100 kilovolts (kV). Just before hitting the anode, the electrons will have a kinetic energy in kiloelectron volts equal in magnitude to the kilovoltage (eg, if the voltage across the x-ray tube is 100 kV, the electron energy is 100 keV). When the electrons smash into the tungsten anode, most of them hit other electrons, and their energy is dissipated in the form of heat. In fact, the anode may become white-hot during an x-ray exposure,

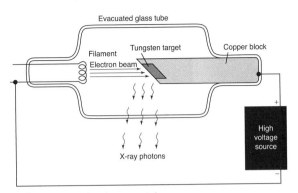

▲ **Figure 2-1.** Simple x-ray tube.

which is one reason for choosing an anode made of tungsten, with a very high melting point. The electrons penetrate the anode to a depth less than 0.1 mm.

A small fraction of the electrons, however, may have a close encounter with a tungsten nucleus, which, because of its large positive charge, exerts a large attractive force on the electron, giving the electron a hard jerk (acceleration) of sufficient magnitude to produce an x-ray photon. The energy of the x-ray photon, which is derived from the energy of the incident electron, depends on the magnitude of the acceleration imparted to the electron. The magnitude of the acceleration, in turn, depends on how closely the electron passes by the nucleus. If one imagines a target consisting of a series of concentric circles, such as a dart board, with the bull's-eye centered on the nucleus, more electrons clearly will impinge at larger distances than in the bull's-eye; hence, a variety of x-ray photon energies will be produced at a given tube voltage (kV) up to a maximum equal to the tube voltage (a hit in the bull's-eye), where the electron gives up all its energy to the x-ray photon. Increasing the voltage will shift the x-ray photon spectrum to higher energies, and higher-energy photons are more penetrating. The radiation produced in this manner is called Bremsstrahlung (braking radiation) and represents only about 1% of the electron energy dumped into the anode by the electron beam; the other 99% goes into heat.

The electron current from filament to anode in the x-ray tube is called the mA, because it is measured in milliamperes. The mA is simply a measure of the number of electrons per second making the trip across the x-ray tube from filament to anode. The rate of x-ray production (number of x-rays produced per second) is proportional to the product of milliamperage and kilovoltage squared. The quantity of x-rays produced in an exposure of duration s (in seconds) is proportional to the product of mA and time and is called the mAs. The quantity of x-rays at a given point is generally measured in terms of the amount of ionization per cubic centimeter of air produced at that point by the x-rays and is measured in roentgens (R) or in coulombs per kilogram of air. This quantity is called exposure, and 1 R of exposure results in 2×10^9 ionizations per cubic centimeter of air.

The electron beam is made to impinge on a small area on the anode of the order of 1 mm in diameter in order to approximate a point source of x-rays. Because a radiograph is a shadow picture, the smaller the focal spot, the sharper the image. By analogy, a shadow picture on the wall (such as a rabbit made with one's hand) will be much sharper if a point source of light such as a candle is used rather than an extended light source such as a fluorescent tube. The penumbra (or unsharpness) of the shadow will depend not only on the source size, but also on the magnification, as can be illustrated by making a shadow of one's hand on a piece of paper using a small light source such as a single light bulb. The closer you bring your hand to the paper (the smaller the magnification), the sharper the edges of the shadow. Similarly, magnification of the x-ray image produced by the point source is less, the closer the patient is to the film and the farther the source is from the film. The magnification factor (M) is defined as the ratio of image size to object size and is equal to the ratio of the focal-to-film distance divided by the focal-to-object distance ($M \geq 1$, and $M = 1$ means no magnification is produced; ie, either the object is right against the film, or the focal spot is infinitely far away). The penumbra, blurring, or unsharpness (Δx) produced on an otherwise perfectly sharp edge of an object and due to the finite focal spot size of dimension a is expressed by the equation

$$\Delta x = a(M - 1)$$

Unfortunately, the smaller the focal spot, the more likely it is that the anode will melt. The power (energy/per second) dumped into the anode is equal to the product of the kilovoltage and milliamperage; ie, at 100 kV and 500 mA, 50,000 watts of heat energy is deposited into an area on the order of a few square millimeters (imagine a 50,000-watt light bulb to get an idea of the heat generated).

▶ Interaction of X-rays with Matter

X-rays primarily interact with matter through interaction of their oscillating electric field with the atomic electrons in the material. Having no electrical charge, the x-rays are more penetrating than other types of ionizing radiation (such as alpha or beta particles) and are therefore useful for imaging the human body. The x-rays may be absorbed or scattered by the atomic electrons. In the absorption process (photoelectric absorption), the x-ray is completely absorbed, giving all its energy to an inner shell atomic electron, which is then ejected from the atom and goes on to ionize other atoms in the immediate vicinity of the initial interaction. In the scattering process (Compton scattering), the x-ray ricochets off an atomic electron, losing some of its energy and changing its direction. The recoiling electron also goes on to ionize hundreds of atoms in the vicinity. Electrons from both processes go on to ionize many other atoms and are responsible for the biological damage produced by x-rays.

The attenuation of the x-ray intensity with thickness of material follows an exponential law due to the random hit-or-miss nature of the interaction. The process is similar to firing a volley of rifle bullets into a forest, where the bullets may either stick in a tree (be absorbed) or ricochet off a tree (scatter). The deeper you go into the forest, the fewer bullets there are; however, a bullet still has a chance of traveling through the forest without hitting a tree. Likewise, an x-ray can make it all the way through a patient's body without touching anything and remain unchanged, as if it had passed through a vacuum instead. These are called primary x-rays. Typically, only about 1% of the incident x-rays penetrate the patient, and only about a third of these are primary x-rays; the rest are scattered x-rays that do not contribute to the anatomic image. An x-ray image is a shadow or projection image which assumes that x-rays reaching the film have traveled in a straight line from the source, but this is true only for the primary x-rays. As Figure 2-2A shows, the film density (blackness) at point P on the film is related to the anatomy along line FP. The scattered photon reaches the film along the path FSP and is relaying information about the anatomy at the random point S to point P on the film. Scatter simply produces a uniform gray background; it does not contribute to the image. Because scatter reduces image contrast, it is desirable that the scatter be removed. This task is accomplished by use of an antiscatter grid (Figure 2-2B). This grid consists of a series of narrow lead strips with radiolucent (low-attenuation) interspace material to remove some of the scatter. With the grid, the scattered photon shown in the figure can no longer reach the film, but the primary x-rays can. More of the scatter than primary x-rays is eliminated by the grid; hence, image contrast increases, but at the cost of an increase of a

factor of 2 to 3 in patient dose. This increase occurs because the scatter, which was previously blackening the film, has been reduced, and therefore, higher x-ray exposure to the front of the patient is necessary to get the requisite number of x-rays through the grid to blacken the film. The grid is usually made to move a few interspaces during the exposure by a motor drive, in order to wash out the grid lines.

The absorption process is more prevalent at lower kilovoltages and in materials with higher atomic numbers. Bones appear white on an x-ray film because photoelectric absorption of x-rays is greater in bone than in soft tissue as a result of the higher atomic number of bone. Lead is a useful shielding material for x-rays because of its high atomic number. The probability of the absorption process decreases rapidly with photon energy (as $1/E^3$) and the scattering process decreases slowly (as $1/E$); hence, the x-ray beam becomes more penetrating as kilovoltage increases. The scattering process is roughly independent of the atomic number of the attenuating material (all electrons look alike to the photon for the scattering process), whereas the absorption process is more probable for tightly bound electrons such as the inner electrons in heavier elements.

Increasing the kilovoltage is therefore beneficial to the patient in that it reduces the radiation dose: that is, fewer x-rays must penetrate the front of the patient to get the requisite number out the back to blacken the film. However, an increase in kilovoltage will reduce image contrast because the absorption process, which is sensitive to atomic number, will decrease and the scattering process is independent of the atomic number of the materials. Even with materials of the same atomic number, contrast improves at lower kilovoltage settings because of higher attenuation, which results in greater differential attenuation between different thicknesses of the same material. Thus there is a tradeoff between image quality (contrast) and patient dose that must be weighed in the selection of kilovoltage.

▶ The Radiographic Image

For production of radiographic images, the x-ray film is placed in a cassette and sandwiched between two fluorescent screens that glow under x-ray exposure, and it is primarily the light from these fluorescent screens that blackens the film. Although x-ray film, which is quite similar to ordinary photographic film, can be blackened by direct x-ray exposure, the film does not absorb the penetrating x-rays very efficiently, because the emulsion consists of silver halide crystals embedded in a low-atomic-number gelatin base. The fluorescent screens, called intensifying screens, are made of high-atomic-number materials, which therefore absorb x-rays very efficiently and also emit hundreds of light photons per x-ray absorbed. These light photons, in turn, are efficiently absorbed by the film. As a result, x-ray exposure to the patient is reduced by a factor on the order of 100 compared to

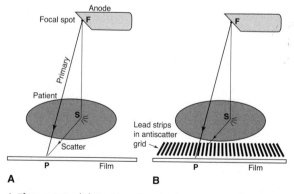

▲ **Figure 2-2.** (**A**) Scattered and primary x-ray photons reaching the same point P on film. (**B**) Scattered photon is removed by antiscatter grid, while primary photon gets through.

direct x-ray exposure of the film. The screens do produce a loss of sharpness of the image due to the spreading out of the light from the point of x-ray absorption before the light reaches the film. This effect can be reduced by making the screen thinner; however, it then absorbs a smaller fraction of the incident x-rays and therefore results in a "slower" system (more patient exposure is required).

In recent years digital image receptors have come into use. One type called CR (computed radiography) utilizes a cassette with a photostimulable phosphor material that stores the x-ray image in the form of trapped electrons for later readout by a scanned laser beam, which releases the electrons from their traps. On release, these electrons cause the phosphor to emit light that has a shorter wavelength than that of the laser beam. This light signal is read out and digitized, thereby forming a digital image. Another type called DR (direct radiography) consists of a flat-panel digital detector plate that is built into the x-ray unit itself. In these, the x-ray image is converted to an electrical signal from a fine matrix of thin-film transistor elements, which creates a digital image having a pixel size of 0.2 mm or less. These digital images, which consist of an array of numbers in a matrix, can be processed to improve image quality; displayed and manipulated on a viewing monitor; and then printed onto film using a laser film printer. The advantage of these digital systems is that the image can be processed to improve contrast and provide edge enhancement, and the film can be printed to the appropriate darkness regardless of the x-ray exposure.

Recall that the quantity of x-rays produced during an exposure is proportional to

$$mAs \cdot kV^2$$

However, because the beam is more penetrating at high kilovoltage, the x-ray exposure that reaches the film through a patient is roughly proportional to

$$mAs \cdot kV^4$$

That is, it depends very strongly on kilovoltage. The exposure time required to blacken the film is thus proportional to

$$s \approx \frac{1}{mA \cdot kV^4}$$

The heat deposited in the anode is proportional to the product of kV and mAs.

Choice of an exposure technique is generally made by first selecting the kilovoltage. A lower kilovoltage gives greater image contrast but also higher patient exposure and requires a longer exposure time at a given milliampere setting, because the x-ray beam is less penetrating and x-ray production is lower at the lower kilovoltages. Thus, for thick body parts, care must be taken not to choose too low a kilovoltage.

Generally, x-ray tubes have two focal spot sizes produced by two different (selectable) filament sizes. That is, they have a large and a small focal spot (eg, 1.25 and 0.6 mm). With the small focal spot, however, the electron energy is deposited in a smaller area, thereby creating a higher anode temperature; hence, at a given kilovoltage, the maximum milliamperage that can be used without melting the anode is limited to a lower value, thereby resulting in a longer exposure time. The small focal spot will result in a sharper image, however, if the longer exposure time required by its selection does not "stop" patient motion; then motion of the patient during the exposure may blur out any sharpness gain realized by use of the small focal spot. In any case, the small focal spot is useful only for looking at fine detail, such as bony detail, and its use does not significantly improve, for instance, an abdominal radiograph in which soft-tissue contrast is the objective. The small focal spot might be used for radiographs of the skull or extremities. The exposure time selected should be short enough to stop the motion of the anatomic part being radiographed. A very short time would be required for the heart and somewhat longer times for the abdomen or chest. Exposure time is less critical for the head or extremities, which are not subject to motion in most cases.

Having selected the kilovoltage and exposure time, one must then select the milliamperage so that the milliampere-seconds (the product of milliamperage and time) is large enough to blacken the film suitably. If the milliamperage required is above 200 mA to 300 mA, a small focal spot generally cannot be used, because it will not allow this high a value of milliamperage without melting the anode.

On many x-ray units, a phototimer sensor (automatic exposure control) is used to automatically terminate the exposure when a given x-ray exposure has been accumulated at the cassette position. In this way, the film is blackened sufficiently regardless of patient thickness and kilovoltage selection. When using this feature, however, the operator loses control of the exposure time. Choosing the highest milliamperage allowable by the tube will ensure the minimum exposure time.

▶ Fluoroscopy

If, instead of using the light from a fluorescent screen to blacken a film, one viewed the fluorescent screen directly with the naked eye, then one would be performing fluoroscopy as it was done in the early days of medical x-ray use. Unfortunately, the image made in this fashion was very dim, even at a high exposure rate to the patient, so modern fluoroscopy uses an image intensifier that amplifies the light from a fluorescent screen. A typical fluoroscopic imaging system is shown in Figure 2-3. The image intensifier tube is an evacuated glass or metal tube with a fluorescent screen (input phosphor) that glows with the image produced by the x-ray pattern that exits the patient. The light from the

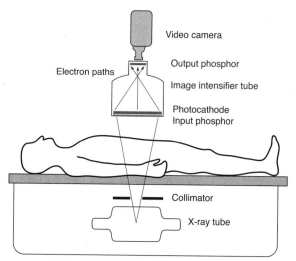

▲ **Figure 2-3.** Fluoroscopic imaging system.

input phosphor causes ejection of electrons from a photoelectric material adjacent to the input phosphor. These electrons are accelerated via a high voltage (30 kV), as well as being focused to preserve the image onto a small (1-inch diameter) screen (the output phosphor), which glows with the image because of the energy deposited by the impact of the accelerated electrons. The output phosphor glows much more brightly than the input phosphor (about 3000 times) because of the energy gain provided by the acceleration of the electrons and also because of minification of the image on the output phosphor. The image on the output phosphor can be viewed with the naked eye, usually with a series of lenses and mirrors, but the image is more commonly viewed by focusing a video camera onto the output phosphor and viewing the image on a TV monitor via a closed-circuit TV system. The fluoroscopic image generally has less contrast and less resolution of fine detail than a radiographic image; however, it is clearly convenient to view the image in real time—particularly when observing the flow of radiopaque contrast agents ingested or injected into the body. (These contrast materials, such as iodine or barium compounds, have a higher atomic number than soft tissue, hence, absorb more x-rays.) During fluoroscopic examinations, the x-ray tube is typically operated below 100 kV and below 3 mA tube current. Even so, entrance exposure rates (at the point where the x-ray beam enters the patient) are about 2 to 5 R/min, depending on patient thickness; hence, fluoroscopic examinations generally result in significantly higher patient exposures than do radiographic examinations.

Fluoroscopic systems generally have an automatic brightness control in which the brightness of the output phosphor is sensed by a light detector. The brightness signal from this detector is compared to a reference level, and the difference signal is used to instruct the x-ray generator to vary milliamperage or kilovoltage (or both) in order to maintain a constant brightness at the output phosphor. For example, after ingestion of barium in a barium-swallow examination, the barium absorbs significantly more x-rays, and the image would tend to go dark without such a system; however, as the brightness falls below the reference level, the automatic brightness control causes the x-ray generator to increase the milliamperage or kilovoltage to maintain a constant brightness on the monitor.

▶ Recording of Fluoroscopic Images

Fluoroscopic images can be recorded for later viewing by several methods. The TV image can be recorded using a videotape recorder or a videodisc recorder, the latter having the advantage of being able to view one frame at a time as well as providing random access rather than the sequential viewing required by videotape.

In addition, some systems have the capability of digitizing the electric signal from a TV frame and storing it in computer memory chips. These systems often have a "last image hold" capability that holds the last TV frame on the monitor. This method is also used in digital subtraction angiography (DSA); that is, the analog signal from the TV camera is digitized and stored frame by frame in a computer memory in a 512 × 512 or 1024 × 1024 image matrix. A short radiographic x-ray pulse is usually used for making the image. Images made just before and after injection of contrast material into the arteries can be subtracted digitally, so that only the vascular system appears in the subtracted image.

▶ Spot Film Devices

The aforementioned image recording methods merely store the image recorded by the TV camera, which is of lower quality than a radiographic image and has even poorer resolution than the image appearing on the output phosphor of the image-intensifier tube because of the limitations of the TV imaging process. In order to record higher quality images during a fluoroscopic examination, spot film devices are used. The most common device transports a conventional radiographic screen/film cassette to a position in front of the image intensifier at the push of a button on the fluoroscopic carriage. The x-ray tube is then switched into a radiographic mode (ie, the milliamperage is increased from low mA to 200 to 400 mA to shorten exposure time), and a conventional radiographic image is obtained on film. Digital spot films can be obtained by digitizing a TV frame from the image intensifier acquired with a short exposure burst at a higher exposure value than that of a single continuous fluoroscopic frame. These produce an image of higher quality (lower noise) than that obtained from the fluoroscopic image.

▶ Computed Tomography

In radiography or fluoroscopy, one is creating a shadow picture or a projection of the attenuation properties of the human body onto a plane. Thus, each ray from the source to a given point on the film, such as ray FP in Figure 2-2, conveys information about the sum of the attenuation along a line in the body; that is, anatomic structures are piled on top of each other and flattened into the radiographic image. In an attempt to give a different perspective, one may obtain projections from two different directions (eg, a lateral and an anteroposterior radiograph), so that the structures that are piled on top of each other differ in each projection. In the late 1960s a British engineer, Geoffrey Hounsfield, concluded that if one obtained projection data from a sufficient number of different angles, one could reconstruct the attenuation properties of each volume element in the body and display these as a cross-sectional image. This required the computational power of a computer to accomplish, and the basic idea is illustrated in Figure 2-4. The x-rays from a source are detected by a series of individual detectors (rather than film) after penetrating the body, and each detector defines a ray from the source through the body, thereby creating a projection. The width of the x-ray beam in the dimension perpendicular to the page is only about 10 mm; hence, only one slice of the body in the longitudinal direction is imaged at a time.

The x-ray tube and the detector bank are rotated 360 degrees about the patient to obtain, for example, 720 projections at 0.5-degree intervals. The computer is then able to reconstruct a cross-sectional image of the slice of the body by dividing the slice into an imaginary matrix. In a matrix of 512×512 pixels in the transverse plane, each pixel represents an area of about 0.5×0.5 mm in a 25-cm diameter body. The computer assigns a numerical value to each pixel, which represents the amount of attenuation contributed by the volume element of the body represented by that pixel, and these numbers are converted into a gray-scale image for viewing. In an axial scan series, after one slice is completed, the patient is advanced via a motorized couch by 10 mm in order to image the adjacent slice, and up to 30 slices (images) may be done to reconstruct the anatomy over a 30-cm length of the patient. Newer scanners, called helical (or spiral) CT scanners, use a continuous advance of the patient through the scan beam rather than the stepping couch motion utilized in axial scans, and axial slices are reconstructed by interpolation of data into the slice from a complete rotation. Multislice helical scanners with subsecond rotation times have been developed that collect data for reconstruction of several slices in each rotation; thus, a 30-cm length of patient anatomy can be imaged in 15 seconds or less.

MAGNETIC RESONANCE IMAGING

The technique called nuclear magnetic resonance, developed by physicists in the 1940s, was first utilized for imaging the human body in the late 1970s. The nuclei of some atoms (notably hydrogen nuclei in the body) have a fundamental angular momentum called spin, which causes them to behave like tiny spinning magnets. When placed in a uniform external magnetic field and excited by a radio pulse tuned to a resonant frequency that is proportional to the externally applied magnetic field strength (Larmor frequency), the axis of rotation of the nuclei will precess around the applied magnetic field direction in a similar fashion to the precession of a leaning gyroscope or top about the gravitational field direction (Figure 2-5). This precession can be detected, because the collection of processing magnets (protons in the body) induces an oscillatory voltage in a pickup or receiver coil. This oscillation at the Larmor frequency can be detected by connecting the pickup coil to a radio receiver, and one could therefore, in effect, hear the protons "singing" in unison into the coil at the Larmor frequency. This provides no imaging information; however, if the external magnetic field is made nonuniform in space in a known fashion (ie, a magnetic field gradient is utilized), then protons at different locations will precess at different frequencies, thereby creating a relationship between location in the body and precessional frequency. With application of such a gradient, the protons no longer sing in unison, but at different frequencies depending on their location, as in a chorus; that is, the sopranos would be located where the magnetic field was largest and the baritones where it was smallest. By listening to different frequencies, one could deduce from the signal strength at a given frequency how many protons were present at the location corresponding to that frequency. This method of imaging allows one to map the density of protons in the body in

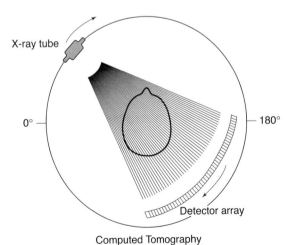

Computed Tomography

▲ **Figure 2-4.** Computed tomographic (CT) scanning geometry. A single projection of the head is illustrated.

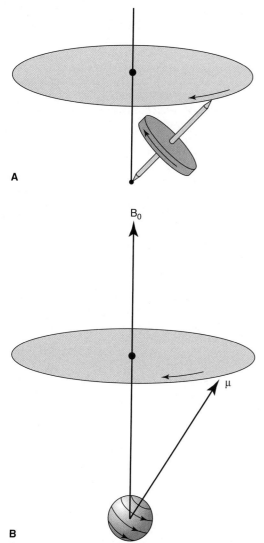

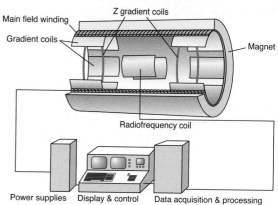

▲ **Figure 2-6.** Magnetic resonance imaging hardware.

▲ **Figure 2-5.** (**A**) Precession of a gyroscope about the earth's gravitational field. (**B**) Precession of the spin axis of a proton of magnetic moment μ about an applied magnetic field B_0.

three dimensions; however, most images are obtained and displayed as planar cross-sectional images similar to those in CT scans and having a slice thickness of 10 mm and a matrix size that is typically 128×256. For greater contrast, the proton density images may also be weighted by the relaxation times (T1, T2), which are measures of the realignment times of protons with respect to the magnetic field direction. This weighting is typically accomplished by varying the radiofrequency pulse durations and spacings in a variety of pulse sequences, the spin-echo pulse sequence being the most commonly used.

The hardware of a (nuclear) magnetic resonance imaging machine (Figure 2-6) consists typically of a cylindrical superconducting coil surrounding the patient to generate a large, static magnetic field; auxiliary coils for generating the magnetic field gradients; radio transmitter/receiver coils in close proximity to the patient; electronics for radiofrequency transmitting and receiving; and a computer to orchestrate the events and to reconstruct the spatial image from the frequency spectra.

ULTRASOUND IMAGING

Sound (or pressure) waves in the 3 MHz to 10 MHz frequency range are used for imaging the body by detecting the intensity of the reflected waves from various organs and displaying this reflected intensity as a gray-scale (or color) image. The sound waves are generated by applying an electrical pulse to a piezoelectric crystal. This crystal also acts as a receiver of the reflected waves after the transmitter pulse is terminated. A typical ultrasound transducer contains a linear array of such crystals, which can be fired in sequence or operated as a phased array to cause the ultrasound beam to rapidly scan across an area 5 to 10 cm in width for real-time imaging. The useful imaging depth is determined by the frequency; the higher frequencies (shorter wavelengths) have less penetrability. For example, at 10 MHz the imaging depth is limited to a few centimeters. Unfortunately, the lower the frequency, the poorer the axial resolution, because objects that are closer together than a wavelength cannot be separated. Hence, there is a tradeoff between axial resolution and penetration depth. Because ultrasound radiation is nonionizing, no adverse biological effects have been observed at diagnostic power levels.

BIOLOGICAL EFFECTS OF X-RAYS

The biological effects of x-irradiation are due to the recoiling electrons produced by the absorption or scattering of the incident x-rays, these electrons having enough kinetic energy to ionize hundreds of atoms along their trajectory. These electrons may damage DNA molecules directly or produce free radicals that can cause chemical damage to genetic material; either effect may result in cell death or mutation. Magnetic resonance imaging and ultrasonic imaging do not utilize ionizing radiation, and there is no significant evidence that any biologic damage results from these imaging modalities.

▶ Effect on the Patient

The primary risk to patients undergoing medical x-ray examinations is radiation-induced cancer, primarily leukemia, thyroid, breast, lung, and gastrointestinal cancer. These relative risks are considered to be related to radiation dose and effective dose, which is essentially the exposure to various critical organs multiplied by an organ-weighing factor (the units of radiation dose or exposure: a rem, a rad, and a roentgen are essentially equivalent for x- and γ-ray irradiation). Table 2-1 lists representative diagnostic procedures and associated typical effective dose in millirem, with the dose translated into relative increase in cancer risk per million persons, as well as the time required to receive the equivalent effective dose from natural background radiation. For example, if 1 million persons received lumbar spine examinations, there would be 51 additional (randomly occurring) cases of cancer above that occurring naturally in this population over their lifetime. In addition, it would take 155 days to receive a dose of radiation from natural background radiation equivalent to one lumbar spine radiograph.

According to a recent report by the National Council on Radiation Protection and Measurements (NCRP), Americans were exposed to greater than seven times the ionizing radiation in 2006, as compared to the early 1980s. This increase was primarily due to the increased utilization of computed tomography, which, when combined with nuclear medicine imaging, constituted 36% of total radiation exposure and 75% of medical-associated radiation exposure received by the US population. Indeed, the NCRP estimated that 67 million CT scans were performed in the United States in 2006. Such markedly increased utilization and associated increase in radiation exposure raise concern about subsequent long-term risk of malignancy. Future research evaluating the diagnostic benefit of imaging compared to the exposure risk to the population will undoubtedly shape the environment and context of medical imaging over the next decade.

▶ The Pregnant Patient

The fetus consists of rapidly dividing cells; hence, it is more sensitive to radiation, particularly in the first trimester. The principal risks to the fetus from in utero irradiation are cancer induction, malformation (eg, small head size), and mental retardation.

Every fertile female patient should be asked if she might be pregnant; if so, the relative risks of the diagnostic x-ray procedure versus the expected benefit should be weighed before the procedure is performed, or alternate imaging procedures such as MR imaging or ultrasound should be considered. It should be noted, however, that the added risk from diagnostic x-ray procedures is generally negligible compared to the normal risks of pregnancy, because fetal doses are typically below 5 rad in these procedures.

Table 2-1. Typical Effective Doses and Resulting Increased Risk of Fatal Cancer for Various X-ray Examinations

X-ray examination	Typical effective dose, mrem (1 mrem = 0.01 mSv)	Lifetime risk of fatal cancer per million persons	Time period for equivalent effective dose from natural background radiation
Chest (PA and lateral)	8	3	10 d
Lumbar spine	127	51	155 d
Upper gastrointestinal tract	244	98	297 d
Barium enema	870	348	2.9 y
Abdomen (KUB)	56	22	68 d
Pelvis	44	18	54 d
Head CT	180	72	219 d
Abdominal CT	760	304	2.53 y

The National Council on Radiation Protection (NCRP) in its report NCRP No. 54 states:

> The risk (to the fetus) is considered to be negligible at 5 rad or less when compared to the other risks of pregnancy, and the risk of malformations is significantly increased above control levels only at doses above 15 rad. Therefore, exposure of the fetus to radiation arising from diagnostic procedures would rarely be cause, by itself, for terminating a pregnancy.

If the x-ray examination involves the abdomen in such a way that the fetus is in the direct x-ray beam, then fetal doses are typically in the 1 to 4 rad (1 rad = 1 cGy) range depending on the number of films and fluoroscopic time (if any). If the examination does not involve the abdomen, and the fetus receives only scatter radiation, the fetal dose is generally small (typically, well below 1 rad).

SUGGESTED READING

1. National Council on Radiation Protection and Measurements. Ionizing radiation exposure of the population of the United States (2009). NCRP Report No. 160. Bethesda, Md: National Council on Radiation Protection and Measurements; 2009.
2. Mettler FA Jr, Huda W, Yoshizumi TT, Mahesh M. Effective doses in radiology and diagnostic nuclear medicine: a catalog. *Radiology.* 2008;248:254-263.

Imaging of the Heart and Great Vessels

3

James G. Ravenel, MD

The heart is often the "forgotten" structure in thoracic imaging studies. Yet a tremendous amount of information regarding cardiac structure and function can be gleaned from careful analysis of studies, regardless of whether they are dedicated to cardiac imaging. This chapter describes the normal radiographic appearance of the heart, pericardium, and great vessels (aorta and pulmonary vessels) and briefly outlines some of the more common pathologic entities in this organ system. Critical evaluation of the findings on the imaging examinations of this region is not possible without paying attention to the lungs, as these two organ systems mirror changes in each other. The most common abnormalities encountered in the cardiovascular system are hypertension, pulmonary arterial hypertension (usually secondary to chronic pulmonary disease), congestive heart failure, atherosclerotic disease, and valvular disease. Less common cardiac and great vessel diseases such as congenital heart disease, neoplasms, and diseases of the pericardium are described in less detail. The last topic, monitoring devices and postoperative changes, is one with which students should be familiar.

It is assumed that the student understands the basic normal anatomy of the cardiovascular system from the basic sci-

ence and clinical years. At the completion of this chapter, the student should have an understanding of the wide range of imaging modalities used, an appreciation for the potential yield from these examinations, a basic knowledge of the normal imaging anatomy on the conventional radiograph, a familiarity with more common postoperative alterations, and the various monitoring devices that may be present in the intensive care unit (ICU).

TECHNIQUES AND NORMAL ANATOMY

A variety of techniques have been developed to evaluate the heart and great vessels (Table 3-1). In this section, we briefly describe the major tests used in imaging this system.

▶ Conventional Radiographs

The most common imaging test for evaluating the heart and great vessels is the chest radiograph, which consists of an upright posterior-to-anterior (PA) and left lateral (LAT) projections. The terms *PA* and *left lateral* refer to the direction the x-ray beam takes through the body before it reaches the

Table 3-1. Imaging Tests for Heart, Great Vessels, and Pericardium

Conventional radiographs
 Posteroanterior (PA) and lateral
 Oblique
 Portable anteroposterior (AP)

Computed tomography (CT)

Echocardiography
 Transthoracic
 Transesophageal

Magnetic resonance (MR) imaging

Angiography
 Coronary arteriography
 Aortography
 Pulmonary arteriography

Radionuclide imaging

Positron emission tomography

radiographic cassette. Chest radiographs are usually obtained with high kilovoltage and milliamperage to minimize exposure time and cardiac motion. When possible, the distance between the x-ray tube source and the film is at least 6 feet to minimize magnification and distortion.

The examination is ideally performed with the patient at maximal inspiration. A good rule of thumb for estimating adequate inspiration is to be able to count 9 to 10 posterior ribs or 5 to 6 anterior ribs from the lung apices to the hemidiaphragms through the aerated lungs (Figure 3-1). When a chest radiograph is taken in the expiratory phase of respiration, the patient may appear to have cardiomegaly, vascular congestion, and even pulmonary edema. This appearance, however, is merely artifactual and caused by the lack of inspiration (Figure 3-2).

Severely ill, debilitated patients or patients who cannot be transported to the radiology department can have their chest radiographs obtained with a portable x-ray machine. Patients in the ICU who have intravascular catheters or who are undergoing mechanical ventilation frequently have chest radiographs performed as a survey for complications that may not be revealed by physical examination or laboratory data. These examinations are done with the cassette placed behind the patient in bed and are therefore anterior-to-posterior (AP) projections. The technical factors, which are controlled by the technologist at the time of the examination, vary with the size of the patient and the distance of the radiographic plate from the x-ray source (or machine). An attempt is still made to obtain the examination during maximum inspiration, but this objective may be difficult to achieve in some patients, especially those who have dyspnea.

With the patient in the supine position, there is normally a redistribution of blood flow to the upper lobe pulmonary veins (cephalization), and the heart may appear enlarged relative to its appearance on the upright PA radiograph, because of magnification (Figure 3-3). Some patients are able to sit for their examinations, whereas others are radiographed in a semiupright position. Ideally, the technologist should mark the exact position of the patient when the radiograph is obtained, and the date and time of the examination should be recorded in all cases. Changes in patient positioning and ventilator settings can have substantial effects on the radiographic appearance and must be taken into account when evaluating any change in the radiograph from a previous study.

The chest radiograph, whether it is obtained in the upright, semiupright, sitting, or supine position, should almost always be the initial screening examination in the evaluation of the cardiovascular system. Because it is essentially a screening study, the chest x-ray must be correlated with the clinical symptoms and physical examination to determine the overall significance of the radiographic findings. This information is also used to decide if other imaging tests are appropriate and which ones will potentially result in the highest diagnostic yield. Decisions regarding further imaging also depend on the impact on the clinical management of the patient, the potential for treatment of any abnormality that may be discovered, the cost and availability of the technique, and the expertise of the interpreting radiologist.

The conventional radiograph is an excellent screening test for the patient suspected of having disease involving the heart and great vessels, because the overall anatomy of these areas is demonstrated well. Whenever possible, all radiographs should be reviewed with all prior relevant imaging studies. Even when a prior chest radiograph is not available, additional information may be ascertained by reviewing other prior images such as thoracic spine or rib-detail image when available. Advanced imaging studies such as computed tomography (CT) and magnetic resonance (MR) imaging can also be used to help clarify complex findings on chest radiographs.

The normal cardiac silhouette size may be determined by the cardiothoracic ratio, a measurement obtained from the PA view. This ratio is calculated by dividing the transverse cardiac diameter (measured from each side) by the widest diameter of the chest (measured from the inner aspect of the right and left lungs near the diaphragm). The average normal value for this ratio in adults is 0.50, although up to 60% may be normal (Figure 3-4). A measurement over 50% is generally considered abnormal in an upright inspiratory-phase PA film, although this may not always be clinically significant. The cardiothoracic ratio cannot be reliably used for the AP projection of the chest, because the heart is magnified (see Figure 3-3). The size of the patient and the degree of lung expansion also should be considered. For instance, in a small person with a petite frame and a small thoracic cage, the heart size may be normal, but the cardiothoracic ratio may

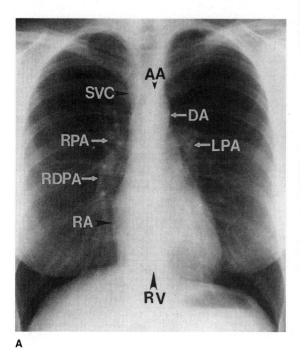

A

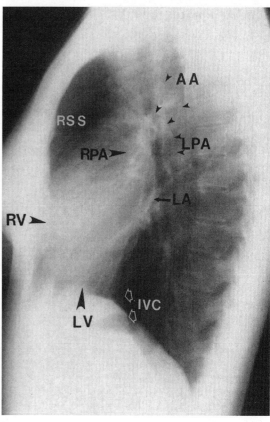

B

▲ **Figure 3-1.** Normal PA and lateral radiographs. **(A)** PA view of normal chest. RA, right atrium; RDPA, right descending pulmonary artery; RPA, right main pulmonary artery; SVC, superior vena cava; AA, aortic arch; DA, proximal descending thoracic aorta; LPA, left pulmonary artery; RV, right ventricle. **(B)** Lateral view of normal chest. RV, right ventricle; RSS, retrosternal clear space; AA, ascending aorta; LPA, left pulmonary artery; RPA, right pulmonary artery en face; IVC, inferior vena cava; LA, left atrium; LV, left ventricle.

measure over 50%. Similarly, if the patient has pulmonary disease such as emphysema, the heart may be enlarged, but because of the overinflation of the lungs, the cardiothoracic ratio may still be normal. In clinical practice, most radiologists do not perform this measurement and rely on experience and "gestalt" to evaluate heart size.

The contours of the heart, mediastinum, and great vessels on the PA view should be evaluated on each chest film (see Figure 3-1A). A reasonable approach is to begin in the upper right side of the mediastinum just lateral to the spine and below the right clavicle. The curved soft-tissue shadow represents the right border of the superior vena cava (SVC). The border of the SVC forms an interface with the lung and should not be confused with the right paratracheal stripe. Below the SVC is the right cardiac border formed by the right atrium. The inferior heart border, or base of the heart,

is the area just above the diaphragm and is composed primarily of the right ventricle, although there is some contribution from the left ventricular shadow. The left ventricle makes up the majority of the apex of the heart, which points to the left of the spine. The origins of the right and left pulmonary arteries are generally well demarcated on the normal PA film as they emerge from the mediastinum. The most prominent and recognizable component of the right pulmonary artery, the right descending pulmonary artery (RDPA), is seen just to the right of the superior cardiac border and descends inferiorly. It can usually be easily followed until it branches. The left main pulmonary artery is less well defined, but its origin can usually be seen above and lateral to the left atrial appendage just before it branches. When enlarged, the main pulmonary artery may be seen superimposed over the left pulmonary artery and filling in the normal space

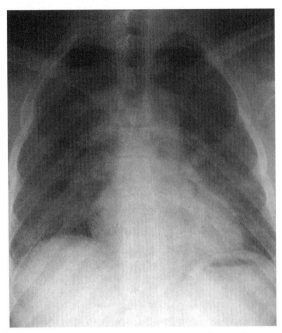

▲ **Figure 3-2.** Expiratory phase on a PA radiograph. Note the low lung volumes, apparent enlargement of the cardiac silhouette, and crowding of bronchovascular structures at the bases. Findings may be misinterpreted as heart failure if analysis of depth of inspiration is not performed.

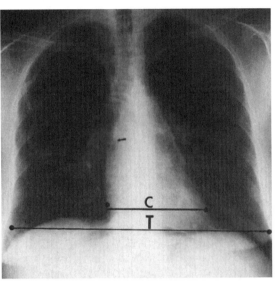

▲ **Figure 3-4.** Upright PA chest radiograph in a patient with leukemia shows normal cardiothoracic (C/T) ratio and how it is measured. Incidentally noted is the tip of an internal jugular triple-lumen catheter in the superior vena cava (arrow).

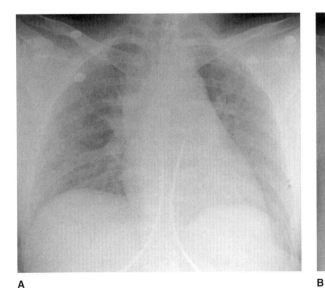

A

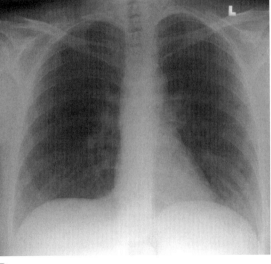

B

▲ **Figure 3-3.** AP (**A**) and PA (**B**) radiographs of the chest in same patient on same day. Note that the cardiac silhouette appears larger on the AP radiograph and may be mistaken for disease if patient position is not considered in the interpretation.

between the left pulmonary artery and transverse aortic arch (the AP window). The aorta originates posterior and to the right of the main pulmonary artery, and the border of the ascending portion of the aorta can usually be seen superimposed on the inferior portion of the SVC. The majority of the transverse arch is not outlined by air and therefore cannot be seen as it crosses the mediastinum. However, the distal transverse and descending aorta can be seen to the left of the mediastinum as it turns inferiorly. The left border of the descending thoracic aorta should be followed down to the aortic hiatus. Any loss of this contour or any contour abnormality may indicate pathology and should be investigated. Dilation or ectasia, localized bulges, and calcification may occur within the aorta as a normal part of the aging process, but should be viewed as abnormal in younger individuals. Of course, the spine, ribs, adjacent soft tissues, and upper abdominal contents should all be scrutinized. The left atrium lies just inferior to the tracheal carina, but it is usually not visualized as a discrete structure on the normal PA view.

The lateral view of the chest also reveals important information regarding the cardiac contour (see Figure 3-1B). Just behind the sternum there is normally a radiolucent area called the retrosternal clear space (RSS). This region represents lung interposed between the chest wall and the anterior margin of the ascending aorta. Any density present within the RSS may be due to an anterior mediastinal mass or postsurgical changes. The anterior border of the cardiac shadow is composed primarily of the anterior wall of the right ventricle. Right ventricular enlargement may also encroach into the retrosternal clear space. The posterior margin of the cardiac silhouette is formed by the left atrium and left ventricle. Just posterior and inferior to the left ventricle is a linear soft-tissue shadow leading into the heart formed by the inferior vena cava (IVC). The left ventricular shadow should not project more than 2 cm posterior to the posterior border of the IVC. The transverse aortic arch can usually be discerned on the normal lateral chest film as a smooth curving shadow originating anteriorly, crossing the mediastinum in a semilunar fashion, and then descending posteriorly as a linear shadow superimposed over the vertebral bodies. The left pulmonary artery (LPA) produces a similar curvilinear shadow just below the aortic arch before it branches. Just below the LPA, the left main/left upper lobe bronchus can be seen (projected end-on) as a round lucency. The right pulmonary artery (RPA) is seen en face down its lumen as an oval soft-tissue structure anterior to the bronchus intermedius and below and anterior to the left pulmonary artery.

▶ Echocardiography

Echocardiography uses high-frequency ultrasound to evaluate the heart and great vessels. The major indications for the technique are listed in Table 3-2. The examination provides a dynamic rendition of cardiac great vessel anatomy and, when

Table 3-2. Indications for Echocardiography

Ventricular function
Congenital heart disease
Valvular heart disease
Cardiomyopathy
Pericardial effusion
Suspected cardiac masses
Aortic disease (proximally)

combined with the Doppler technique, yields information regarding cardiac and great vessel blood flow (hemodynamics) as well. Because of the high frame rates inherent in ultrasonography, echocardiography can image the heart in a dynamic real-time fashion, so that the motion of cardiac structures can be reliably evaluated. Echocardiography is useful in assessing ventricular function, valvular heart disease, myocardial disease, pericardial disease, intracardiac masses, and aortic abnormalities (Figures 3-5 and 3-6). With Doppler technology, cardiac chamber function, valvular function, and intracardiac shunts frequently seen in congenital heart disease can be assessed. Combined Doppler echocardiography is a commonly performed procedure because it is relatively inexpensive and widely available, provides a wealth of information, is noninvasive, has no risk of ionizing radiation, and can also be performed at the bedside in critically ill patients. Furthermore, the results are immediately available because no special postexamination image processing is required. However, this technique is technically challenging and requires a great deal of operator expertise. Also, a small percentage of patients have poor acoustic windows that can severely degrade image quality. This disadvantage can be obviated by placing the sonographic probe in the esophagus, a procedure called transesophageal echocardiography (TEE). Transesophageal echocardiography yields consistently excellent images of the heart and great vessels, but involves a small amount of discomfort and risk to the patient. More recently, echocardiography has been combined with stress-testing modalities to assess inducible myocardial ischemia using wall motion analysis of left ventricular function.

▶ Radionuclide Imaging (Nuclear Medicine)

Cardiac radionuclide imaging, primarily used for the patient with suspected myocardial ischemia or infarction, requires an intravenous injection of radioactively labeled compounds that have an affinity for the myocardium. These compounds localize within the myocardium in diseased or damaged areas, and a radioactivity detector such as a gamma camera can image their distribution. These tests are most commonly

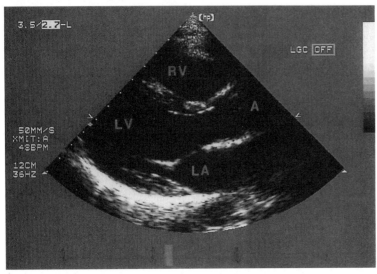

A

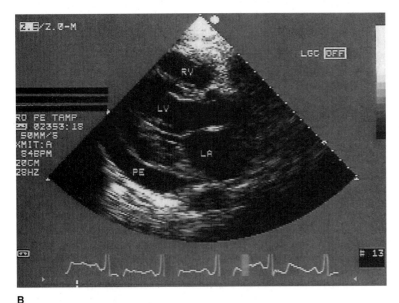

B

▲ **Figure 3-5. (A)** Normal transthoracic echocardiogram from a healthy subject. Views are taken from the left midparasternal region through an intercostal space. The structure closest to the apex of the screen is the chest wall. The mitral valve, separating the left atrium and left ventricle, is partially open in this image from early systole. A, aorta; LA, left atrium; LV, left ventricle; RV, right ventricle. **(B)** Transthoracic echocardiogram, left parasternal view, from a patient with a moderate-sized posterior pericardial effusion (PE), visualized as a sonolucent space between the epicardium and pericardium. RV, right ventricle; LV, left ventricle; LA, left atrium.

used in the evaluation of patients with angina and atypical chest pain (Figure 3-7). Gallium scans are occasionally used to assess for intrinsic myocardial disease such as myocardial sarcoidosis. Positron emission tomography (PET) with ^{18}F-FDG (^{18}F-fluorodeoxyglucose) is a problem-solving tool that has shown promise in assessing myocardial viability in patients with known coronary artery disease and to assess for metabolically active infiltrative disease (Figure 3-8). In addition, rubidium-82 and nitrogen-13 ammonia have been used as PET agents to evaluate myocardial perfusion.

▶ Computed Tomography

Cardiac computed tomographic angiography has undergone a revolution over the past decade. Owing to improved detectors, increased detector rows, and decreased scan times, breath-hold imaging of the heart can now be performed in many cases without pharmaceutical intervention (Figure 3-9). The major indications for cardiac CT are to evaluate the coronary arteries in subjects with indeterminate nuclear stress tests, to characterize or confirm coronary or cardiac

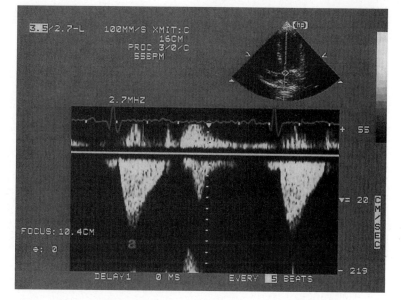

▲ **Figure 3-6.** Transthoracic spectral Doppler tracing taken from an intercostal space over the cardiac apex. The Doppler sample is placed in line with the left ventricular outflow and aorta (shown in miniature echocardiogram image at top right). Velocity of flow is denoted along left edge of tracing in cm/s. The Doppler tracing shows that aortic peak velocity (a) is normal (140 cm/s). This technique can reliably assess the presence of and quantitate the severity of aortic stenosis.

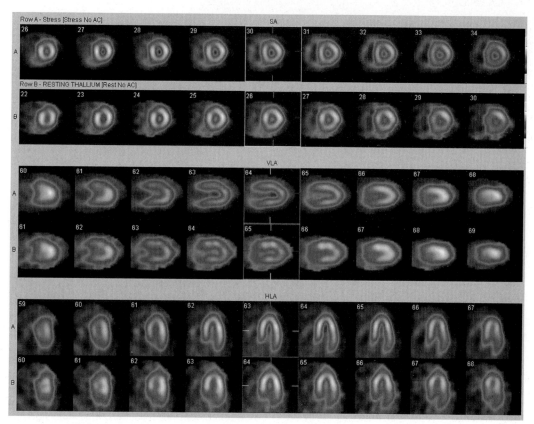

▲ **Figure 3-7.** Normal myocardial stress/rest study. Stress imaging performed with technetium-99m tetrofosmin following treadmill exercise achieving target heart rate. Resting images performed using thallium-201. Homogeneous perfusion of the left ventricular cavity is seen with both stress images (top of image pairs) and rest images.

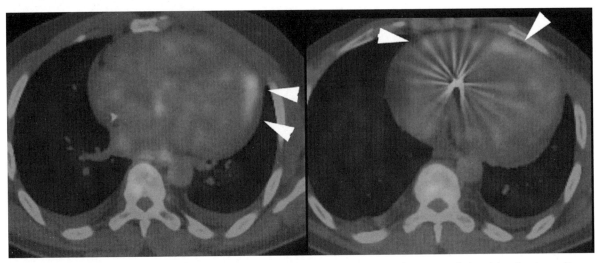

▲ **Figure 3-8.** ^{18}F-FDG-PET cardiac study performed after 24-hour fast shows patchy myocardial activity due to cardiac sarcoidosis (arrowheads). Normal myocardium is suppressed because of glucose deprivation and change in metabolism to free fatty acids.

anomalies, to assess location and patency of bypass grafts, and, in some cases, to assess for the presence of atherosclerotic disease in subjects presenting to the emergency department with atypical chest pain. The last is often performed with an extended coverage of the chest to concomitantly evaluate for pulmonary embolism and aortic dissection (triple rule-out). At the present time, some physicians also use the measurement of calcium in the coronary arteries detected at unenhanced ECG-gated CT to stratify the risk of future cardiovascular events (Figure 3-10). Contrast administration is mandatory when there are questions related to intrinsic cardiac anatomy or abnormalities of the thoracic aorta such as dissection or for evaluation of the pulmonary arteries for pulmonary embolism. For many of these applications, rapid administration of contrast is necessary (up to 4–5 mL per second), and a well-functioning large-bore (at least 18- to 20-gauge) IV catheter must be present to ensure a high-quality study.

The major drawback to CT for cardiac imaging at present is the use of ionizing radiation, which without careful management can be 4 to 5 times higher than for a standard chest CT. Fortunately, many techniques have been developed that lower radiation exposure. These include, but are not limited to, limiting scan distance, pulsing the x-rays to limit exposure during systole, prospectively gating rather than retrospectively reconstructing oversampled data, and modulating the x-ray beam based on patient size.

Magnetic Resonance Imaging

MR imaging has also gained rapid acceptance for cardiac evaluation, as it does not use ionizing radiation, can provide mor-

phologic and physiologic data, and can be performed to give cine-loop images. MR cardiac imaging remains a challenge because of the inherent difficulty of simultaneously dealing with respiratory and cardiac motion, the competing needs for spatial and temporal data, and the hands-on approach to tailor the examination to the specific clinical question. Thus, MR imaging is largely a problem-solving tool, rather than a screening study. The major indications for MR imaging are congenital heart disease and suspected intracardiac masses, valvular dysfunction, pericardial disease, and aortic abnormality. From a functional standpoint, MR has the ability to asses cardiac function and motion, distinguish infarct from ischemia and help determine the advisability of revascularization (Figure 3-11), and measure flow across valves or coarctations. On the research side, MR imaging has also shown some promise in measuring the degree of damage from coronary artery atherosclerosis and evaluating the composition of atherosclerotic plaque.

Angiography

Conventional angiography is one of the most commonly performed imaging tests for evaluating the heart and great vessels. After the introduction of a catheter into a peripheral vessel (usually, the femoral or axillary vein or artery), the angiographer, under fluoroscopic visualization, positions the catheter in the region of interest, injects contrast material to confirm the location of the catheter, and then injects larger amounts of contrast material for diagnostic purposes. This injection of contrast material can be videotaped, recorded as standard or digital radiographs, or digitally stored for later review. There are four major types of angiography:

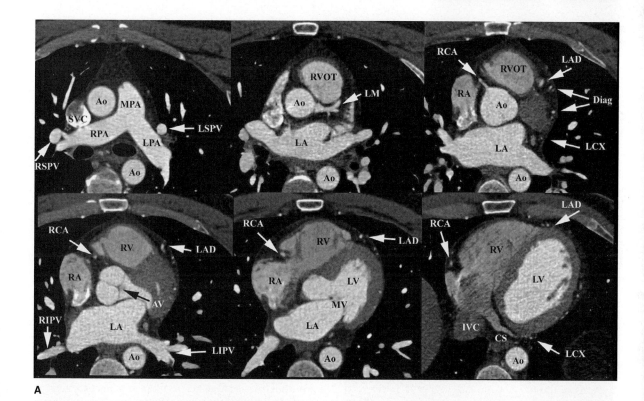

A

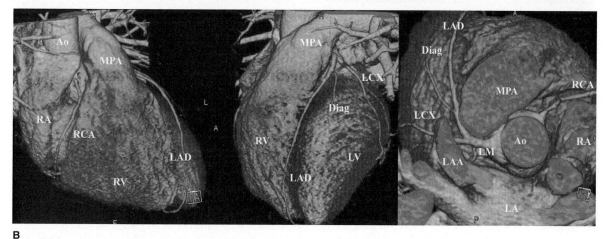

B

▲ **Figure 3-9.** Normal anatomy at cardiac CT angiography. **(A)** Axial composite image and **(B)** 3D volume rendered images in right anterior oblique, left anterior oblique, and cephalad projections (from left to right). Ao, aorta; AV, aortic valve; CS, coronary sinus; Diag, diagonal branch; IVC, inferior vena cava; LA, left atrium; LAA, left atrial appendage; LAD, left anterior descending artery; LCX, left circumflex artery; LM, left main coronary artery; LIPV, left inferior pulmonary vein; LPA, left pulmonary artery; LSPV, left superior pulmonary vein; LV, left ventricle; MV, mitral valve; MPA, main pulmonary artery; RA, right atrium; RCA, right coronary artery; RIPV, right inferior pulmonary vein; RPA, right pulmonary artery; RSPV, right superior pulmonary vein; RV, right ventricle; RVOT, right ventricular outflow tract; SVC, superior vena cava.

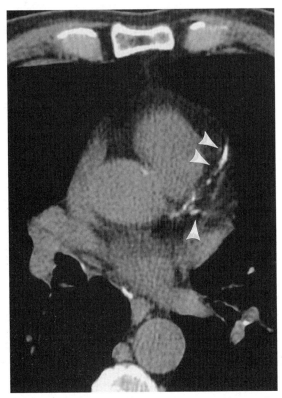

▲ **Figure 3-10.** Axial CT image shows atherosclerotic disease in the left anterior descending and left circumflex arteries (arrowheads) as evidenced by the presence of calcium.

angiocardiography (heart), coronary arteriography (coronary arteries) (Figure 3-12), aortography (aorta) (Figure 3-13), and pulmonary angiography (pulmonary arteries and lungs). Techniques developed by radiologists, angiocardiography and coronary arteriography, are now almost exclusively performed by cardiologists.

TECHNIQUE SELECTION

There is a wide array of imaging tests that can be used to evaluate the cardiovascular system (see Table 3-1). After a thorough history and physical examination, the initial screening study should always be a chest radiograph. Ideally, the PA and lateral views should be obtained with maximum inspiration. This study gives important information about the cardiac contour and the status of the lungs, and it is a good examination for excluding disorders that would require immediate treatment, such as pneumothorax. Furthermore, evaluation of the chest radiograph can often lead to a specific diagnosis and treatment, such as in congestive heart failure, or can help determine the need for another imaging study.

Depending on the history and physical examination findings, echocardiography, nuclear cardiac imaging, CT, MR, or conventional coronary angiography may follow. Echocardiography is a good screening test to assess cardiac and great-vessel valvular motion and structural abnormalities, cardiac chamber morphology, and flow. Angiography delineates the structural status of the coronary arteries and can give information on blood flow through the cardiac chambers, valves, and proximal great vessels, mainly in patients with suspected atherosclerosis. It is also used to guide interventions such as stent placement in the coronary arteries. Because of its inherent risks, coronary arteriography is usually reserved for patients with signs and symptoms of myocardial ischemia or infarction on the basis either of history or of results of electrocardiography, echocardiography, or radionuclide myocardial imaging.

In patients with suspected pulmonary emboli, helical CT is the most appropriate test in the setting of an abnormal chest x-ray (Figure 3-14). The ventilation-perfusion (V/Q) scan can be performed if the chest radiograph is normal and is also the preferred examination in young females because of the radiation dose to the breast by CT. Both of these tests can confirm the clinically suspected diagnosis of pulmonary embolic disease and often provide a useful "map" of the most suspicious regions of the lung for the angiographer if an angiogram is required for the definitive diagnosis of pulmonary embolism. CT can also detect important alternative diagnoses not detected by either V/Q scan or pulmonary angiography. More frequently, patients with atypical chest pain are being referred for the triple rule-out examination. This test is not appropriate for patients with clear signs or symptoms of myocardial ischemia and should be reserved for intermediate- to low-risk patients with a nondiagnostic ECG and negative first set of troponins.

Echocardiography, MR imaging, or CT or cardiac angiography may be selected for patients with suspected congenital heart disease. The advantages of MR imaging in this setting is that it is noninvasive, generally needs no contrast material administration, and uses no ionizing radiation, an important consideration in the pediatric patient. For these reasons, MR imaging has become the preferred imaging test in the pediatric population. As dose reduction techniques have improved, the use of CT for congenital heart disease has also increased.

Suspected aortic dissection (either atherosclerotic or traumatic in origin) can be evaluated by helical CT, TEE, aortography, or MR imaging. Helical CT is the imaging modality of choice for acute dissection because of its accuracy and availability (Figure 3-15). With multislice technology, CT angiography can provide images in multiple planes to show the relation of the dissection to key branch vessels. TEE has the advantages of being quick and noninvasive, and the examination can be performed expediently at the bedside. MR imaging is noninvasive, uses no ionizing radiation, is less operator-dependent, and can be performed in multiple planes. It is limited by availability and imaging time and because it cannot be used in patients with certain implanted

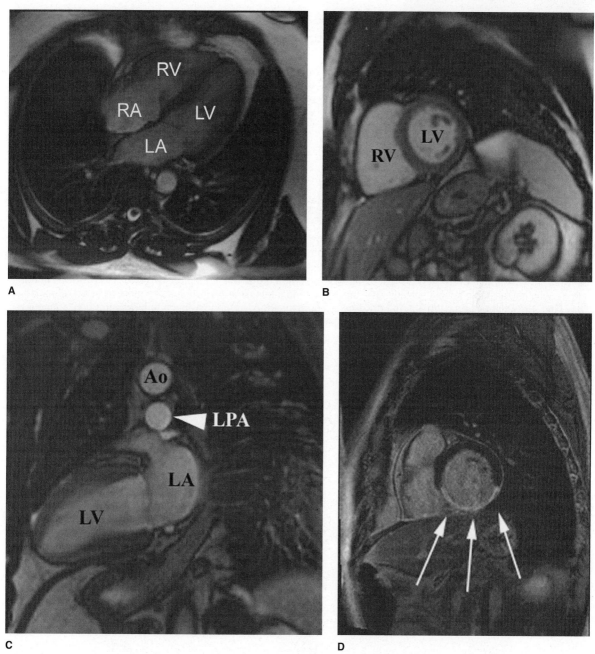

▲ **Figure 3-11.** Axial (**A**), short-axis (**B**), and long-axis (**C**) gradient echo "white blood" MR images with normal anatomy. (**D**) Delayed gadolinium enhancement study in a different case reveals extensive delayed enhancement of inferior wall (arrows) indicating infarct that is not amenable to revascularization. Ao, aorta; LA, left atrium; LPA, left pulmonary artery; LV, left ventricle; RA, right atrium; RV, right ventricle.

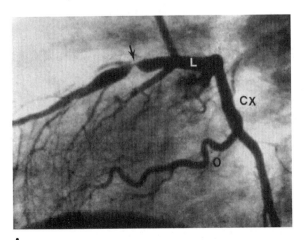
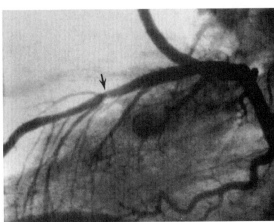

A   **B**

▲ **Figure 3-12. (A)** Coronary arteriogram. Images were obtained from the left lateral projection with contrast injection into the left main coronary artery. The left anterior descending (L), left circumflex (CX), and first obtuse marginal (O) branches are visualized. Severe stenosis is seen in the midportion of the left anterior descending artery (arrow) in this patient, who had unstable angina pectoris. **(B)** Coronary arteriogram, same projection and patient as in (A), obtained 1 day later. The stenosis in the left anterior descending coronary artery (arrow) has been reduced after percutaneous balloon angioplasty.

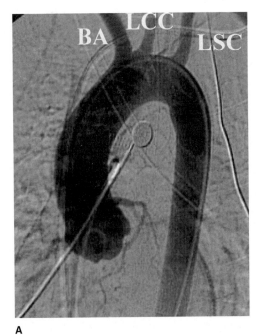
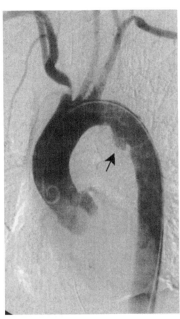

A   **B**

▲ **Figure 3-13. (A)** Normal aortogram of transverse arch in patient suspected of having traumatic aortic injury. Note the normal origins of the brachiocephalic artery (BA), left common carotid artery (LCC), and left subclavian artery (LSC) from the arch of the aorta. **(B)** Aortogram in a patient with acute traumatic aortic injury. The site of injury is the focal outpouching at the insertion of ductus arteriosus (arrow).

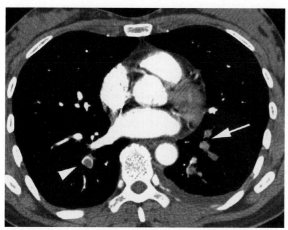

▲ **Figure 3-14.** Axial CT image shows filling defect (arrowheads) in right lower lobe artery and absence of flow in left lower lobe arteries (arrow) from pulmonary embolism.

devices, particularly pacemakers. Angiography has mostly been relegated to minimally invasive treatments such as stent-graft placement. Because survival rates often depend on early surgical intervention, availability and timeliness of the examinations is important.

In patients whose chest radiographs suggest intrinsic pulmonary or mediastinal processes, a standard chest CT is currently the preferred modality. The use of contrast depends on the indication, the preference of the radiologist, and any possible contraindications to administration of intravenous contrast for individual patients.

Finally, regardless of the situation, it is reasonable for the clinician and radiologist to decide together which imaging tests are most appropriate. In many instances, the choice of the next most efficacious and least costly imaging examination is not always clear-cut. In fact, in some circumstances, it is not necessary to perform another test because of the limited potential yield from the examination or because there is no adequate therapy for the suspected abnormality. It is hoped that future recommendations for test selection will be determined by well-designed prospective unbiased outcome studies comparing all of these modalities in various clinical scenarios. In the meantime, a commonsense approach, taking into consideration the history and physical examination findings, the information gleaned from the conventional radiograph, and the potential yield from the array of other available imaging tests, is the most appropriate. In all instances, communication between the clinician and radiologist is critical for the best patient care.

▶ Monitoring Devices

In clinical hospital practice, particularly in the ICU setting, a variety of catheters and tubes are used to monitor various

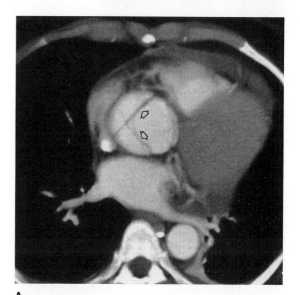

A

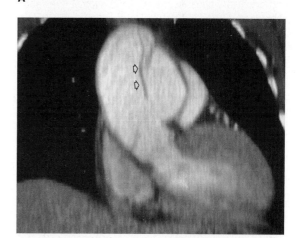

B

▲ **Figure 3-15.** Axial (**A**) and coronal (**B**) CT images show intimal flap of type A dissection (arrows).

parameters in patients (Figure 3-16). The student should be familiar with the normal routes and positions of these devices, as well as inappropriate positions and complications. Table 3-3 lists the most common monitoring devices.

Table 3-3. Common Monitoring Devices

Central venous catheters
Flow-directed pulmonary arterial catheters (Swan-Ganz catheters)
Intraaortic counterpulsation balloon
Cardiac pacemakers

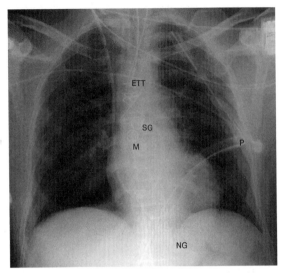

▲ **Figure 3-16.** Frontal radiograph immediately after coronary artery bypass surgery shows typical lines and tubes encountered in the ICU. Endotracheal tube (ETT), nasogastric tube (NG), Swan-Ganz catheter (SG), mediastinal drain (M), and left pleural drain (P) are present.

The basic venous anatomy of the upper mediastinum should be reviewed and kept in mind when evaluating catheter placement. The most common routes of catheter insertion in the chest include the internal jugular and subclavian veins. Radiographs obtained after insertion show the catheter following the course of either the internal jugular or subclavian vein and passing through the brachiocephalic vein. It then curves gently downward to terminate in the superior vena cava proximal to the right atrium (Figure 3-17). One normal variation of venous anatomy is the persistent left superior vena cava. In this situation the catheter descends down the left mediastinum terminating in the left SVC. The left SVC ultimately drains into the coronary sinus, which then enters the right atrium.

Intrathoracic central venous catheters are used mainly for monitoring central venous pressure (CVP), maintaining proper nutrition, delivering medication, and hemodialysis. It is standard practice to request a chest radiograph after catheter placement to verify its location (Figure 3-18) and to check for potential complications, such as pneumothorax (Figure 3-19) or hemothorax. Measurement of CVP is optimally obtained when the tip of the catheter is proximal to the right atrium and distal to the most proximal valves of the large veins. A catheter tip proximal to the veins gives an inaccurate

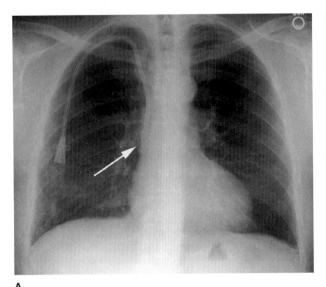

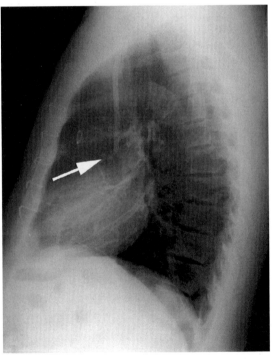

A   B

▲ **Figure 3-17.** PA (**A**) and lateral (**B**) view of a patient whose tunneled central venous catheter placement is normal with its tip in the superior vena cava above the right atrium (arrows).

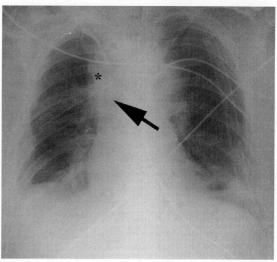

A

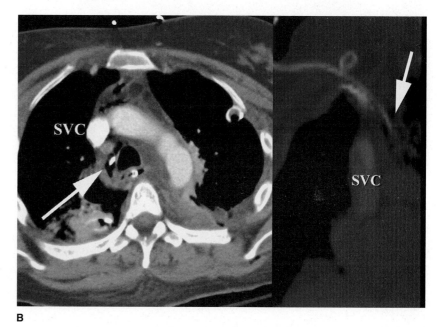

▲ **Figure 3-18.** Malposition of central venous catheter. **(A)** Portable frontal radiograph reveals central venous catheter overlying the expected region of superior vena cava (arrow). Because of lack of blood return, CT with contrast was obtained. Note also the widening of the right paratracheal stripe (*). **(B)** Axial and curved planar reformation reveal catheter has perforated the posterior wall of the superior vena cava with the tip residing in the mediastinum (arrows). SVC, superior vena cava.

B

reading of CVP, and a tip too close to the right atrium may cause arrhythmias from irritation of the right atrial myocardium. The reason for catheter insertion is critical for identifying its appropriate position. If it has been placed just for fluids and/or medications, a termination in the brachiocephalic vein is satisfactory. Conversely, a plasmapheresis catheter should never be located in the right atrium because of the risk of complications. More frequently, central venous catheters are being placed centrally via a peripheral vein. These

catheters have minimal risk, can remain in place for longer periods of time without being exchanged, and are primarily used for the delivery of fluids and long-term antibiotics.

The major potential complications from catheter placement are outlined in Table 3-4. A malpositioned central venous catheter may result in inaccurate CVP measurement, thrombosis, catheter knotting, and infusion of substances into the mediastinum or pleura. Catheter tips against the wall of the SVC may erode into the mediastinum or may extend

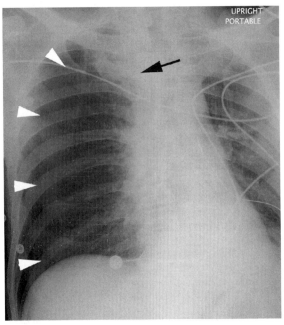

▲ **Figure 3-19.** Upright AP chest radiograph obtained after placement of right internal jugular (arrow) catheter shows a large right pneumothorax (arrowheads).

retrograde into tributary veins, particularly the azygous vein (Figure 3-20).

Flow-directed arterial catheters are also regularly used in cardiac and ICU patients to monitor cardiac output. The most common flow-directed catheter is the Swan-Ganz (SG) catheter (see Figure 3-16). It is usually inserted percutaneously

Table 3-4. Potential Complications of Intrathoracic Catheters

Malposition
Catheter knotting/fragmentation
Pneumothorax
Vascular injury
Thrombosis (venous)
Infarction (pulmonary arterial)
Infection/septic emboli/endocarditis
Air embolism
Cardiac arrhythmias

Fistulas
    Arteriovenous
    Venobronchial
    Arteriobronchial

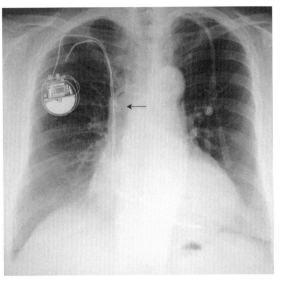

A

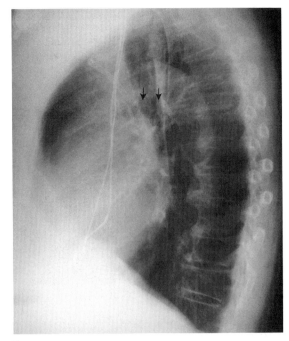

B

▲ **Figure 3-20.** PA (**A**) and lateral (**B**) views show central venous catheter with tip in azygous vein (arrows).

into the left or right subclavian vein and threaded through the brachiocephalic vein, superior vena cava, right atrium, tricuspid valve, right ventricle, pulmonic valve, and directed out into the main pulmonary artery. Usually terminating in the right or left pulmonary arteries, the SG tip should be distal to the pulmonary valve and proximal to the smaller pulmonary arterial vessels so it will not cause occlusion and, potentially, thrombosis. A simple rule of thumb is that the catheter should not extend past the mediastinal borders. It may then be intermittently "wedged" into a distal pulmonary artery branch to obtain a pulmonary capillary wedge pressure.

Complications of SG catheter placement are similar to those with other central venous catheters. The tip may be positioned in a number of inappropriate vessels or locations, and a chest radiograph should be obtained after catheter insertion to confirm its position (Figure 3-21). Introduction of any catheter into the subclavian vein, because of its close proximity to the lung apex, can cause pneumothorax (see Figure 3-19). A catheter tip position in the right ventricle can lead to ventricular arrhythmias, and leaving the catheter tip too distal may result in a pulmonary artery pseudoaneurysm or pulmonary infarct.

An intraaortic counterpulsation balloon pump (IABP) is occasionally used in patients with cardiogenic shock. This catheter measures approximately 26 cm in length and is surrounded by a balloon, which inflates with helium or carbon dioxide gas during diastole and deflates during systole. Deflation during systole decreases afterload and results in dimin-

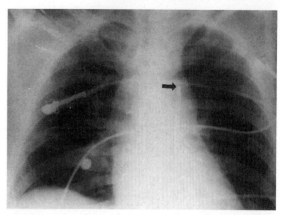

▲ **Figure 3-22.** Supine AP radiograph of patient 6 hours following coronary artery bypass surgery shows an IABP in normal position distal to the origin of the left subclavian artery (arrow).

ished left ventricular work and oxygen requirements, while the inflation of the balloon during diastole increases cardiac pressure to help ensure adequate perfusion of the coronary arteries. The catheter, introduced percutaneously into the thoracic aorta via the common femoral artery or placed into the ascending aorta at the time of surgery, should be positioned so that its tip is just distal to the origin of the left subclavian artery. The tip of the catheter has a small radiopaque marker so that this position can be ascertained on the chest radiograph (Figure 3-22). The major complications of the IAPB result from positioning of its tip proximal to the left subclavian artery, which may cause occlusion of the left subclavian vessel orifice, cerebral artery embolization, or aortic tear. If positioned too low, the balloon may occlude the celiac, superior mesenteric, and renal arteries.

Unipolar or bipolar pacemakers are most common and are usually implanted in the chest wall with leads inserted into the subclavian vein. The unipolar pacemaker tip is normally situated at the apex of the right ventricle. The bipolar pacemaker has a proximal lead that terminates in the right atrium and a distal lead that terminates within the right ventricle (similar to the unipolar pacemaker position). Biventricular pacemakers have a third lead present in the coronary sinus, appearing superior to the right ventricular lead (Figure 3-23). Its posterior position can be confirmed on the lateral view. Pacemakers that also have the ability to act as defibrillators have larger leads with a coil spring appearance. Leads are usually placed from a transvenous approach, although in certain circumstances they can be placed directly on the epicardium through the chest wall. The purpose of the chest radiograph after the pacemaker insertion is to document the appropriate placement of these leads, to check for complications from placement,

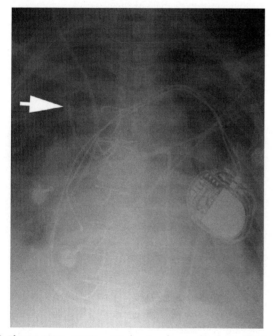

▲ **Figure 3-21.** Supine AP chest radiograph of a patient in the ICU in congestive failure shows a Swan-Ganz catheter tip positioned too far distally within the right upper lobe pulmonary artery (arrow).

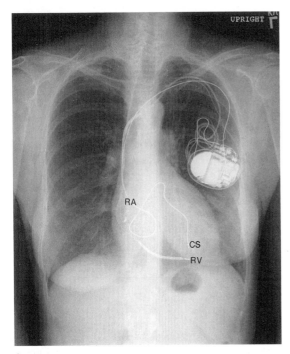

RA

CS
RV

A

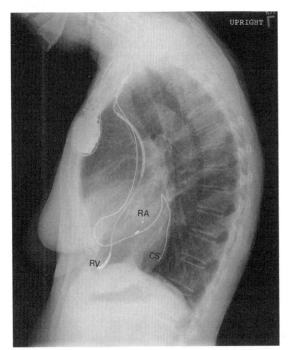

RA

RV   CS

B

▲ **Figure 3-23.** PA (**A**) and lateral (**B**) views show the most common locations of pacing leads: RA, right atrium; RV, right ventricle; and CS, coronary sinus.

and to establish a baseline examination to compare with future chest radiographs.

EXERCISE 3-1. INCREASED HEART SIZE

3-1. The most likely diagnosis in Case 3-1 (Figure 3-24) is
A. congestive heart failure.
B. pericardial effusion.
C. intracardiac shunt.
D. expiratory phase of respiration.
E. pulmonic stenosis.

3-2. The most likely diagnoses in Case 3-2 (Figure 3-25) is
A. mediastinal mass.
B. intracardiac shunts (atrial septal defect [ASD] and ventricular septal defect [VSD]).
C. pericardial effusion or cardiomyopathy.
D. combined aortic and pulmonary arterial disease.
E. technical aberrations.

3-3. The most likely diagnosis in Case 3-3 (Figure 3-26) is
A. mediastinal mass.
B. intracardiac shunts (ASD and VSD)
C. pericardial effusion or cardiomyopathy
D. combined aortic and pulmonary arterial disease.
E. technical aberrations.

3-4. The most likely diagnosis in Case 3-4 (Figure 3-27) is
A. Ebstein's anomaly.
B. mediastinal mass.
C. intracardiac shunt.
D. pericardial effusion.
E. mitral and aortic stenosis.

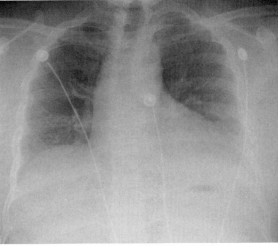

▲ **Figure 3-24.** Case 3-1: 20-year-old uncooperative man with minimal chest pain.

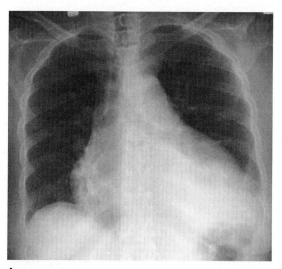

A

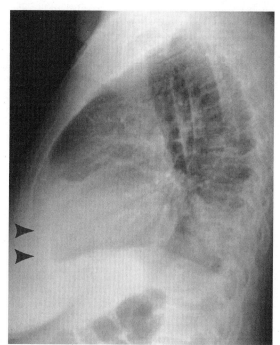

B

▲ **Figure 3-25.** (**A,B**) Case 3-2: 70-year-old man with uremia.

3-5. The most likely diagnosis in Case 3-5 (Figure 3-28) is
   A. congenital heart disease.
   B. congestive heart failure.
   C. pericardial effusion.
   D. acute pneumonia.
   E. aortic dissection.

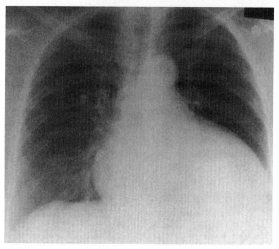

▲ **Figure 3-26.** Case 3-3: 60-year-old alcoholic man with shortness of breath.

Radiologic Findings

3-1. This case (Figure 3-24) represents an apparent "enlarged heart" due to an expiratory phase of respiration in an uncooperative patient (D is the correct answer to Question 3-1). Note the decreased lung volumes and the elevation of the hemidiaphragms. The resultant crowding of vessels obscures much of the cardiac border. The technique of inspiratory PA radiograph is preferred to avoid "diagnosing" diseases that a patient does not have.

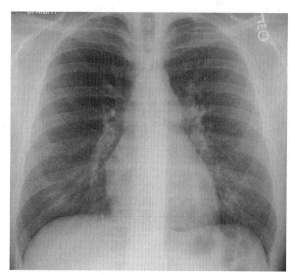

▲ **Figure 3-27.** Case 3-4: 28-year-old woman with a loud systolic murmur and without cyanosis.

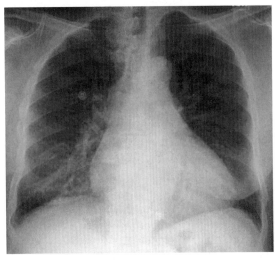

A

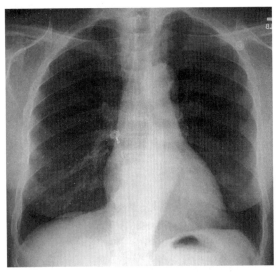

B

▲ **Figure 3-28.** **(A,B)** Case 3-5: **(A)** 55-year-old woman with an acute shortness of breath. **(B)** Chest radiograph of the same patient obtained 1 month earlier.

3-2. This case (Figure 3-25) is an example of pericardial effusion (arrowheads) (C is the correct answer to Question 3-2). The conventional radiograph findings on the frontal view are the so-called globular or water-bottle configuration of the heart.

3-3. This case (Figure 3-26) shows similar radiographic findings as in Case 3-2. This is the case of cardiomyopathy (C is the correct answer to Question 3-3).

3-4. This patient (Figure 3-27) has cardiomegaly, increased pulmonary vascularity, and prominent pulmonary

arteries, findings suggestive of an intracardiac shunt, which in this case was an atrial septal defect (ASD) (C is the correct answer to Question 3-4). The lateral radiograph (Figure 3-29) shows the enlarged central pulmonary arteries and right ventricular prominence due to increased flow.

3-5. This case (Figure 3-28A) illustrates cardiomegaly, increased pulmonary vascularity, redistribution of blood flow to the upper lobes, and Kerley's B-lines typical of pulmonary edema (B is the correct answer to Question 3-5). Note the normal radiograph 1 month prior (Figure 3-28B).

Discussion

Pericardial effusion and cardiomyopathy have similar appearances on PA chest radiographs (Cases 3-2 and 3-3). This appearance is often referred to as a globular shape or a water-bottle heart. When this appearance is observed, an echocardiogram is the next best imaging test to differentiate between these two entities. However, this diagnosis may be suggested on the lateral radiograph by a separation of the pericardial and epicardial fat by pericardial fluid, as exhibited in Figure 3-25B (arrowheads). Additionally, the presence or absence of pulmonary edema may sometimes assist in the diagnosis. As a rule of thumb, pericardial effusions do not result in pulmonary edema, and therefore the

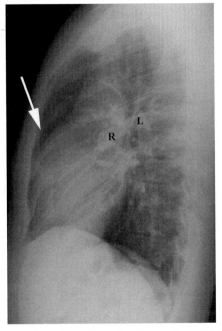

▲ **Figure 3-29.** Lateral view of patient in Case 3-4 shows filling in of the retrosternal space by the enlarged right ventricle (arrow) and large right (R) and left pulmonary arteries (L) from the pulmonary arterial hypertension.

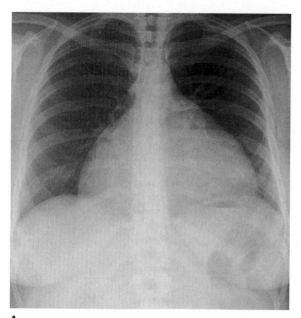

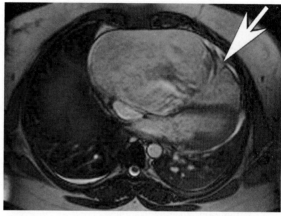

A   B

▲ **Figure 3-30.** **(A)** Upright PA view of chest in patient with Ebstein's anomaly reveals the globular-shaped heart characteristic of this disorder. **(B)** Axial gradient echo MR image reveals markedly enlarged right atrium with low-lying tricuspid valve (arrow) and small right ventricular chamber.

presence of edema should lead one to favor dilated cardiomyopathy. Mediastinal masses may occur in a location or a distribution that makes the heart appear enlarged on the chest radiograph. CT is the next best test to confirm a clinical suspicion of a mass and to evaluate mediastinal adenopathy.

Ebstein's anomaly, mentioned in Question 3-4, is an uncommon type of congenital heart disease that may also result in a globular appearance of the heart on the chest radiograph (Figure 3-30A). In these patients, the tricuspid valve is displaced downward, resulting in tricuspid regurgitation (Figure 3-30B). There is usually an associated ASD. The tricuspid insufficiency results in a massively enlarged right atrium, and the pulmonary vascularity is usually diminished due to decreased flow through the pulmonary arteries. These patients often present with congestive failure early in life, and echocardiography, MR imaging or cardiac angiography is necessary to make this diagnosis.

Increased heart size is a common clinical problem that may be caused by a variety of abnormalities. Cardiac enlargement may be diagnosed if the cardiothoracic ratio is greater than 60%. Often the lateral view is helpful for confirming left atrial and left ventricular enlargement. The most common cause of enlargement is atherosclerotic disease, although a number of other entities may cause an increased cardiac silhouette. In congestive heart failure (CHF), hydrostatic forces result in fluid collection in the interlobular septa, those connective tissue sheaths, veins, and lymphatics surrounding the secondary pulmonary lobule (Figure 3-31, arrows). As

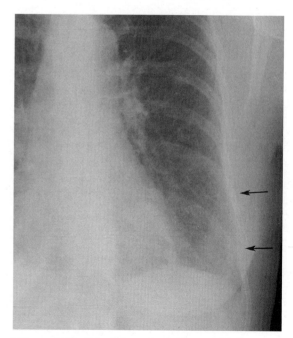

▲ **Figure 3-31.** Coned down frontal image of left hemithorax reveals fine reticular opacities extending to the pleural surface. These are Kerley B-lines (thickened interlobular septae) (arrows).

hydrostatic pressures increase, fluid may then accumulate in the alveoli giving an air-space pattern of disease. Intracardiac shunts, especially ventricular septal defect (VSD), can also cause cardiac enlargement because of the increased flow from the internal shunting. VSD is the most common congenital cardiac anomaly, and the intracardiac shunt must be at least 2 to 1 for the radiograph to show recognizable changes.

EXERCISE 3-2. ALTERATIONS IN CARDIAC CONTOUR

3-6. In Case 3-6 (Figure 3-32), the most likely cause of the radiographic abnormality is
   A. syphilis.
   B. cystic medial necrosis.
   C. aortic stenosis.
   D. congenital heart disease.
   E. drug abuse.

3-7. In Case 3-7 (Figure 3-33), the abnormality is due to
   A. mitral valve disease.
   B. left ventricular hypertrophy.
   C. pulmonic stenosis.
   D. right atrial enlargement.
   E. mediastinal mass.

3-8. In Case 3-8 (Figure 3-34), what is the cardiac contour abnormality?
   A. Left atrial enlargement
   B. Left ventricular enlargement
   C. Right atrial enlargement
   D. Left ventricular aneurysm
   E. Right ventricular aneurysm

3-9. The diagnosis in Case 3-9 (Figure 3-35) is
   A. situs inversus.
   B. dextrocardia.
   C. technical aberration.
   D. tetralogy of Fallot.
   E. pulmonary atresia.

3-10. The configuration of the heart in Case 3-10 (Figure 3-36) has been called the
   A. boot-shaped heart.
   B. third mogul of the heart.
   C. snowman appearance.
   D. double contour sign.
   E. water-bottle heart.

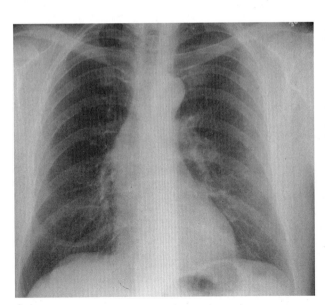

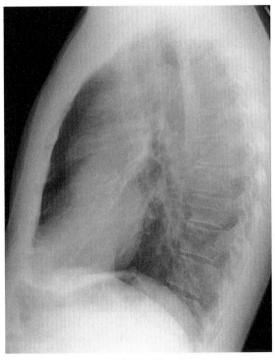

A   B

▲ **Figure 3-32.** Case 3-6: 68-year-old man with a long history of elevated blood pressure and systolic murmur.

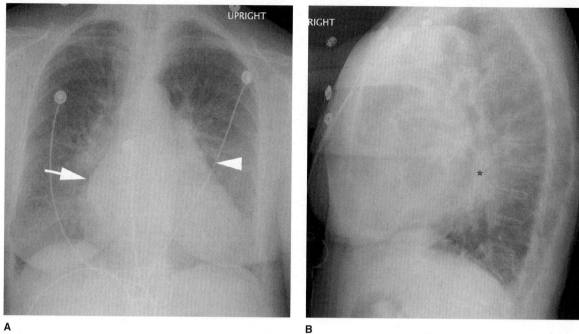

▲ Figure 3-33. Case 3-7: 77-year-old woman with systolic and diastolic murmurs and a history of rheumatic fever as a child.

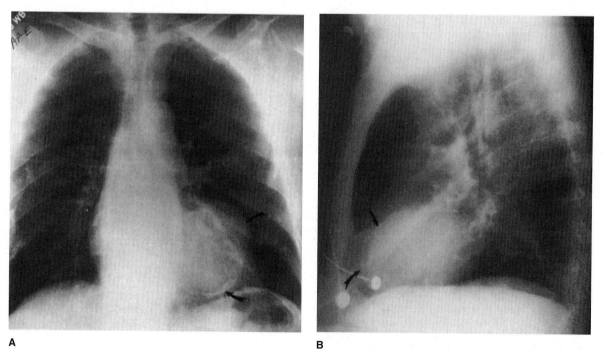

▲ Figure 3-34. Case 3-8: 75-year-old man with a history of a myocardial infarction 10 years earlier had this study done as a routine screening examination.

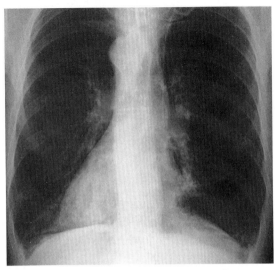

▲ **Figure 3-35.** Case 3-9: 24-year-old man with recurrent pulmonary infections.

Radiographic Findings

3-6.   In this case (Figure 3-32), the classical findings of enlargement of the left ventricle, characteristic of left ventricular hypertrophy, are seen on both the PA and the lateral radiograph as well as deviation of the ascending aorta contour to the right. This pattern is often the result of long-standing aortic stenosis (C is the correct answer to Question 3-6).

3-7.   In this case (Figure 3-33), a double density to the right side of the heart is seen on the PA radiograph (arrow).

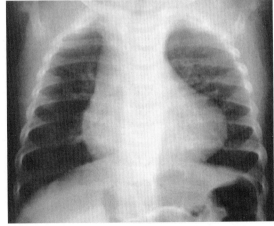

▲ **Figure 3-36.** Case 3-10: 3-year-old child with a history of cardiac complications since birth.

There is also an enlarged left atrial appendage (arrowhead). The lateral radiograph shows enlargement of the left atrial shadow, the superior and posterior region of the cardiac contour (*), and posterior displacement of the left main bronchus and enlargement of the right ventricle (A is the correct answer to Question 3-7). Along with increased pulmonary vascularity, the constellation of findings is characteristic of left atrial enlargement due to mitral valve insufficiency.

3-8.   The PA and lateral radiographs in this case (Figure 3-34) show an enlargement of the left ventricular contour with a focal bulge containing calcification within its wall (arrows). The lateral radiograph confirms the calcification (curved arrows). Given the history of myocardial infarction 10 years earlier, the most likely diagnosis is a left ventricular aneurysm (D is the correct answer to Question 3-8).

3-9.   The patient in this case (Figure 3-35) shows the apex of the heart to be on the right side of the chest and the descending aorta to be in its correct position on the left. These findings are diagnostic of dextrocardia, which in this case is secondary to Kartagener syndrome (B is the correct answer to Question 3-9).

3-10. In this case (Figure 3-36), tetralogy of Fallot, the apex of the left ventricle is elevated by right ventricular hypertrophy. These findings are sometimes referred to as a boot-shaped heart (A is the correct answer to Question 3-10).

Discussion

Alterations of the normal cardiac contour are common clinical scenarios. The most common contour abnormality is probably enlargement of the left ventricle from long-standing hypertension, as exhibited by the 68-year-old man in Case 3-6 (Figure 3-32). Cardiac enlargement is first suggested on the PA view by an increase in the CT ratio to over 50%. Left ventricular enlargement is suggested by prominence of the apex of the cardiac contour. On the lateral projection, the left ventricle should not project more than 2 cm posterior to the IVC measured 2 cm above the diaphragm. If the left ventricle projects more than 2 cm behind this landmark, left ventricular enlargement should be suspected. The configuration of the left ventricle and ascending aorta has been likened to the Schmoo from Al Capp's Li'l Abner.

Left atrial enlargement (LAE), as shown in Case 3-7 (Figure 3-33), occurs mainly with left-sided obstructive lesions such as mitral stenosis or mitral regurgitation, often the result of rheumatic heart disease. The major sign of LAE on the PA view is a double density centrally caused by the dilated left atrium extending to the right of the spine projected behind the right atrium (Figure 3-33A, arrow). Another sign of LAE is enlargement of the left atrial appendage. The left atrial appendage is immediately adjacent and inferior to the left main bronchus.

When enlarged, there is an extra bump along the left heart border, the so-called third mogul of the left cardiac border (Figure 3-33A, arrowhead). LAE also causes a separation and widening of the carinal angle that can be seen on the PA chest radiograph, although this is a late sign of LAE. The carinal angle normally measures between 60 and 120 degrees. Widening of this angle may occasionally be caused by subcarinal adenopathy and therefore should be correlated with other signs of LAE.

The left atrium makes up the posterior cardiac shadow just above the left ventricle (LA in Figure 3-1). Left atrial enlargement is recognized on the lateral film by enlargement and posterior displacement of the left atrial shadow (Figure 3-33B, *). As further enlargement occurs, the left atrium displaces the left main and left lower lobe bronchus posteriorly. Ultimately the elevated left heart pressures can be transmitted back across the pulmonary circulation, leading to pulmonary arterial hypertension and subsequent right heart enlargement (see later discussion).

Right ventricular enlargement (RVE) or hypertrophy (RVH) results most commonly from right-sided heart failure from a variety of disorders resulting in pulmonary hypertension (Table 3-5). In this cardiac contour abnormality there is an increase in the soft-tissue density within the retrosternal clear space that is best seen on the lateral radiograph (Figure 3-37). On the PA film, uplifting of the cardiac apex may be also seen. Anterior mediastinal masses may also cause retrosternal soft tissue density and should be included in the differential diagnosis (Figure 3-38); however, the majority of anterior mediastinal masses fill the RSS from superior to inferior and may not obscure right sided cardiac structures. When the cause is not clear from the conventional radiograph, CT is the next most appropriate test to differentiate between these two considerations.

Cardiac aneurysms, as shown in the patient in Case 3-8 (Figure 3-34), are almost always the sequelae of myocardial

Table 3-5. Causes of Pulmonary Hypertension

Pulmonary arterial hypertension
Idiopathic
Familial
Associated
Collagen vascular disease
Congenital systemic-pulmonary shunt
Portal hypertension
HIV
Drugs and toxins
Associated with venous or capillary involvement
Persistent pulmonary hypertension of newborn
Pulmonary hypertension with left heart disease
Pulmonary hypertension with lung disease or hypoxemia
Pulmonary hypertension due to chronic thrombotic/embolic disease
Miscellaneous

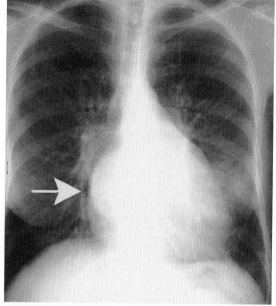

A

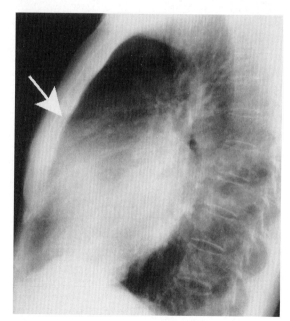

B

▲ **Figure 3-37.** PA (**A**) and lateral (**B**) views of patient with long-standing mitral stenosis show the double contour (arrow) on the PA view and filling in of the retrosternal space (arrow) on the lateral view. Right ventricular hypertrophy will be manifested as soft-tissue density in the retrosternal space on the lateral view.

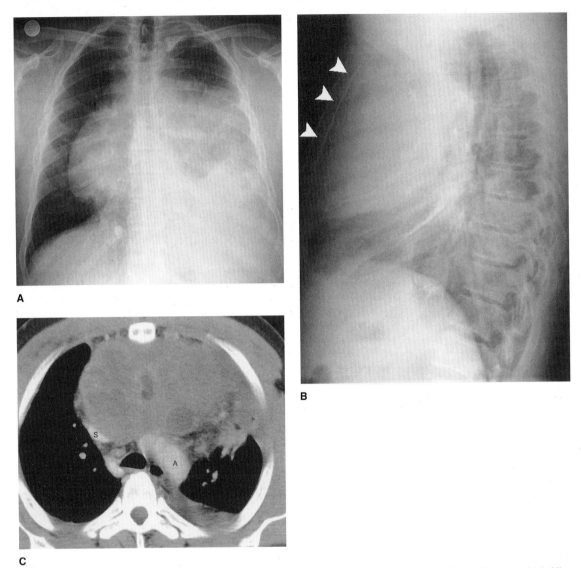

▲ **Figure 3-38.** PA (**A**) and lateral (**B**) views of patient with night sweats show an anterior mediastinal mass, which fills in the retrosternal space on the lateral view (arrowheads). A CT scan (**C**) in the same patient shows the location of the anterior mediastinal mass adjacent to the aortic arch (A). S, superior vena cava. Biopsy of the mass revealed germ-cell neoplasm.

infarction. There are two types of cardiac aneurysms: true and false aneurysms. True aneurysms most frequently occur at the cardiac apex and contain all three layers of myocardium. False aneurysms or pseudoaneurysms occur with disruption of the endocardium, with dissection of blood into the cardiac wall. Pseudoaneurysms, therefore, are not bound by all three layers of the heart wall. Pseudoaneurysms most frequently occur along the free walls of the heart (inferior and lateral walls). Aneurysms are usually diagnosed on the PA chest radiograph

as localized soft-tissue outpouchings or irregularities at the apical or anterolateral segments of the left ventricular cardiac contour. A linear rim of dystrophic calcification may develop within the nonviable myocardium after the infarction. With echocardiography, aneurysms show paradoxical enlargement during systole. Because there is stasis of blood in the aneurysm, blood clots can develop and may be a source of distal systemic arterial emboli. Echocardiography, CT, and MR imaging can all be used to make the diagnosis of cardiac aneurysm and distinguish between true and false aneurysms. The distinction is important because false aneurysms are at higher risk for rupture and require surgical repair.

Dextrocardia, as shown in Case 3-9 (Figure 3-35), is usually recognized easily on the PA chest radiograph. However, this finding may be overlooked if the left and right designations on the film are marked incorrectly or are misinterpreted. In most cases of dextrocardia, the aorta descends on the left side and the patient is asymptomatic. If the aorta descends on the right side, a number of other abnormalities should be considered. The references provide more in-depth discussion of this topic.

The boot shape of the cardiac shadow in Case 3-10 (Figure 3-36) is secondary to tetralogy of Fallot. The four components of this congenital cardiac anomaly are an overriding aorta, ventricular septal defect, pulmonic stenosis, and right ventricular hypertrophy. It is the right heart enlargement that results in the upturned cardiac apex. The degree of shunt and pulmonary stenosis dictate the presentation. In cases where the stenosis is severe, infants are cyanotic and there is generalized decrease in pulmonary vasculature. If the pulmonary stenosis and degree of left-to-right shunt is mild, the abnormality may not manifest itself until childhood (Figure 3-39).

EXERCISE 3-3. PULMONARY VASCULARITY

3-11. The most likely cause of the patient's symptoms in Case 3-11 (Figure 3-40) is
  A. pneumonia.
  B. pulmonary edema.
  C. interstitial lung disease.
  D. panic attack.
  E. pneumothorax.

3-12. The curved arrow in Case 3-12 (Figure 3-41A) is directed to the
  A. right atrium.
  B. ascending aorta.
  C. right descending pulmonary artery.
  D. main pulmonary artery.
  E. pneumonia.

3-13. The most likely diagnosis in Case 3-13 (Figure 3-42) is
  A. aortic stenosis.
  B. pulmonic stenosis.
  C. VSD.
  D. pulmonary edema.
  E. normal chest radiograph.

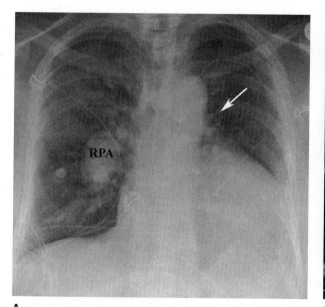

A

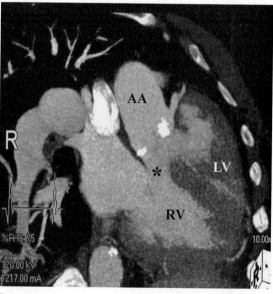

B

▲ **Figure 3-39.** Frontal radiograph (**A**) and oblique coronal reformatted CT (**B**) of an adult patient with uncorrected tetralogy of Fallot. On chest radiograph, note enlarged right pulmonary artery (RPA). Left pulmonary artery is diminutive because of long-standing stenosis (arrow). CT image reveals characteristic features including ventricular septal defect (*), overriding aorta, and right ventricular hypertrophy secondary to pulmonary stenosis. AA, ascending aorta; LV, left ventricle; RV, right ventricle.

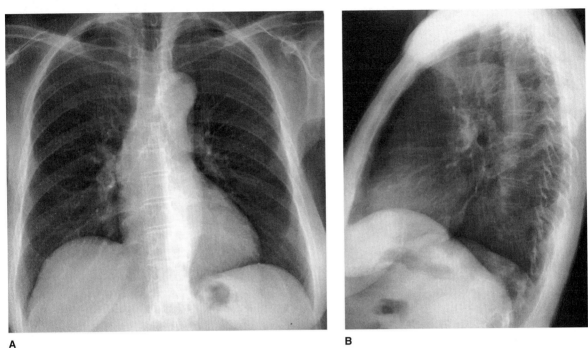

A   B

▲ **Figure 3-40.** Case 3-11: 53-year-old woman examined in the emergency department for chest pain, tachycardia, and shortness of breath with normal ECG.

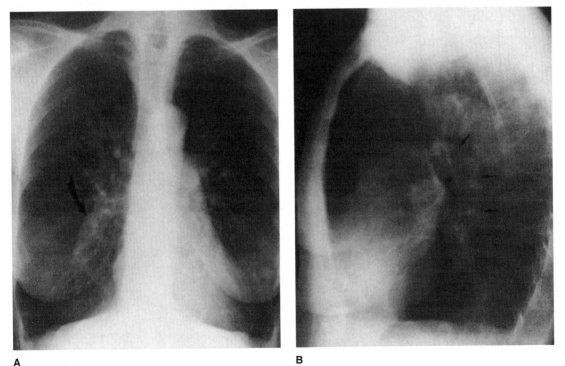

A   B

▲ **Figure 3-41.** Case 3-12: 65-year-old woman with a 100-pack-a-year history of smoking.

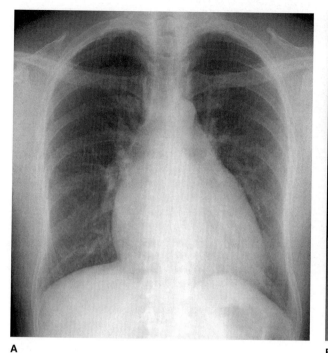
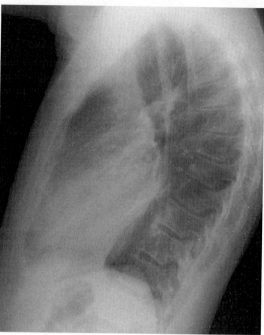

A   B

▲ **Figure 3-42. A,B.** Case 3-13: An acyanotic 40-year-old man with a systolic murmur.

3-14. The appearance of the pulmonary vasculature indicates that the diagnosis in Case 3-14 (Figure 3-43) is

    A. enlarged atrial appendage.
    B. partial anomalous pulmonary venous return.
    C. right ventricular hypertrophy.
    D. left atrial enlargement.
    E. pulmonary arteriovenous malformation.

3-15. The most likely etiology of the radiographic findings in Case 3-15 (Figure 3-44) is

    A. cardiac failure with pulmonary edema.
    B. pulmonic stenosis with pneumonia.
    C. pulmonary embolism.
    D. pneumomediastinum.
    E. pneumothorax.

Radiologic Findings

3-11. In this case (Figure 3-40), the chest radiograph was normal in a 53-year-old woman seen in the emergency department for left-sided chest pain. The electrocardiogram was also normal, and there was no obvious cause for the patient's pain. (D is the correct answer to Question 3-11). Note the well-defined pulmonary vessels in the perihilar region and normal branching of these vessels into the lungs. There is a gradient of pulmonary vascular markings from the bases to the apices on an upright radiograph due to the increased perfusion to the lower lobes. No

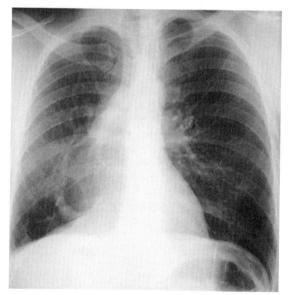

▲ **Figure 3-43.** Case 3-14: 36-year-old man with asthma.

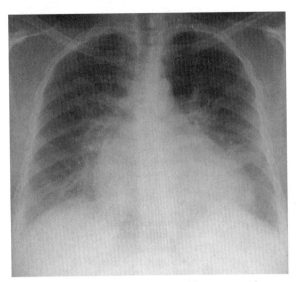

▲ **Figure 3-44.** Case 3-15: 50-year-old woman with acute shortness of breath.

pulmonary parenchymal abnormalities are present to support the other diagnoses. It should be noted that the chest radiograph is often normal in myocardial infarction, and a normal chest x-ray does not exclude intrinsic cardiac disease per se.

3-12. This case (Figure 3-41) is an example of chronic obstructive pulmonary disease. The large central pulmonary arteries indicate pulmonary arterial hypertension. The curved arrow in Figure 3-41A identifies the enlarged right descending pulmonary artery (C is the correct answer to Question 3-12). The generalized proximal pulmonary artery enlargement is confirmed on the lateral radiograph by the large left pulmonary artery (arrows in Figure 3-41B). Note the attenuation of vessels in the periphery of the lungs. This constellation of findings is typical of emphysema. There are also large bullae, which result in an absence of pulmonary vessels and hyperlucency of the lungs.

3-13. This case (Figure 3-42) shows increased pulmonary vascularity in a 40-year-old patient with VSD (C is the correct answer to Question 3-13). Note the large central pulmonary arteries, the increased linear opacities radiating out into the lungs, and the relatively uniform distribution of the pulmonary vascular shadows. In individuals with long-standing intracardiac shunts and pulmonary hypertension, the pulmonary arterial resistance may exceed systemic pressures, resulting in Eisenmenger's physiology, a reversal of an intracardiac shunt from L > R to R > L.

In these individuals, the central pulmonary arteries are quite large, but the peripheral pulmonary arteries are markedly attenuated.

3-14. This case (Figure 3-43) shows the characteristic appearance of venolobar (scimitar) syndrome (B is the correct answer to Question 3-14). The scimitar vein is the result of partial anomalous pulmonary venous return.

3-15. This case (Figure 3-44) is an example of a pulmonary edema due to fluid overload and congestive heart failure (A is the correct answer to Question 3-15). Note the increased size of the cardiac silhouette, the ill-defined reticular perihilar air-space opacities, the enlargement of the vascular pedicle, and the redistribution of blood flow to the upper lung zones.

Discussion

The main pulmonary arteries are large, the lobar arteries smaller, and each branching segment becomes progressively smaller. As the vasculature tree ramifies, the arteries are closely related to the adjacent bronchus and are approximately the same size. On the chest radiograph, this pattern is manifest by linear opacities or shadows that are much more prominent in the central portion of the chest and gradually become less prominent toward the periphery of the lung, as in the normal person in Case 3-11. The right descending pulmonary artery is one important landmark on the PA chest film (see Figure 3-1). In the normal chest, the lateral border of the RDPA is usually well demarcated, and the artery usually measures less than 15 mm in its widest diameter.

Enlargement of the pulmonary vessels is caused by a variety of abnormalities (see Table 3-5). Chronic obstructive pulmonary disease, with resultant pulmonary hypertension, is the most common cause of pulmonary arterial hypertension and is shown in the patient in Case 3-12 (Figure 3-41).

Intracardiac shunts that result in increased pulmonary arterial flow can also enlarge the pulmonary vascular system. The most common lesions causing increased vascularity without cyanosis are ASD, VSD, and patent ductus arteriosus (PDA). Case 3-13 (Figure 3-42) is an example of a VSD with increased vascularity. The main cardiac lesions with cyanosis and increased pulmonary vascularity are transposition of the great vessels, truncus arteriosus, and total anomalous pulmonary venous return (TAPVR). The standard texts listed at the end of the chapter can provide more in-depth discussions of these entities.

One other common cause of pulmonary artery enlargement is mitral disease (either stenosis or regurgitation). In this case, increasing left atrial pressures are transmitted to the pulmonary veins. In time, this raises pulmonary capillary wedge pressures and eventually right heart pressures, similar to cor pulmonale from left heart failure (see Case 3-7).

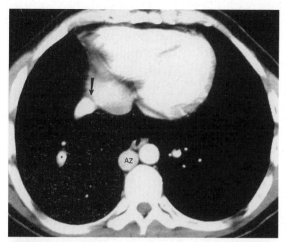

▲ **Figure 3-45.** Axial CT with contrast shows anomalous right pulmonary vein descending (*) and entering (arrow) inferior vena cava. AZ, azygous vein.

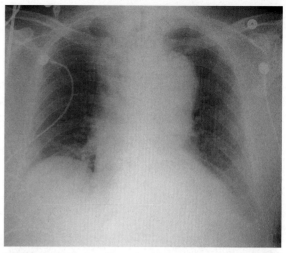

▲ **Figure 3-46.** Case 3-16: 74-year-old man with a long history of hypertension and ripping pain between the scapulae.

Venolobar syndrome is a form of partial anomalous pulmonary venous return. Note the right inferior pulmonary vein descending in a curvilinear fashion to empty into the inferior vena cava (Figures 3-43 and 3-45). Right lung hypoplasia causes the small size of the right hemithorax and results in shift of the heart and mediastinum to the right. Other congenital anomalies may be present.

Pulmonary edema, as exhibited in Case 3-15 (Figure 3-44), regardless of the cause, is another process that causes the increase in the pulmonary vascularity seen on chest radiograph (discussed further in the next chapter). Perihilar indistinctness, caused by interstitial edema, may obliterate the borders of the pulmonary vessels. Associated findings are redistribution of blood flow to the apices, engorgement of the central veins, Kerley's B-lines, and pleural effusions (see Figure 3-31).

EXERCISE 3-4. VASCULAR ABNORMALITIES

3-16.   The most likely diagnosis in Case 3-16 (Figure 3-46) is
   A. pericardial cyst.
   B. adenopathy.
   C. aortic dissection.
   D. pulmonary artery aneurysm.
   E. enlarged azygous vein.

3-17.   The abnormality outlined by arrows in Case 3-17 (Figure 3-47) is
   A. substernal goiter.
   B. innominate artery aneurysm.
   C. lung cancer.
   D. right aortic arch.
   E. mediastinal adenopathy.

3-18.   Causes for the appearance of the chest in Case 3-18 (Figure 3-48) include all of the following except
   A. ascending aortic aneurysm.
   B. anterior mediastinal mass.
   C. pleural mass.
   D. lung cancer.
   E. Ewing's sarcoma of the rib.

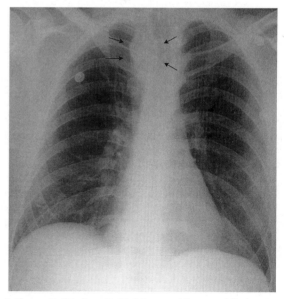

▲ **Figure 3-47.** Case 3-17: 25-year-old man with chest fullness.

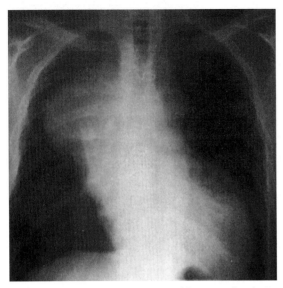

▲ **Figure 3-48.** Case 3-18: 76-year-old man with substernal chest pain.

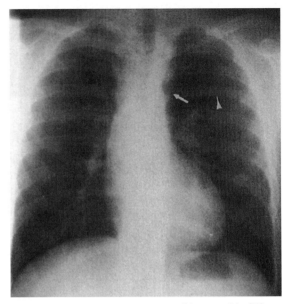

▲ **Figure 3-49.** Case 3-19: 22-year-old man with differential pulses in the legs and arms.

3-19. The arrow in Figure 3-49 is showing
    A. aortic ectasia.
    B. aortic constriction.
    C. pulmonary artery dilatation.
    D. adenopathy.
    E. embolic changes.

3-20. The abnormality shown by the arrow in Figure 3-50 is most likely a(n)
    A. enlarged main pulmonary artery.
    B. descending thoracic aorta aneurysm.
    C. patent ductus arteriosus.
    D. pulmonary vein stenosis.
    E. left superior vena cava.

Radiographic Findings

3-16. In this case (Figure 3-46), there is marked enlargement of the distal ascending and transverse thoracic aorta with shift of the trachea to the right. In association with the clinical symptoms, the most worrisome diagnosis is dissection of the aorta (C is the correct answer to Question 3-16).

3-17. This case (Figure 3-47) is an example of a right-sided aortic arch in an asymptomatic individual (D is the correct answer to Question 3-17).

3-18. This case (Figure 3-48) is a radiograph of the patient in Case 3-16 (Figure 3-46) 9 years later and shows a localized mass in the region of the ascending aorta.

The CT image (Figure 3-51) confirmed the large ascending aorta aneurysm (E is correct answer to Question 3-18).

3-19. This case (Figure 3-49) shows rib notching (arrowhead) and a localized constriction of the proximal descending aorta (arrow) (B is the correct answer to Question 3-19). These findings are diagnostic of coarctation of the aorta.

3-20. This case (Figure 3-50) is an example of a chronic pseudoaneurysm of the proximal descending aorta (arrow) in a patient with remote major trauma (B is the correct answer to Question 3-20).

Discussion

Anomalies of the major vessels are commonly encountered on the chest radiograph. The aortic arch is an easily recognized shadow. On the PA projection, the aorta originates in the middle of the chest and then arches superiorly and slightly to the left (hence the term *aortic arch*), then curves, crosses the mediastinum at an oblique angle, and continues as the descending thoracic aorta (see Figure 3-1). The configuration of the aorta changes during life. In the young person, the aortic arch is narrow and smooth and the descending thoracic segment very straight. In the older individual with atherosclerotic disease or aortic stenosis, the ascending aorta becomes more prominent along the right heart border and may have an undulating pattern in the descending thoracic portion.

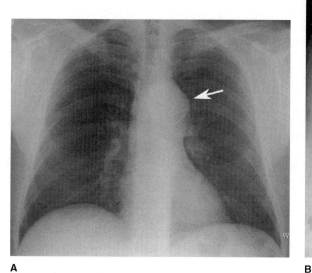
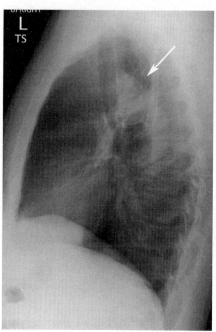

A   B

▲ **Figure 3-50.** Case 3-20: 38-year-old man with atypical chest pain.

Aortic dissection as seen in Case 3-16 (Figure 3-46) can be a life-threatening diagnosis. This is often the result of atherosclerosis and/or medial layer necrosis. In this disorder, blood dissects into the aortic wall through a tear of the intima. This process may begin anywhere along the course of the thoracic aorta, but the exact location is very impor- tant because it has therapeutic implications. Aortic dissec- tion is most easily classified by the Stanford system. This di- vides dissections into type A, those involving the ascending aorta, and type B, those that begin distal to the left subcla- vian. When associated with symptoms, type A dissections are considered surgical emergencies, whereas symptomatic

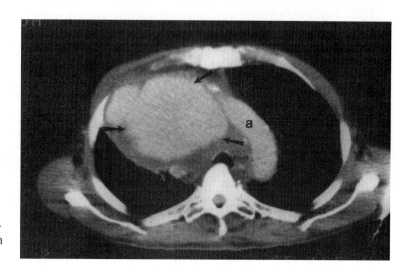

▲ **Figure 3-51.** Axial CT image shows large aortic aneurysm (arrows) originat- ing from the proximal ascending portion of the aortic arch (a).

type B dissections often can be managed medically. In the acute setting, the diagnosis is best established by CT because it can rapidly define the entire scope of the dissection as well as show the relationship to other major vessels (see Figure 3-15). Echocardiography can also rapidly detect dissection but provides less anatomic detail. MR imaging is often not used in the acute setting because of time and availability issues. The role of angiography as a diagnostic procedure for dissection has virtually disappeared; however, intravascular therapy including placement of stent-grafts and fenestration of the dissection flap can be performed for treatment in many instances, including medically inoperable individuals.

Other abnormalities of the aortic arch are uncommon. Congenital aortic anomalies include left aortic arch with aberrant branching, right aortic arch, and double aortic arch. The most prominent of these aberrations is the right aortic arch, which occurs in 1 in 2500 people. It can be diagnosed on the conventional radiograph by noting an indentation to and slight deviation of the right side of the trachea and displacement of the SVC shadow, as shown in Case 3-17 (Figure 3-47, arrows). In many individuals, the right arch is discovered incidentally and in these cases, is usually associated with an aberrant left subclavian artery (Figure 3-52). The barium swallow can also demonstrate mass effect on the esophagus by the aberrant subclavian and aorta as it crosses from right to left in the chest. When associated with congenital anomalies (tetralogy of Fallot, truncus arteriosus, etc), the great vessel branching pattern is a mirror image of that seen in a normal left aortic arch.

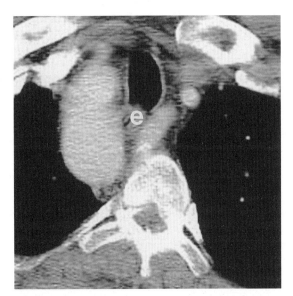

▲ **Figure 3-52.** Axial CT shows aberrant left subclavian artery coursing posterior to the esophagus (e).

Aneurysms of the aorta, shown in Cases 3-18 and 3-20 (Figure 3-48 and 3-50), are most often caused by atherosclerosis. Trauma, infection, and connective tissue disorders such as Marfan and Ehlers-Danlos syndrome are other causes. Aneurysms may be saccular or fusiform in shape, and symptoms include chest pain, hoarseness from compression of the recurrent laryngeal nerve, postobstructive atelectasis from compression of a bronchus, and dysphagia from esophageal compression. However, aneurysms are most commonly discovered as an incidental finding on an imaging study done for other reasons. An aneurysm of the ascending or transverse aortic segments shows a focal enlargement of the aortic shadow, usually with curvilinear calcification in its wall. A saccular aneurysm of the descending aorta may be misdiagnosed as a lung, mediastinal, or pleural mass, especially if it does not contain linear calcification. In these cases, as mentioned previously, CT is the next best imaging modality to perform (see Figure 3-51). The lack of rib destruction in Case 3-18 strongly argues against a chest wall sarcoma.

The abnormality in Case 3-19 (Figure 3-49) is coarctation of the aorta. This congenital anomaly results in partial or complete obstruction of the aorta at the junction of the aortic arch and descending aorta near the ligamentum arteriosum (the in utero connection between the aorta and pulmonary arteries). About one half of these individuals also have a bicuspid aortic valve. The obstruction to flow due to the coarctation results in elevated upper-extremity blood pressure and decreased lower-extremity blood pressure. A systolic ejection murmur may also be heard. Because of the partial aortic obstruction, collateral flow through the intercostal arteries results in the rib notching seen (Figure 3-53).

EXERCISE 3-5. HEART AND GREAT VESSEL CALCIFICATIONS

3-21. In Case 3-21 (Figure 3-54) the calcific density (straight arrow) is due to calcification of the
   A. mitral annulus.
   B. tricuspid valve.
   C. aortic valve.
   D. pulmonary embolus.
   E. pericardium.

3-22. In Case 3-22 (Figure 3-55) the calcifications are related to
   A. pulmonary arteries.
   B. pericardium.
   C. myocardium.
   D. ascending aorta.
   E. descending thoracic aorta.

3-23. In Case 3-23 (Figure 3-56) the calcifications on the chest radiograph are related to which structure?
   A. Pericardium
   B. Mitral valve
   C. Aortic valve

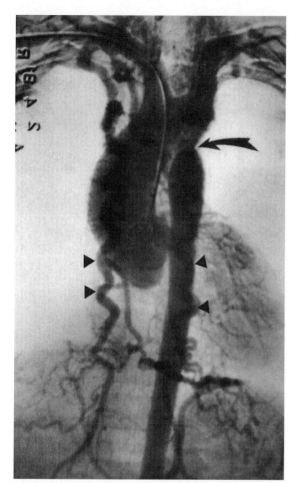

▲ **Figure 3-53.** Aortogram of the patient in Case 3-19 shows the characteristic constriction in the descending aorta (curved arrow) and the dilated intercostal veins (arrowheads).

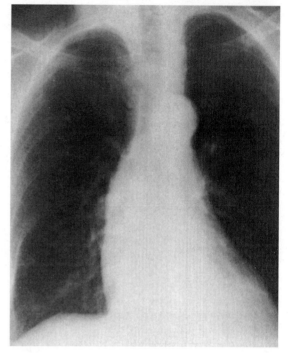

A

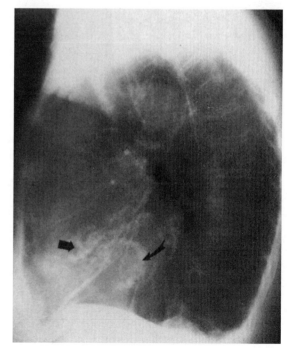

B

▲ **Figure 3-54.** Case 3-21: 75-year-old woman with rheumatic fever as a young adult.

D. Descending aorta
E. Left ventricle

3-24. In Case 3-24 (Figure 3-57) the curved arrows point to calcification within the region of which cardiac structure?
  A. Aortic valve
  B. Mitral valve
  C. Pericardium
  D. Coronary artery
  E. Aortic aneurysm

3-25. In Case 3-25 (Figure 3-58) the arrows and arrowheads point to a(n)
  A. calcified mediastinal mass.
  B. calcified left atrial myxoma.

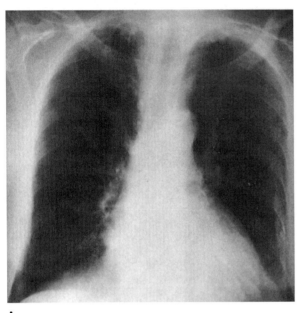
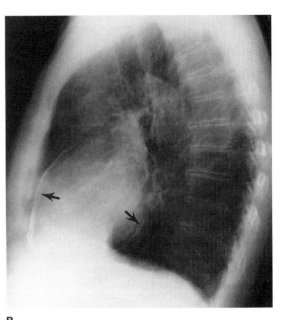

A
B

▲ **Figure 3-55.** Case 3-22: 70-year-old woman who has peripheral edema and jugular venous distention.

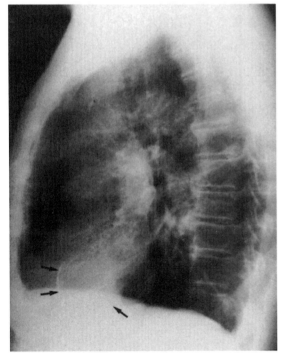
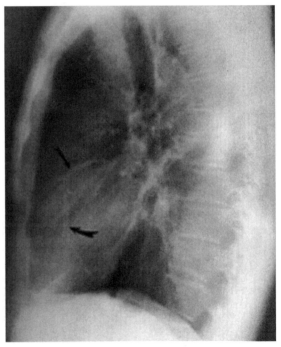

▲ **Figure 3-56.** Case 3-23: Lateral chest radiograph in a 65-year-old man with a long history of hypertension hospitalized 6 years ago with an acute illness.

▲ **Figure 3-57.** Case 3-24: Lateral chest radiograph in a 66-year-old man with long-standing diabetes mellitus.

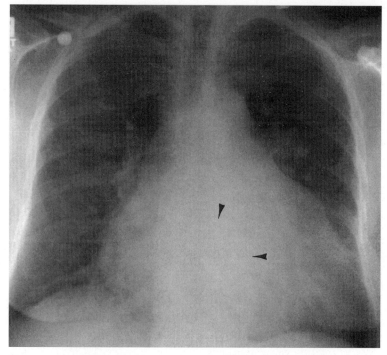

A

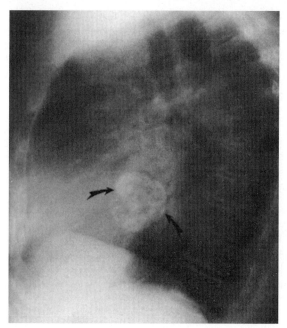

B

▲ **Figure 3-58.** Case 3-25. PA and lateral chest radiographs in a woman with shortness of breath and decreased exercise tolerance.

C. pulmonary embolus calcification.
D. aortic valve calcification.
E. mitral valve calcification.

Radiographic Findings

3-21. The PA and lateral chest radiographs (Figure 3-54) show curvilinear coarse calcifications in the mitral annulus (curve arrow) and linear calcification (straight arrow) reside in the aortic value, best seen on the lateral projection (C is the correct answer to Question 3-21).

3-22. This case (Figure 3-55) shows pericardial calcification in a woman who had viral pericarditis as a young child (B is the correct answer to Question 3-22). Note that the calcification is seen much better on the lateral view.

3-23. The chest radiograph in this case (Figure 3-56) shows linear calcification (arrows) in a focal area overlying the left ventricle. This calcification resides in a left ventricular aneurysm that this man developed after a myocardial infarction 6 years earlier (E is the correct answer to Question 3-23).

3-24. The lateral chest radiograph in this case (Figure 3-57) shows linear tram-track calcifications overlying the course of the coronary arteries. These calcifications represent coronary artery atherosclerosis in a patient with long-standing diabetes (D is the correct answer to Question 3-24).

3-25. In this case (Figure 3-58), a circular, heavily calcified area overlying the left atrium is seen in both the PA (arrowheads) and lateral (curved arrows) projections. These calcifications resided within a left atrial myxoma that was causing the patient's symptoms of shortness of breath and decreased exercise tolerance (B is the correct answer to Question 3-25).

Discussion

Calcifications, present in almost any area of the cardiovascular system, may be either metastatic or dystrophic in origin. Metastatic calcifications are usually caused by soft-tissue deposition of calcium due to hypercalcemia of any cause. Dystrophic soft-tissue calcifications are responses to tissue injury or degeneration and have no metabolic cause. They can be seen in practically any of the soft-tissue components of the cardiovascular system. We concentrate here on calcifications that can be seen on the conventional radiograph, although CT is a more sensitive test for detecting calcium. Calcium scoring has become an accepted way of assessing the degree of atherosclerosis in the coronary arteries, but provides mainly risk stratification rather than site-specific information on stenosis. This technique has been shown to provide risk stratification data that are additive to traditional clinical data. The most common site of calcification seen on the conventional chest radiograph is within the aorta, usually in eld-

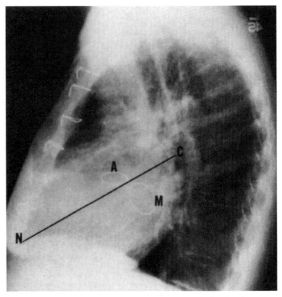

▲ **Figure 3-59.** Lateral view of a patient who had undergone replacement of the aortic (A) and mitral (M) valves. The line C to N connects the carina and the anterior cardiophrenic angle. Aortic valves usually lie above this line and mitral valves below it.

erly patients with long-standing atherosclerotic disease or diabetes. In this instance, the calcification is linear and is associated with the aortic wall. These calcifications may also be present in aneurysms (see Figure 3-34).

The aortic valve and mitral valve annulus are the most common intracardiac regions to demonstrate dystrophic calcification, usually secondary to long-standing stenosis or insufficiency from rheumatic fever. Bicuspid valves may also show this type of calcification. The lateral film is best for deciding which valve is calcified. A line drawn from the hilum (C) obliquely and downward to intersect the anterior cardiophrenic angle (N) will project behind aortic calcifications (A) (Figure 3-59). Calcifications that lie in back of this line are usually mitral annulus calcifications (M) (Figure 3-59). The presence of mitral annular calcification has been shown to predict the presence of carotid atherosclerosis and therefore may be associated with stroke.

Pericardial calcification as in Case 3-22 (Figure 3-55) is seen in approximately 50% of patients with constrictive pericarditis. It has a characteristic curvilinear appearance outlining the location of the pericardium and is most often seen along the right heart border (Figure 3-55).

Myocardial calcification, as is seen in left ventricular aneurysms, was discussed in the exercise on altered cardiac contour and is shown in a slightly different form in Case 3-23 (Figure 3-56). Thin, focal, linear calcifications overlying the left ventricle should be considered as aneurysms, and echocardiography, CT, and MR imaging are all useful examinations to confirm this diagnosis.

Calcifications within the wall of the coronary arteries, as exhibited in Case 3-24 (Figure 3-57), are recognized on conventional radiographs as thin, linear, calcific deposits corresponding to the course of the coronary arteries. When discovered by conventional radiographs, it is a late finding of atherosclerosis, and these patients have a high incidence of obstructive coronary artery disease.

Case 3-25 (Figure 3-58) is an example of the rare primary cardiac neoplasm that may calcify and be detected initially on the plain film. The cardiac tumor that most commonly calcifies is the left atrial myxoma, and calcification occurs in about 10% of these lesions (Figure 3-58). Rarely, myocardial metastatic disease (such as osteosarcoma) or other primary cardiac tumors may calcify. Finally, primary mediastinal neoplasms such as teratomas may rarely show calcification. In these patients, CT should be performed for diagnosis.

EXERCISE 3-6. MONITORING DEVICES

3-26. The complication of Swan-Ganz catheter placement in Case 3-26 (Figure 3-60) is
A. malposition of the tip.
B. pneumothorax.
C. perforation.
D. catheter coiling.
E. catheter thrombosis.

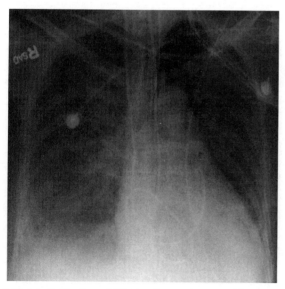

▲ **Figure 3-60.** Case 3-26: Routine supine portable chest radiograph obtained after SG catheter placement.

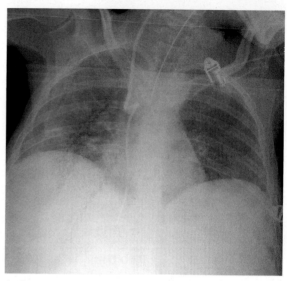

▲ **Figure 3-61.** Case 3-27: Supine chest radiograph obtained after difficult CVP placement.

3-27. The tip of the central venous catheter in Case 3-27 (Figure 3-61) is in the
A. inferior vena cava.
B. right ventricle.
C. azygous vein.
D. hemiazygous vein.
E. middle hepatic vein.

3-28. The malpositioned catheter in Case 3-28 (Figure 3-62) is a(n)
A. tracheostomy tube.
B. intraaortic balloon pump.
C. Swan-Ganz catheter.
D. nasogastric tube.
E. Blakemore tube.

3-29. The complication with the pacemaker shown in Case 3-29 (Figure 3-63) is
A. right atrial lead dislodgement.
B. right ventricular perforation.
C. pneumothorax.
D. right ventricular lead dislodgement.
E. diaphragmatic pacing.

3-30. The catheter in Case 3-30 (Figure 3-64, arrow) is in the
A. lung parenchyma.
B. left superior vena cava.
C. left upper lobe pulmonary vein.
D. descending thoracic aorta.
E. left pulmonary artery.

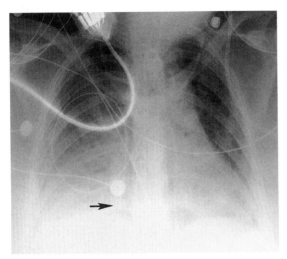

▲ **Figure 3-62.** Case 3-28: Routine supine chest radiograph in ICU patient after placement of several lines and tubes.

Radiographic Findings

3-26. The supine portable chest radiograph obtained after SG catheter placement in this case (Figure 3-60) is coiled within the right ventricle before it terminates in the proximal main pulmonary artery (D is the correct answer to Question 3-26). This coiling of the catheter in the right ventricle may cause thrombosis or arrhythmia, and it is necessary to reposition this catheter.

3-27. The supine chest radiograph in this case (Figure 3-61) shows two turns in the course of the catheter after a difficult CVP placement. The catheter turns posteriorly into the azygous vein and then descends on the right in the hemiazygous system (D is the correct answer to Question 3-27).

3-28. In this case (Figure 3-62), the chest radiograph obtained shows a nasogastric tube extending down the right main bronchus into the right lung (Figure 3-62, arrow) (D is the correct answer to Question 3-28).

3-29. In this case (Figure 3-63), the tip of the right ventricular pacemaker lead does not extend to the expected border of the myocardium. Usually a slight shouldering is encountered as the lead crosses the tricuspid valve. In some cases, the right ventricular lead may be positioned higher along the interventricular septum and may take a more horizontal course. A vertical course, as in this case, indicates the tip is not lodged in the myocardium. This positioning results in a lack of normal pacing function. The right atrial lead is in an appropriate position. (D is the correct answer to Question 3-29.)

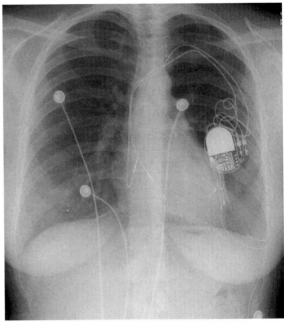

▲ **Figure 3-63.** Case 3-29: Chest radiograph obtained following pacemaker insertion.

3-30. This case (Figure 3-64) is a patient who has anomalous venous return from the upper lobe. The catheter placed in the left internal jugular vein courses into the left brachiocephalic vein and, rather than crossing the

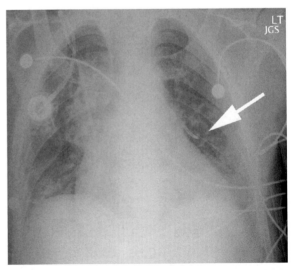

▲ **Figure 3-64.** Case 3-30: Chest radiograph obtained following central venous catheter placement with return of low-pressure oxygenated blood.

midline to the superior vena cava, extends into the left superior pulmonary vein (C is the correct answer to Question 3-30). Because it is carrying blood returning from the pulmonary capillary bed, it is oxygenated like systemic arterial blood, but comes from a low-pressure system.

Discussion

As mentioned in the subsection on monitoring devices within the chapter, a variety of catheters can be inserted into the heart and great vessels to monitor various hemodynamic parameters, particularly in the ICU setting. Table 3-3 lists the most common monitoring devices, and Table 3-4 shows the most common complications from placement of these devices. It is important to trace out and account for each catheter individually. For instance, the nasogastric tube might have initially been mistaken for an ECG lead. The result of instilling fluid through this tube could have been disastrous. Even so, the result of this placement was a pneumothorax. We have reviewed the normal placement of catheters and some of the more common related complications. The student should be familiar with this aspect of radiography in the ICU setting, and the references cited at the end of the chapter will provide further in-depth learning.

CONCLUSION

The heart and great vessels present an interesting and demanding diagnostic challenge to the physician. A thorough history and physical examination are the initial steps to gen-erate a differential diagnosis and to decide which imaging tests are necessary to limit these possibilities. The choice of imaging tests should ideally be made in consultation with the radiologist, taking into consideration potential morbidity, cost, availability of the technology, and the interest and expertise of the radiologist. Students should be aware that careful decision making has the potential to decrease the cost of medical care in the United States.

Acknowledgments *Special thanks to my colleague Gregory Braden, MD, for providing Figure 3-12 for use in this chapter.*

SUGGESTED READING

1. Bastarrika G, Lee YS, Huda W, Ruzsics B, Costello P, Schoepf UJ. CT of coronary artery disease. *Radiology.* 2009;253:317-338.
2. Bengel FM, Takahiro H, Javadi MS, Lautamaki R. Cardiac positron emission tomography. *J Am Coll Cardiol.* 2009;54:1-15.
3. Chen JT: *Essentials of Cardiac Imaging.* Philadelphia: Lippincott-Raven; 1997.
4. Finn JP, Nael K, Deshpande V, Ratib O, Laub G. Cardiac MR imaging: state of the art technology. *Radiology.* 2006;241:338-354.
5. Higgins CB: *Essentials of Cardiac Radiology and Imaging.* Philadelphia: Lippincott; 1992.
6. Lee VS: *Cardiovascular MR Imaging: Physical Principles to Practical Protocols.* Philadelphia: Lippincott Williams & Wilkins; 2005.
7. Miller SW, Abbara S, Boxt L: *Cardiac Radiology: The Requisites.* 3rd ed. St. Louis, Mo: Mosby; 2009.
8. Remy-Jardin M, Remy J, Baert AL: *Integrated Cardiothoracic Imaging with MDCT.* New York: Springer; 2008.
9. Vitola JV, Delbeke D: *Nuclear Cardiology and Correlative Imaging: A Teaching File.* New York: Springer; 2004.
10. Warnes CA: *Adult Congenital Heart Disease.* Hoboken, NJ: Wiley-Blackwell; 2009.

Radiology of the Chest

Caroline Chiles, MD
Shannon M. Gulla, MD

INTRODUCTION

The chest radiograph is the most frequently performed radiographic study in the United States. It should almost always be the first radiologic study ordered for evaluation of diseases of the thorax. The natural contrast of the aerated lungs provides a window into the body to evaluate the patient for diseases involving the heart, lungs, pleurae, tracheobronchial tree, esophagus, thoracic lymph nodes, thoracic skeleton, chest wall, and upper abdomen. In both acute and chronic illnesses, the chest radiograph allows one to detect a disease and monitor its response to therapy. For many disease processes (eg, pneumonia and congestive heart failure) the diagnosis can be established and the disease followed to resolution with no further imaging studies. There are limitations to the chest radiograph, and diseases may not be sufficiently advanced to be detected or may

not result in detectable abnormalities. Other imaging methods are needed to complement the conventional chest radiograph. These imaging methods include computed tomography (CT), positron emission tomography/computed tomography (PET/CT) and other radionuclide studies, magnetic resonance (MR) imaging, and ultrasound (US). These techniques, their clinical uses, and case studies are included in this chapter.

TECHNIQUES

▶ Conventional Radiography

The Posteroanterior and Lateral Chest Radiograph

The simplest conventional study of the chest is a posteroanterior and lateral chest radiograph taken in a radiographic unit specially designed for these studies. The x-rays travel through the patient and expose a receptor from which the image is recorded. Most commonly, digital receptors are used, although a receptor utilizing an intensifying screen and radiographic film remains in some use as well. Computed radiography and large field-of-view image intensifiers are two types of digital receptors. The digital images may be printed on film by laser printers but are generally viewed on monitors. The two views of a chest radiograph are taken in projections at 90 degrees to each other with the patient's breath held at the end of a maximum inspiration. The first view is obtained as the patient faces the receptor with the x-ray beam source positioned 6 feet behind him. Because the x-ray beam travels in a posterior-to-anterior direction, this view is called a posteroanterior (PA) chest radiograph. Another view is then obtained with the patient turned 90 degrees and the left side against the receptor and arms overhead. The x-ray beam travels from right to left through the patient, and this is called a left lateral view. Anatomic features of the chest that are readily identifiable on conventional radiographs are shown in Figures 4-1 and 4-2.

Other Radiographic Projections

In some clinical situations, patients may not be able to stand or sit upright for the conventional PA and lateral radiographs, and an image must be taken with the patient's back turned to the receptor and the x-ray beam traversing the patient in an anterior-to-posterior direction. These radiographs are called anteroposterior (AP) radiographs. They may be taken in the x-ray department but are more commonly obtained as portable studies at the patient's bedside.

Images may also be obtained with the patient lying on one side in a decubitus position with the x-ray beam traversing the patient either PA or AP along a horizontal plane. These images are designated as lateral decubitus images (see Figure 4-63c). A left lateral decubitus radiograph indicates that the left side of the patient is dependent against the table. A right lateral decubitus radiograph indicates that the right side of the patient is dependent against the table.

The Portable Chest Radiograph

If the clinical situation prevents the patient from coming to the radiology department, a chest radiograph may be obtained at the patient's bedside, and these are almost always AP radiographs. The AP portable radiograph does not provide as much information as PA and lateral chest radiographs for a number of reasons. Because it is a single view, lesions are not as easily or accurately localized along the AP axis of the thorax. The patients for whom these images are obtained are usually quite ill and cannot be positioned as well as patients traveling to the x-ray department. An ill patient may not be able to cooperate by holding his breath at full inspiration. A mobile x-ray generator is typically not as powerful as a fixed x-ray generator, and longer exposure times therefore are necessary to obtain sufficient exposure. The quality of portable chest radiographs, therefore, is often inferior to that of PA and lateral radiographs, as a result of both respiratory and cardiac motion. X-ray grids are used to reduce scatter radiation and improve image quality. Grids are used for most conventional chest radiographs done in radiology departments where fixed equipment is present. Grids are not usually used for portable radiographs, and the result is a high proportion of scattered x-rays, which degrade the image. Paradoxically, the portable radiograph may be more expensive than a conventional PA and lateral chest radiograph, owing to extra labor and equipment costs in obtaining a bedside radiograph.

▶ Computed Tomography of the Chest

Computed tomography is described in detail in Chapter 1. For CT examinations of the chest, intravenous contrast material is frequently administered for opacification of arteries and veins within the mediastinum and hila to facilitate the recognition of abnormal masses or lymph nodes. Anatomic features of the chest that are readily identifiable on CT scans are shown in Figures 4-3 and 4-4.

▶ Nuclear Medicine Perfusion Imaging of the Chest

Nuclear medicine techniques used in evaluating diseases of the thorax include ventilation-perfusion (V/Q) scanning and scanning with tumor-seeking radiopharmaceuticals for tumor staging. The V/Q scan may be used for patients with suspected pulmonary thromboembolism and who have contrast allergy or renal failure. The V/Q scan is noninvasive, and when results are negative, fewer than 10% of patients have pulmonary thromboembolism. The ventilation study is typically performed with the patient inhaling 10 to 30 mCi of xenon-133 while images are obtained with a scintillation camera (Figure 4-5A). Wash-in images are obtained for two consecutive 120-second periods, an equilibrium image is obtained, and then wash-out images are obtained over 30- to 60-second periods in posterior and left and right posterior oblique projections. This portion of the study takes about 15 minutes. The perfusion scan is obtained by intravenously injecting 2 to 4 mCi of technetium-99m-labeled macroaggregated albumin containing 200,000 to 700,000 particles. The particles range in size from 10 to 100 μm, and they lodge in capillaries and capillary arterioles, accurately reflecting pulmonary blood flow (Figure 4-5B). The scintillation camera is

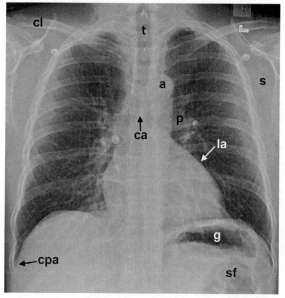

A

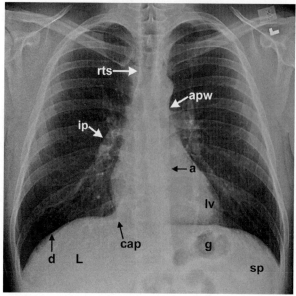

B

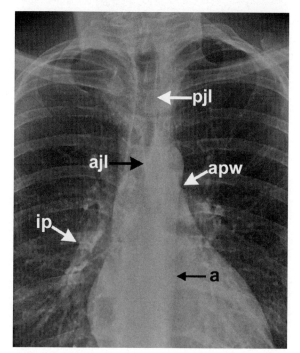

C

▲ Figure 4-1. (A–C) Normal radiographic anatomy. Posteroanterior chest radiographs. a, aorta; ajl, anterior junction line; apw, aortopulmonary window; ca, carina; cap, cardiophrenic angle; cl, clavicle; cpa, costophrenic angle; d, diaphragm; g, gastric air bubble; ip, interlobar (or descending) pulmonary artery; L, liver; la, left atrium; lv, left ventricle; p, main pulmonary artery; pjl, posterior junction line; rts, right tracheal (or paratracheal) stripe; s, scapula; sf, splenic flexure of colon; sp, spleen; t, trachea.

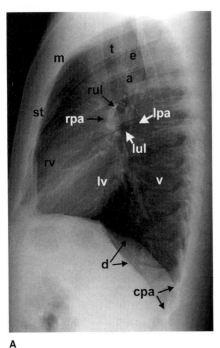
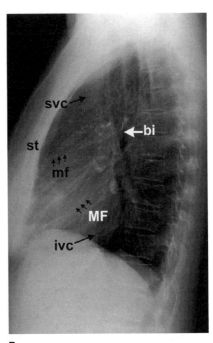

A   B

▲ **Figure 4-2. (A,B)** Normal radiographic anatomy. Lateral chest radiographs. a, aorta; bi, bronchus intermedius; cpa, costophrenic angle; d, diaphragm; e, esophagus; ivc, inferior vena cava; lpa, left pulmonary artery; lul, left upper lobe bronchus; lv, left ventricle; m, manubrium; mf, minor fissure; MF, major fissure; rpa, right pulmonary artery; rul, right upper lobe bronchus; rv, right ventricle; st, sternum; svc, superior vena cava; t, trachea; v, vertebral body.

set so that it obtains anterior, posterior, both posterior oblique, and both anterior oblique projections for 750,000 counts per image. The perfusion study takes about 30 minutes to perform.

▶ **Positron Emission Tomography/Computed Tomography Imaging of the Chest**

Tomography is also available for radionuclide imaging. A PET scanner resembles a CT scanner and uses positron emitters (fluorine-18 [F-18] or carbon-11 [C-11]). Today, the most widely used positron emitter is F-18-fluoro-deoxyglucose (FDG), which is used as a metabolic tracer. The raised metabolic rate can be used to distinguish neoplasm and inflammation from normal tissue. Although PET provides tomographic images, the spatial resolution (0.7 to 1.0 cm) is somewhat inferior to that of CT. This spatial resolution is improved by utilizing PET/CT fusion imaging in which a patient receives both a PET scan with F-18 FDG as well as a CT with or without contrast. These images can then be overlaid, or fused (Figure 4-6), to combine the spa-

tial resolution of CT with the localization power of radionuclide imaging.

▶ **Magnetic Resonance Imaging of the Chest**

The principles and applications of MR are described in Chapter 1. Anatomic features of the chest that are readily identifiable on MR images are shown in Figures 4-7 and 4-8.

▶ **Ultrasonography of the Chest**

Ultrasound is described in detail in Chapter 1. Ultrasound of the chest is typically performed to evaluate fluid collections within the pleural space. Ultrasound may be used to guide thoracentesis, especially when the fluid collection is small or loculated. Less frequently, ultrasound is utilized to guide percutaneous biopsy of mediastinal or peripleural lung lesions. Advances in image fusion also allow fusion of ultrasound images with a separately performed CT examination, which can be useful for ultrasound-guided biopsies in the thorax.

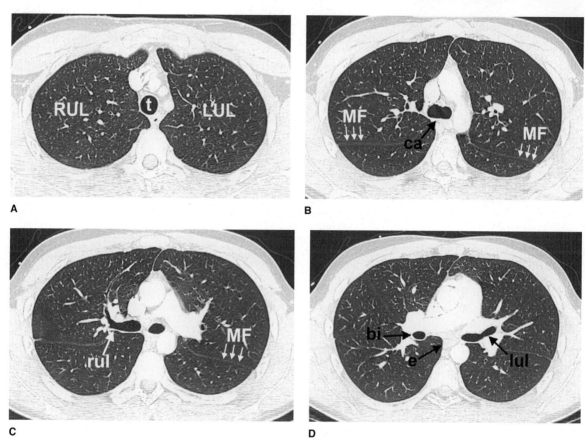

▲ **Figure 4-3.** **(A–H)** Normal CT anatomy. Axial scans of the chest, contiguous slices at approximately 1 cm collimation, lung window settings. bb, basilar segmental bronchi of lower lobes; bi, bronchus intermedius; ca, carina; e, esophagus; Li, lingula segment of the left upper lobe; LLL, left lower lobe; lul, left upper lobe bronchus; LUL, left upper lobe; MF, major fissure; RLL, right lower lobe; RML, right middle lobe; rml, right middle lobe bronchus; RUL, right upper lobe; rul, right upper lobe bronchus; ss, bronchus to superior segment of lower lobe; t, trachea.

TECHNIQUE SELECTION

The number of diseases and clinical situations for which a chest radiograph may be indicated is so large that an exhaustive listing of individual indications is prohibitive. As a general rule, however, conventional radiographs should be obtained for any patient with symptoms suggesting disease of the heart, lungs, mediastinum, or chest wall. In addition, a chest radiograph is indicated for patients with systemic diseases that have a high likelihood of secondary involvement of those structures. Examples of the former are pneumonia and congestive heart failure and of the latter are a primary extrathoracic neoplasm and connective tissue disease.

In an acutely ill patient, the portable chest radiograph is an invaluable tool for monitoring the patient's cardiopulmonary status. These radiographs are also used for monitoring of life-support hardware, such as central venous access catheters, nasogastric tubes, and endotracheal tubes.

Fluoroscopy provides real-time imaging of the chest. Fluoroscopy may be used to evaluate the motion of the diaphragm in a patient with suspected diaphragmatic paralysis. A paralyzed hemidiaphragm has sluggish motion as the patient breathes, and as the patient takes in a quick breath of air, it moves paradoxically upward as the normal hemidiaphragm moves downward ("sniff test"). Fluoroscopy and fluoroscopically positioned spot images are also useful for

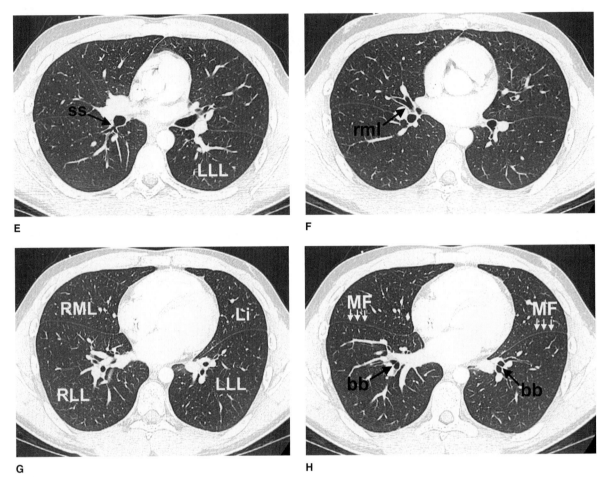

E

F

G

H

▲ **Figure 4-3.** *(Continued)*

identification of calcification within a pulmonary nodule, within coronary arteries, or within cardiac valves. Fluoroscopic guidance can also be used for percutaneous transthoracic needle biopsy of lung masses.

Because the three dimensions of the thorax are captured on a single two-dimensional chest radiograph, superimposition of structures within the thorax may result in confusing shadows. Because CT provides images without this overlap, it is frequently used to clarify confusing shadows identified on conventional radiographs (Table 4-1). These examinations are also used to detect disease that is occult because of small size or a hidden position. Because of its wider range of density discrimination, CT can demonstrate mediastinal and chest wall abnormalities earlier than is possible with conventional chest radiography. Abnormalities of hilar structures can be identified on CT scans because of the decreased overlap of the complex structures of the hilum. CT scans of the chest are routinely ordered for oncology pa-

tients, both for evaluation of the extent of disease at presentation and for monitoring response to therapy or progression of disease. CT is useful for evaluation of the lung

Table 4-1. Major Indications for CT of the Chest

Clarification of abnormal chest radiograph findings
Staging of lung cancer and esophageal cancer
Detecting metastatic disease from extrathoracic malignancy
Evaluation of a solitary pulmonary nodule
Suspected mediastinal or hilar mass
Suspected pleural tumor or empyema
Determining source of hemoptysis (eg, bronchiectasis)
CT-guided percutaneous needle aspiration of lung and mediastinal masses
CT-guided pleural drainage

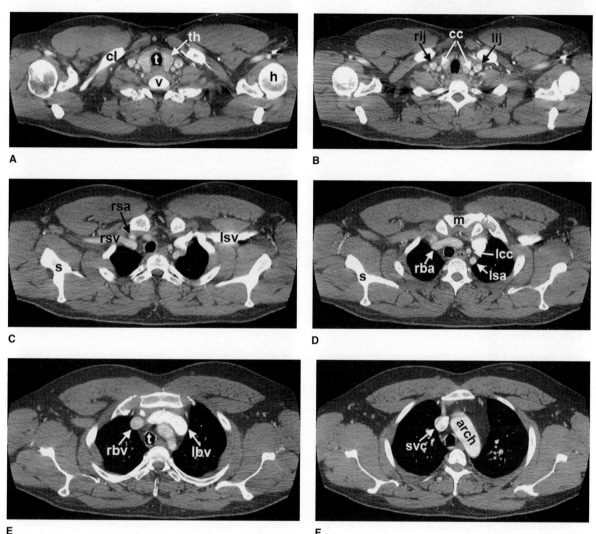

▲ **Figure 4-4.** **(A–N)** Normal CT anatomy. Axial scans of the chest, contiguous slices at approximately 1 cm collimation, soft-tissue (mediastinal) window settings. aa, ascending aorta; arch, transverse section of the aortic arch; azv, azygos vein; cc, common carotid artery; cl, clavicle; cs, coronary sinus; da, descending aorta; e, esophagus; hazv, hemiazygos vein; h, humerus; im, internal mammary artery and vein; ip, interlobar (or descending) pulmonary artery; ipv, inferior pulmonary vein; ivc, inferior vena cava; ivs, interventricular septum; L, liver; la, left atrium; LAD, left anterior descending coronary artery; lbv, left brachiocephalic vein; lcc, left common carotid artery; lij, left internal jugular vein; lpa, left pulmonary artery; lsa, left subclavian artery; lsv, left subclavian vein; lv, left ventricle; lvot, left ventricular outflow tract; m, manubrium; mpa, main pulmonary artery; pc, pericardium; r, rib; ra, right atrium; rba, right brachiocephalic artery; rbv, right bronchiocephalic vein; rij, right internal jugular vein; rpa, right pulmonary artery; rsa, right subclavian artery; rsv, right subclavian vein; rv, right ventricle; rvot, right ventricular outflow tract; s, scapula; sp, spleen; st, sternum; svc, superior vena cava; t, trachea; th, thyroid; v, vertebral body.

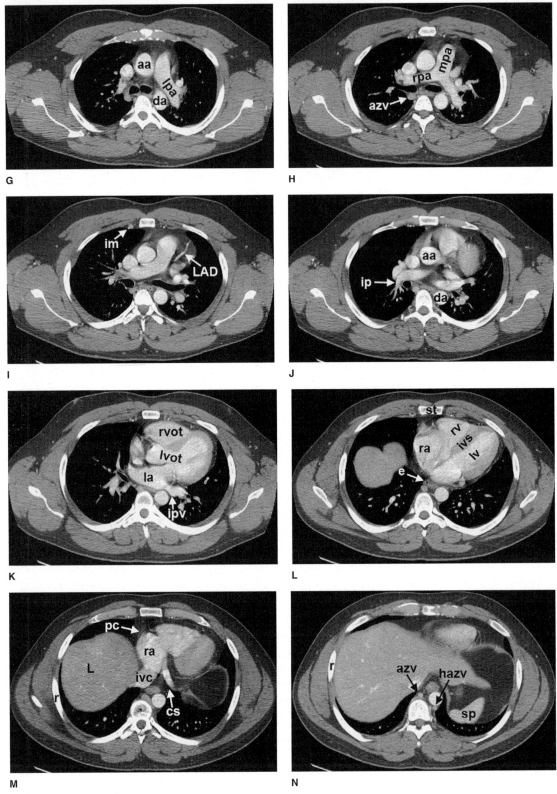

▲ Figure 4-4. *(Continued)*

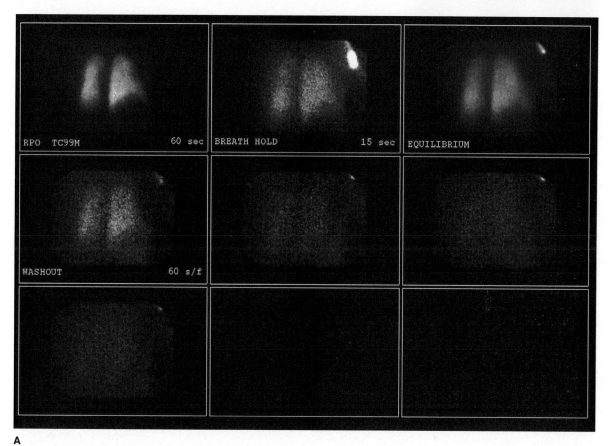

| RPO   TC99M   60 sec | BREATH HOLD   15 sec | EQUILIBRIUM |
| WASHOUT   60 s/f | | |

A

▲ **Figure 4-5.** **(A)** Ventilation scan performed in the right posterior oblique projection shows normal wash-in of the xenon-133 gas and no retention of gas in any regions on the wash-out views.

parenchyma, as thin sections (1 to 2 mm thick) reveal great anatomic detail. Thin-section CT (or high-resolution CT [HRCT]) may enable detection of occult pulmonary parenchymal disease and may be used for following the course of known pulmonary disease (Table 4-2). HRCT is especially useful in the diagnosis of interstitial lung diseases. Additionally, CT angiography (CTA) of the chest is particularly useful for the evaluation of vascular pathology as well as pulmonary embolus (Table 4-3). Because intravenous contrast material can be administered, vascular structures

may be evaluated and the technique may be useful in patients with aortic dissection, aortic aneurysm, and superior vena caval obstruction. Because the cost of CT is approximately 10 to 20 times that of a PA and lateral chest radiograph, CT is not practical for monitoring the course of diseases on a daily basis.

The diseases and situations for which nuclear medicine techniques are helpful are determined for the most part by the radioactive tracer, and these have been outlined in the technique section (Table 4-4).

Table 4-2. Major Indications for High-Resolution CT of the Chest

| Evaluation of acute and chronic pulmonary disease |
| Evaluation of occult parenchymal disease |

Table 4-3. Major Indications for CTA of the Chest

| Suspected pulmonary embolism |
| Suspected aortic dissection |
| Superior vena cava syndrome |

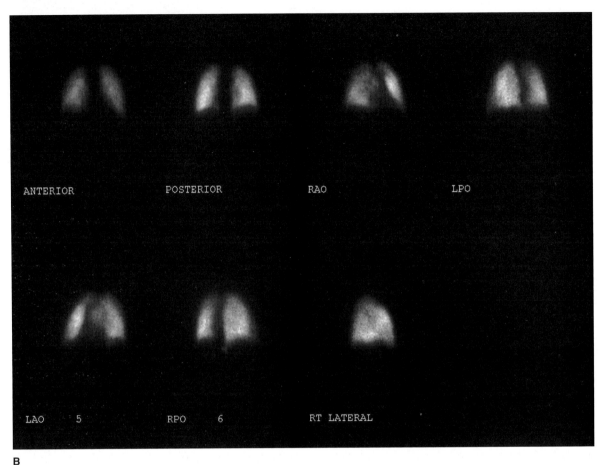

ANTERIOR   POSTERIOR   RAO   LPO

LAO 5   RPO 6   RT LATERAL

B

▲ **Figure 4-5.** *(Continued)* (**B**) Normal perfusion scan performed in seven projections, shows equal perfusion of radionuclide throughout all segments of the lungs. RAO, right anterior oblique; LAO, left anterior oblique; RPO, right posterior oblique; LPO, left posterior oblique.

MR imaging of the thorax is most commonly used for cardiovascular imaging, but there are indications for MR imaging in mediastinal and pulmonary parenchymal imaging as well (Table 4-5). MR is helpful when bronchogenic carcinoma is suspected of invading vascular structures, including the cardiac chambers, pulmonary arteries and veins, and the

Table 4-4. Major Indications for Nuclear Medicine Imaging of the Chest

Suspected pulmonary thromboembolism (V/Q scan)
Differentiation of benign and malignant pulmonary nodule (PET)
Staging of thoracic malignancy (eg, lung, breast, esophagus) (PET)
Detecting recurrent or metastatic tumor (PET)

Table 4-5. Major Indications for MR Imaging of the Chest

Evaluation of a mediastinal mass
Suspected Pancoast (superior sulcus) tumor
Superior vena cava syndrome
Staging of lung cancer, when CT suggests invasion of the heart, great vessel, chest wall, diaphragm
Suspected aortic dissection
Evaluation for central pulmonary embolus in patients with allergy to iodinated contrast media or renal failure
Evaluation of the mediastinum and hilum in patients with allergy to iodinated contrast media or renal failure
Congenital and acquired heart disease

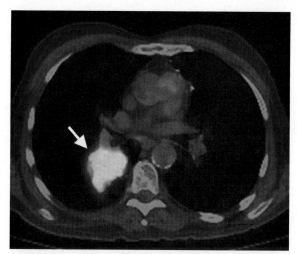

▲ **Figure 4-6.** PET-CT fused image demonstrates hypermetabolic activity in a tumor in the superior segment of the right lower lobe. Hypermetabolic activity (arrow) on fused imaging is demonstrated as a bright spot overlying the tumor.

superior vena cava. In a patient with suspected Pancoast's (superior sulcus) tumor (Figure 4-9), MR imaging is preferred to CT because of the ability to obtain images in coronal and sagittal planes. The apex of the lung can be difficult to evaluate on axial images alone because of partial-volume effects.

Ultrasonography is useful for imaging the soft tissues of the chest wall, heart, and pericardium, as well as fluid collections within the pleural space. Large, mobile pleural effusions are usually aspirated without sonographic guidance, because these collect predictably within dependent areas of the thorax. On the other hand, loculated pleural fluid collections may be difficult to aspirate without guidance, and the most appropriate entrance site may be marked with sonography for easier access. Ultrasonography has been used for guidance for biopsy of peripheral lung lesions as well.

EXERCISE 4-1. THE OPAQUE HEMITHORAX

4-1. The most likely diagnosis for Case 4-1 (Figure 4-10) is
 A. massive right pleural effusion.
 B. total atelectasis of the right lung.
 C. left pneumothorax.
 D. aplasia of the right lung.
 E. mediastinal hematoma.
4-2. The most likely diagnosis for Case 4-2 (Figure 4-11) is
 A. left pleural effusion.
 B. collapse of the left lung.

 C. right pneumothorax.
 D. collapse of the right lung.
 E. mediastinal hematoma.

Radiologic Findings

4-1. In this case, a frontal chest radiograph (Figure 4-10) shows that the right hemithorax is opaque. Signs of mass effect are present and suggest a space-occupying lesion in the right hemithorax. There is shift of the mediastinum toward the *contralateral* hemithorax, as evidenced by shift of the trachea and left heart border to the left. If a nasogastric tube were in place, esophageal shift could be inferred from the shift of the nasogastric tube. Space-occupying lesions also cause inferior displacement of the hemidiaphragm. Although the diaphragm itself is not visible, when the process is on the left, one can infer that the diaphragm is depressed by the inferior displacement of the gastric air bubble. Mass effect may also widen the distance between ribs. In this patient, the space-occupying lesion was a large right pleural effusion resulting from tuberculous empyema. A chest CT scan (Figure 4-12) in this patient shows the large pleural effusion and complete collapse of the underlying right lung against the medial aspect of the right hemithorax (A is the correct answer to Question 4-1).

4-2. In this case, a frontal chest radiograph (Figure 4-11) shows that the left hemithorax is opaque. In contrast to the patient in Figure 4-10, the patient in Figure 4-11 has signs of volume loss within the left hemithorax. There is mediastinal shift toward the *ipsilateral* hemithorax, as evidenced by shift of the trachea and the right heart border into the left hemithorax. The gastric air bubble is higher in the left upper quadrant of the abdomen than is normally seen, because of elevation of the left hemidiaphragm. The mediastinal window of the chest CT examination (Figure 4-13A) shows the mediastinal shift to the left and consolidation of the left lung. The lung window of the chest CT examination (Figure 4-13B) shows that the right lung is aerated. In this patient, the left lung collapse is due to a bronchogenic carcinoma in the left main bronchus (asterisk). This case exhibits the signs of volume loss, as opposed to mass effect (B is the correct answer to Question 4-2).

Discussion

This exercise reviews the principal signs that allow one to distinguish mass effect from volume loss. The mass effect caused by a tumor or by a large pleural effusion expands the hemithorax and displaces the trachea, mediastinum, and

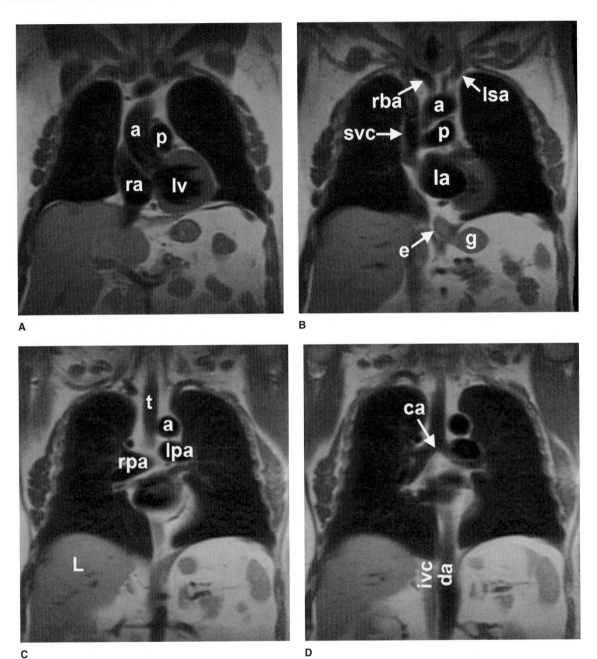

▲ **Figure 4-7.** (**A–E**) Normal MR anatomy. Coronal spin-echo images of the thorax. a, aorta; azv, azygos vein; ca, carina; da, descending aorta; e, esophagus (seen distally); g, gastric fundus; h, humerus; ivc, inferior vena cava; k, kidney; L, Liver; la, left atrium; lpa, left pulmonary artery; lsa, left subclavian artery; lv, left ventricle; p, pulmonary artery; ra, right atrium; rba, right brachiocephalic artery; rpa, right pulmonary artery; sp, spleen; svc, superior vena cava; t, trachea; v, vertebral body.

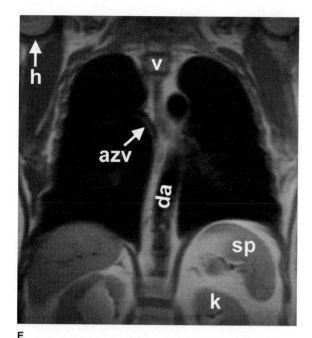

E

▲ **Figure 4-7.** *(Continued)*

diaphragm away from the mass. There may be a subtle increase in the distance between ribs. Volume loss, on the other hand, decreases the size of the hemithorax, and the trachea, mediastinum, and diaphragm move toward the involved hemithorax. The distance between the ribs on the abnormal side will be slightly decreased. In Figure 4-10, the opacification of the right hemithorax occurs as a result of massive right pleural effusion, and the right lung is collapsed as a result of both compression by the fluid present within the right pleural space and a loss of the negative intrapleural pressure that keeps the lung in close juxtaposition to the chest wall. In Figure 4-11, the collapse is due to obstruction of the left main bronchus, resulting in atelectasis (airlessness) of the left lung.

EXERCISE 4-2. LOBAR ATELECTASIS

4-3.   In Figure 4-14 A,B, the inferior margin of the opacity in the right upper thorax is due to
   A. the major fissure in right upper lobe (RUL) collapse without a hilar mass.
   B. the minor fissure in RUL collapse with a hilar mass.
   C. the minor fissure in RUL collapse without a hilar mass.
   D. the major fissure in RUL collapse with a hilar mass.

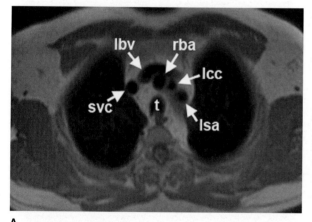

A

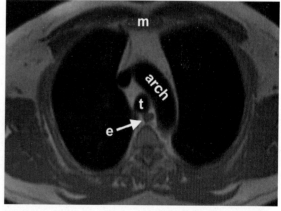

B

▲ **Figure 4-8. (A–L)** Normal MR anatomy. Axial spin-echo images of the thorax. aa, ascending aorta; arch, transverse section of the aortic arch; azv, azygos vein; bi, bronchus intermedius; ca, carina; cs, coronary sinus; da, descending aorta; e, esophagus; g, gastric fundus; hazv, hemiazygos vein; im, internal mammary artery and vein; ip, interlobar (or descending) pulmonary artery; ipv, inferior pulmonary vein; ivc, inferior vena cava; ivs, interventricular septum; L, Liver; la, left atrium; laa, left atrial appendage; lbv, left brachiocephalic vein; lcc, left common carotid artery; LM, left main coronary artery; lpa, left pulmonary artery; lsa, left subclavian artery; lv, left ventricle; m, manubrium; pc, pericardium; ra, right atrium; rba, right brachiocephalic artery; rpa, right pulmonary artery; rv, right ventricle; rvot, right ventricular outflow tract; spv, superior pulmonary vein; st, sternum; svc, superior vena cava; t, trachea; v, vertebral body.

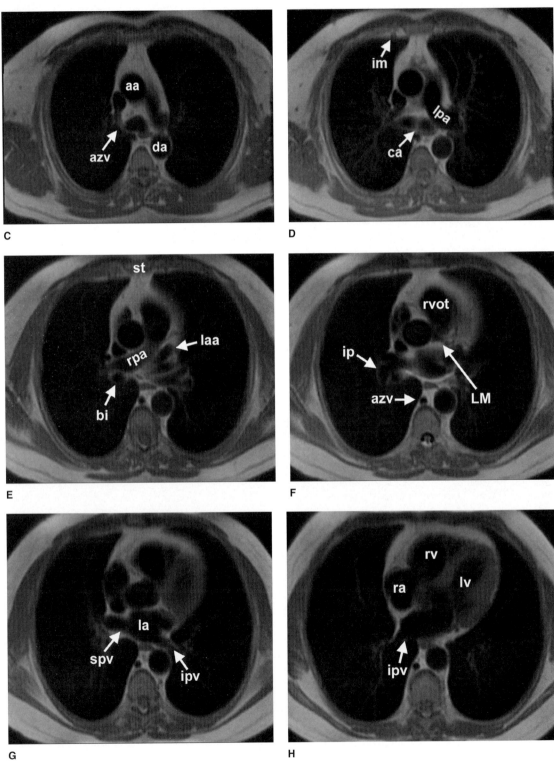

▲ Figure 4-8. *(Continued)*

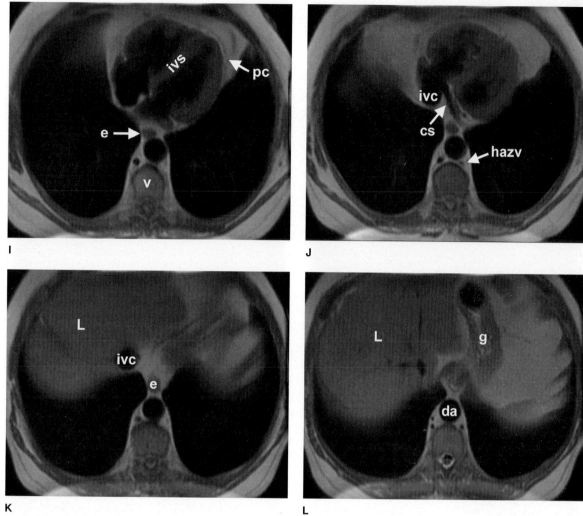

I   J

K   L

▲ **Figure 4-8.** *(Continued)*

4-4. In Figure 4-15 A,B, which of the following is true re-
      garding right middle lobe collapse?
      A. A triangular opacity is superimposed on the heart
          on the frontal radiograph.
      B. The right heart border is obscured.
      C. The minor fissure is superiorly displaced.
      D. The right heart border is shifted to the left.

4-5. In Figure 4-16 A,B, a sign of left lower lobe collapse in
      this patient is which of the following?
      A. Obscuration of the lateral wall of the ascending
          thoracic aorta
      B. Superior displacement of the left hilum
      C. Obliteration of the anterior aspect of the left
          hemidiaphragm on the lateral view

D. Triangular opacity in the left retrocardiac area on
    the frontal view
E. Shift of the major fissure toward the anterior
    chest wall on the lateral view

4-6. In Figure 4-17 A,B, signs of left upper lobe collapse
      seen in this patient include which of the following?
      A. Crescent of air around the transverse section of
          the aortic arch resulting from hyperexpansion of
          the superior segment of the left lower lobe
      B. Posterior displacement of the left major fissure on
          the lateral view
      C. Obscuration of the right heart border
      D. Tracheal deviation to the right
      E. Inferior displacement of the left hilum

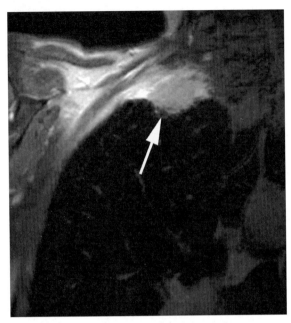

▲ **Figure 4-9.** Coronal post-gadolinium MRI image demonstrates an enhancing mass (arrow) in the right lung apex extending superiorly into the soft tissues of the chest wall.

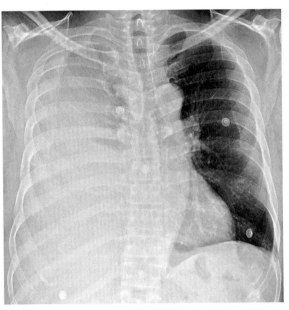

▲ **Figure 4-10.** Case 4-1: 40-year-old man with fever and dyspnea.

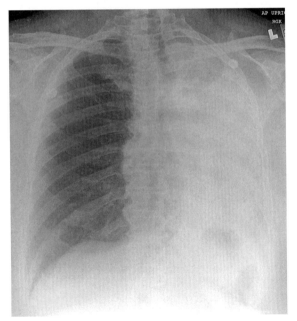

▲ **Figure 4-11.** Case 4-2: 62-year-old man with dyspnea, increased over the past several months.

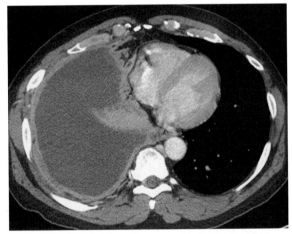

▲ **Figure 4-12.** Axial CT scan of the chest of the same patient as in Figure 4-10 shows filling of the right pleural space by fluid, with compression of the right lung and displacement of the mediastinal contents into the left hemithorax. The pleural fluid in this case represented tuberculous empyema.

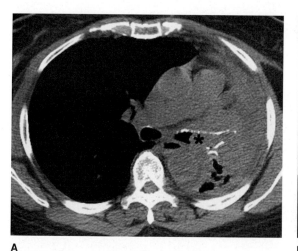
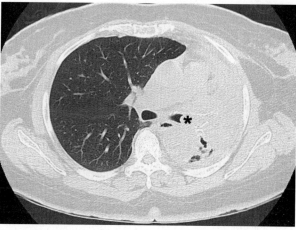

A   B

▲ **Figure 4-13.** (**A**) CT scan of the same patient as in Figure 4-11 shows mediastinal shift to the left, consolidation of the entire left lung, and an endobronchial lesion in the left mainstem bronchus (asterisk). (**B**) Lung window shows that the right lung is overexpanded to compensate for the left lung atelectasis.

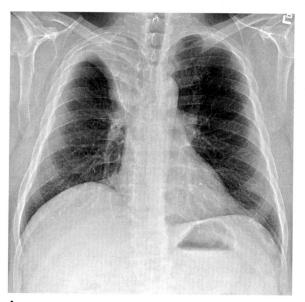
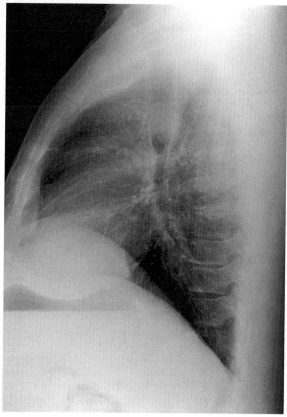

A   B

▲ **Figure 4-14.** (**A,B**) Case 4-3: 61-year-old man with dyspnea.

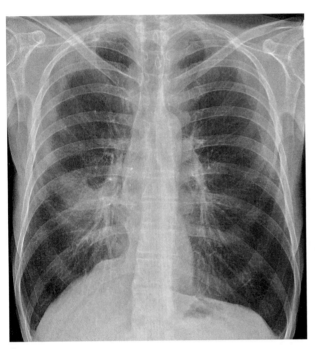

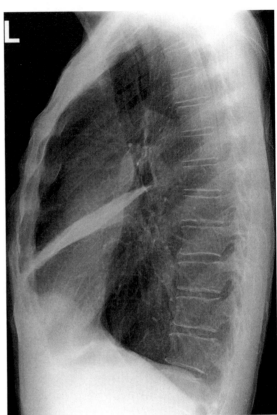

A   **B**

▲ **Figure 4-15.** (**A,B**) Case 4-4: 45-year-old man with chronic cough.

Radiologic Findings

4-3.   In Figure 4-14, there is opacity in the right upper lung that is sharply marginated on its inferior border. Volume loss is evidenced by the slight displacement of the trachea into the right hemithorax, the position of the right heart border further to the right of the thoracic spine than normal, and the slight elevation of the right hemidiaphragm, which is normally 1 to 1.5 cm higher than the left hemithorax. The pulmonary vessels of the right hilum are obscured by opacity in the right upper thorax. The configuration of the inferior margin of the opacity is that of a reverse S or S on its side. The "S-sign of Golden" describes the appearance of the minor fissure in right upper lobe collapse, which is due to bronchogenic carcinoma. In this case, bulky right hilar lymph-node enlargement has caused extrinsic compression of the right upper lobe bronchus and has resulted in right upper lobe collapse. The right hilar mass tethers the medial aspect of the minor fissure to

its normal midthoracic position, whereas the lateral aspect of the minor fissure moves freely and collapses superiorly. In patients in whom the minor fissure is incomplete, collateral air drift across the canals of Lambert and the pores of Kohn may allow a lobe to remain aerated despite complete obstruction of its bronchus. In Figure 4-14 A, hyperexpansion of the superior segment of the right lower lobe produces the ovoid lucency on the medial aspect of the collapsed right upper lobe. On the lateral radiograph, a V-shaped opacity is seen at the lung apex. A mass-like opacity is superimposed on the suprahilar area, corresponding to a combination of tumor and atelectatic lung (B is the correct answer to Question 4-3). In patients with right upper lobe collapse without a hilar mass, the fissure is able to rotate in a straighter line and does not result in the reverse S sign. The major fissure is oriented in a coronal plane and is not normally visualized on the frontal chest radiograph. Therefore, the major fissure would

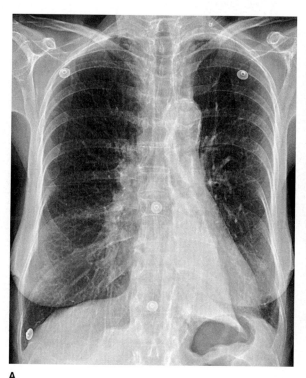
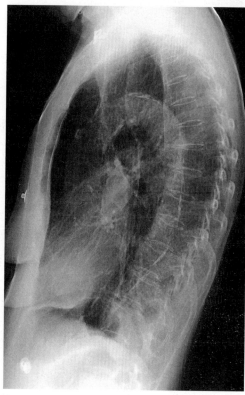

A   **B**

▲ **Figure 4-16. (A,B)** Case 4-5: 62-year-old man with a cough productive of blood-tinged sputum.

not account for the opacity seen on the frontal chest radiograph, either with or without a hilar mass.

4-4. In Figure 4-15 A,B, the right heart border is obscured by adjacent opacity on the PA radiograph. The lungs are hyperinflated. The heart is in the midthorax in approximately its normal position. The heart border has not been displaced to the left. On the lateral radiograph, a narrow triangular opacity is superimposed on the heart. The apex of the triangle points toward the hilum, and the base of the triangle is against the anterior chest wall. This is a collapsed right middle lobe. The right hemidiaphragm is slightly elevated, but there are no other signs of significant volume loss. Right middle lobe collapse may have minimal impact on the overall volume in the right hemithorax because it is the smallest of the pulmonary lobes, and the upper and lower lobes can expand to compensate for its volume loss. Right middle lobe collapse, unlike other lobar collapse, is often due to benign causes, such as extrinsic pressure by enlarged lymph nodes, which totally surround the bronchus. This enlarge-

ment is most frequently due to granulomatous disease of an infectious or noninfectious nature (B is the correct answer to Question 4-4).

4-5. When the left lower lobe collapses, the result is a triangular opacity, which can be quite subtle, behind the heart. Secondary signs of volume loss, however, should prompt one to look closely for the collapse. These signs include shift of the trachea and heart to the left (note that the right heart border is now superimposed on the thoracic spine), inferior displacement of the left hilum, and elevation of the left hemidiaphragm. On the lateral radiograph, the right hemidiaphragm is visible along its entire contour. However, the left hemidiaphragm is obscured posteriorly because it is "silhouetted" by the collapsed left lower lobe. Because it is tethered medially by the inferior pulmonary ligament, the left lower lobe collapses posteriorly and medially (Figure 4-18). The major fissure is displaced *posteriorly*, as well as rotated into a more sagittal orientation than the normal coronal orientation (D is the correct answer to Question 4-5). You may have noted the large

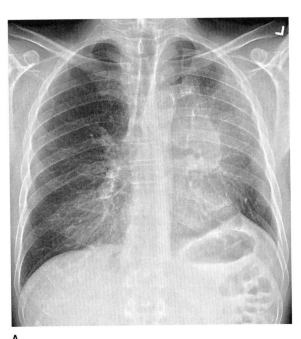 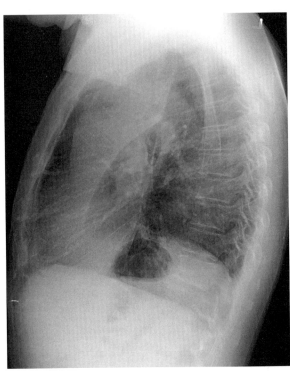

A   B

▲ **Figure 4-17.** (**A,B**) Case 4-6: 49-year-old man with cough.

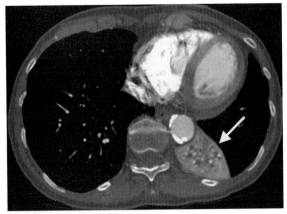

▲ **Figure 4-18.** Axial CT scan of the same patient as in Figure 4-16 shows a lenticular mass (arrow) within the posteromedial aspect of the left hemithorax. This represents the collapsed left lower lobe. Note the shift of the heart toward the left hemithorax.

lung volumes in this patient, which are due to centrilobular emphysema. In this patient, who has a long history of cigarette smoking, a squamous-cell carcinoma in the left lower lobe bronchus was responsible for the collapsed left lower lobe.

4-6.   The primary sign of volume loss in Figure 4-17 B is anterior displacement of the left major fissure on the lateral radiograph. The collapsed left upper lobe is opaque as a result of both airlessness and postobstructive pneumonitis. When there is little pneumonitis within the obstructed lobe, the left upper lobe can collapse completely behind the anterior chest wall, so that only a narrow band of opacity is visible behind the sternum. In this situation, the diagnosis may be suggested by the secondary signs of volume loss. Note the shift of the trachea to the left and the slight elevation of the left hemidiaphragm. The left lower lobe is hyperexpanded. The hyperexpanded superior segment of the left lower lobe produces a crescent of air around the transverse section of the aortic arch on the PA radiograph. A thin opaque line is visible at the apex of the left hemidiaphragm on the PA radiograph. Presence of this line, called a juxtaphrenic peak, should prompt one to look for upper lobe collapse. The hilum may be displaced anteriorly in left upper lobe collapse, but it is never displaced inferiorly. Option E, inferior displacement of the left hilum, is therefore false (A is the correct answer to Question 4-6). Because the lingular bronchus arises from the left upper lobe bronchus, the lingular segment of the left upper lobe is collapsed as well in this patient. The lingula is adjacent to the left heart border and is responsible for the obscuration of the left heart border in left upper lobe collapse.

Discussion

The term *atelectasis* refers to volume loss, or airlessness, within the lung. The term *collapse* is often used to describe complete atelectasis of an entire lobe or an entire lung. Atelectasis can occur as a result of several pathophysiologic processes. Obstruction of a bronchus by bronchogenic carcinoma should always be considered in an adult with lobar atelectasis. The tumor may be within the bronchus (endobronchial), as occurs with squamous-cell carcinoma or small-cell undifferentiated carcinoma. The tumor may be outside the bronchus, and enlarged lymph nodes may cause extrinsic compression of the bronchus. In a child, aspiration of a foreign body is a more likely cause of obstruction of a bronchus. Complete obstruction of a lobar bronchus may not always result in lobar collapse because pathways of collateral ventilation are present within the lung. The pores of Kohn and the canals of Lambert allow collateral air drift between adjacent areas of lung but do not extend across pleural surfaces. The visceral pleural surface that covers the lung creates the interlobar fissures (minor fissure, major fissure) that separate lobes of the lungs. These fissures are not always complete, however, and may not extend entirely across the lung. When the right upper lobe bronchus is occluded, for example, the right upper lobe may remain partially aerated as a result of collateral air drift from the right middle lobe, around an incomplete minor fissure. Obstruction of smaller airways can occur as a result of mucous plugs, which are often present in intubated patients and in patients with chronic small airway disease.

Passive atelectasis (see Figure 4-10) occurs as a result of a space-occupying process within the pleural space. This is also called relaxation atelectasis, because the lung is no longer exposed to the negative intrapleural pressure that normally keeps the lung apposed to the chest wall. Any space-occupying pleural process, including a large pneumothorax (air in the pleural space), pleural effusion, hemothorax (blood in the pleural space), or pleural tumor, can cause atelectasis within the underlying lung. *Compressive atelectasis* is the term used to describe atelectasis caused by a space-occupying process within the lung itself. *Cicatrization atelectasis* describes the volume loss that occurs as a result of pulmonary scarring. *Adhesive atelectasis* occurs when there is a loss of the pulmonary surfactant that maintains the surface tension that keeps alveoli open. Adhesive atelectasis occurs with pulmonary embolism, and with respiratory distress syndrome of the newborn. Atelectasis of small areas of lung is often referred to as *subsegmental atelectasis* and may be recognized as linear bands of opacity, often at the lung bases (Figure 4-19).

It is helpful to remember the normal positions of the hemidiaphragms, trachea, mediastinum, and hila so that displacement of these structures can be readily noted. In most patients, the left hilum appears slightly higher than the right, because the left hilar opacity is predominantly due to the left pulmonary artery arching over the left main bronchus. The right hemidiaphragm is usually 1.0 to 1.5 cm higher than the left hemidiaphragm. The trachea should be in the midline, and the spinous processes of the upper thoracic vertebrae should be superimposed on the center of the tracheal air column. The right heart border normally lies just to the right of the thoracic spine. Subtle signs of volume loss may be more readily appreciated by comparison of the patient's radiograph with baseline radiographs taken previously.

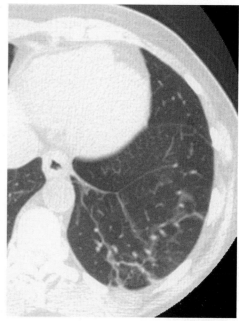

▲ **Figure 4-19.** Axial CT image of the left lung base demonstrates linear bandlike opacities extending to the pleural surface in the periphery. This is an example of subsegmental atelectasis.

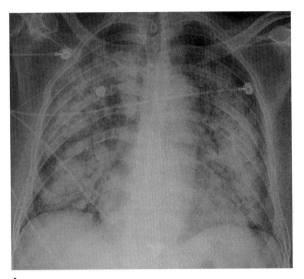

A

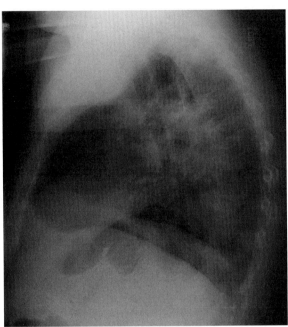

B

▲ **Figure 4-20. (A,B)** Case 4-7: 65-year-old man with cough, and hemoptysis.

EXERCISE 4-3. AIRSPACE DISEASES

4-7. Which of the following is the best descriptor of Figure 4-20 A,B?
 A. Diffuse airspace disease
 B. Lobar airspace disease
 C. Interstitial pattern
 D. Unilateral airspace disease

4-8. For Figure 4-21, which one of the following best explains the opacity in the right hemithorax?
 A. Collapse of the right upper lobe due to bronchial obstruction
 B. Airspace consolidation of the right middle lobe
 C. Empyema loculated within the right major fissure
 D. Carcinoma in the right upper lobe

Radiologic Findings

(Both of these patients have airspace opacities)

4-7. In this case (Figure 4-20), the opacity involves multiple lobes bilaterally (A is the correct answer to Question 4-7.).

4-8. In this case (Figure 4-21), the opacity is in the right middle lobe and obscures the medial margin of the heart. On the lateral view of this patient, the margins are sharply demarcated by the fissures, indicating the

lobar nature of the process. Radiolucent structures that exhibit a branching pattern are noted to arborize through both opacities (B is the correct answer to Question 4-8.).

Discussion

The patient in Figure 4-20 has pulmonary hemorrhage as a consequence of underlying Wegener's granulomatosis, manifested as multilobar airspace disease bilaterally, also seen on CT (Figure 4-22). The patient in Figure 4-21 has pneumococcal pneumonia (*Streptococcus pneumoniae*) in the right middle lobe. The opacity seen on both radiographs is best described as airspace disease. The alveoli, or airspaces, that are normally filled with air have become filled with exudate. The exudate-filled alveoli surround the bronchi, so that the air-filled bronchi are visible as radiolucent branching structures within the more radiopaque background (Figure 4-23). Airspace disease is often lobar (Figure 4-21), multilobar, or diffuse (Figure 4-20) in distribution. The process may initially appear as multiple ill-defined nodules that rapidly coalesce. These nodules are the shadows of fluid-filled acini. They are 6 to 10 mm in diameter and always have ill-defined margins. The margins of these coalescing opacities are difficult to outline. Although there can be associated volume loss as the surfactant within the alveoli is lost, the signs of volume loss are

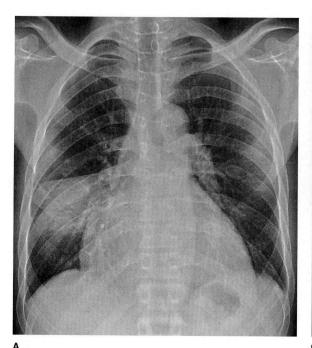
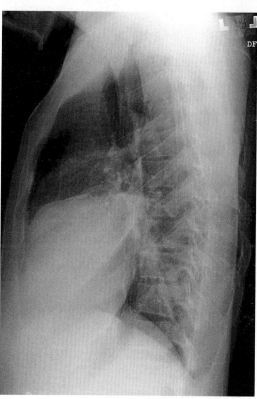

A   **B**

▲ **Figure 4-21.** **(A,B)** Case 4-8: 38-year-old man with fever and a cough productive of purulent sputum.

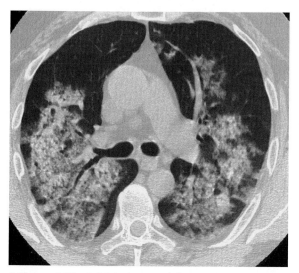

▲ **Figure 4-22.** Axial CT image of the patient in Figure 4-20 shows diffuse airspace opacities representing blood-filled alveoli in this patient with hemoptysis.

often subtle and do not account for the opacity seen within the lung. Once airspace disease is identified, an attempt should be made to determine its cause. Airspace disease that appears suddenly or exhibits change over hours to days is due either to pulmonary hemorrhage or to contusion, pneumonia, or pulmonary edema (blood, pus, or water). The patient's clinical history, physical examination, and laboratory data help to determine the most likely diagnosis. In patients likely to have infectious disorders, the responsible organism is usually not identified at first treatment, and the patient is just given antibiotics. In patients who do not respond to this initial treatment, an attempt should be made to identify the organism.

In a patient with fever and productive cough, pneumonia is likely. On the other hand, a patient with rib or sternal fractures as a result of blunt chest trauma is more likely to have pulmonary contusion. Pulmonary edema, which may occur as a result of either cardiogenic or noncardiogenic disease, is discussed later in this chapter.

A reticular pattern is one in which the opacities are linear in nature and the lines range from quite thin to several millimeters thick. The opacities are oriented in multiple directions and

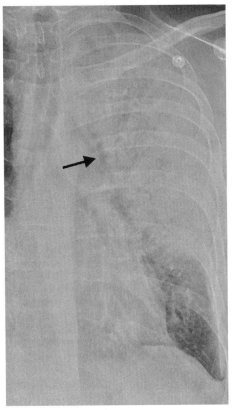

▲ **Figure 4-23.** Close-up view of the left upper lobe shows a radiopaque opacity. Arborizing through this opacity are radiolucent branching structures (arrow) representing the air-filled bronchi (air bronchograms).

appear to overlap so as to create the appearance of a net. This pattern is not present.

EXERCISE 4-4. DIFFUSE LUNG OPACITIES

4-9.   Which of the following best describes the chest radiograph in Figure 4-24?
   A. Alveolar pulmonary edema
   B. Interstitial pulmonary edema, and small bilateral pleural effusions
   C. Unilateral interstitial disease
   D. Oligemia in the right lung

Radiologic Findings

4-9.   Frontal chest radiograph (Figure 4-24) shows mild enlargement of the heart and indistinct vascularity, particularly at the lower lungs. Interlobular septal

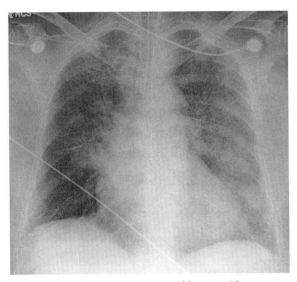

▲ **Figure 4-24.** Case 4-9: 57-year-old man with progressive dyspnea, orthopnea, and pedal edema and a history of hypertension.

lines are visible adjacent to both lower costophrenic angles. (B is the correct answer to Question 4-9)

Discussion

Pulmonary edema can be divided into two major categories: cardiogenic edema and noncardiogenic edema. Cardiogenic edema occurs as a result of elevation of pulmonary capillary pressure, which is usually due to pulmonary venous hypertension. Noncardiogenic edema occurs as a result of disorders that increase pulmonary capillary permeability. With both types of edema, there is a net movement of fluid out of the microvasculature and into the pulmonary interstitium and alveoli. The most common cause of pulmonary edema is left ventricular failure, which may be due to atherosclerotic coronary artery disease, mitral or aortic valvular disease, myocarditis, or cardiomyopathy. Cardiogenic edema is preceded by pulmonary venous hypertension, which is associated with redistribution of pulmonary blood flow from dependent regions of the lung to nondependent regions. In the erect patient, the radiographic sign of this redistribution is an increase in size of vessels in the upper lungs and a decrease in the caliber of pulmonary vessels in the lung bases. Radiographically, it is often difficult to distinguish pulmonary arteries from pulmonary veins, but for purposes of determination of flow redistribution, the distinction is ignored and multiple vessels are measured at equal distances from the hilum or chest wall.

When seen end-on, normal bronchoarterial bundles may appear as adjacent circles of equal diameter, with the artery opaque and the bronchus lucent. The pulmonary arteries and bronchi are located together in the same interstitial space and arborize adjacent to each other. The pulmonary veins return blood to the heart in a separate interstitial space and have a slightly different arborization pattern. As the pulmonary venous pressure increases, fluid leaks from the pulmonary capillaries into the adjacent interstitium. This interstitial pulmonary edema may be identified by peribronchial cuffing, indistinctness of the perivascular margins, perihilar haziness, and thickening of the interlobular septa and interlobar fissures. Septal thickening results in Kerley A (arrow) and Kerley B (arrowhead) lines on chest radiograph (Figure 4-25). As the pulmonary capillary pressure increases further, fluid spills into the alveoli, producing a symmetrical appearance of airspace filling that is predominantly perihilar (central) and basilar in distribution. Cardiogenic edema is greatest in dependent regions of the lungs. In supine patients, the dependent regions are the posterior segments of the upper lobes, and the superior and posterior basilar segments of the lower lobes. The central pattern of pulmonary edema has been called "bat-wing" edema (Figure 4-26). As the pulmonary edema worsens, the pulmonary and pleural lymphatics clear fluid from the lungs, and pleural effusions will develop. In congestive heart failure, the pleural effusions are generally small to moderate in size, and there is typically more fluid within the right pleural space than the left. Isolated left pleural effusion is

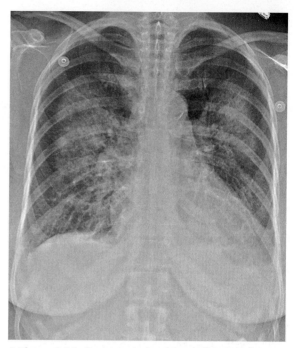

▲ **Figure 4-26.** Posteroanterior chest radiograph demonstrates "bat-wing" or central pulmonary edema with opacities focused around the hila.

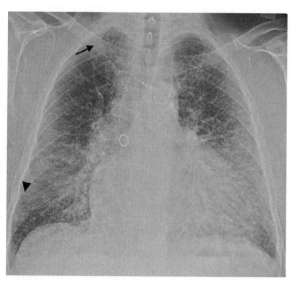

▲ **Figure 4-25.** Posteroanterior chest radiograph of a patient with pulmonary edema demonstrates septal thickening known as Kerley A (arrow) and B (arrowhead) lines. The cardiac silhouette is enlarged, and the patient has had median sternotomy for coronary artery bypass graft as evidenced by sternal wires and graft marker projecting over the midline.

unlikely to be due to congestive heart failure. In cardiogenic edema, the heart size will be increased. The cardiothoracic ratio is a guide to determining cardiac enlargement. The transverse dimension of the heart is divided by the transverse diameter of the thorax at the same level. When the cardiothoracic ratio is greater than 0.5, cardiomegaly is often (but not always) present. When possible, both the PA and lateral projections should be used to determine cardiac volume. Cardiomegaly may be more readily recognized when comparison is made with prior radiographs. Comparison requires a similar depth of inspiration and similar positioning of the patient (AP versus PA, supine versus erect).

Noncardiogenic edema (Figure 4-27), or "capillary leak" edema, may be due to a number of conditions, including adult respiratory distress syndrome, fat embolism, amniotic fluid embolism, drug overdose, near drowning, and acute airway obstruction. The cause of pulmonary edema in patients with intracranial injury or tumor (neurogenic pulmonary edema) is uncertain. Similarly, the etiology of high-altitude pulmonary edema is incompletely understood. The common radiographic findings in noncardiogenic edema are symmetric, diffuse areas of airspace filling that is often patchier in appearance and more peripheral in distribution. The heart size is usually normal; pleural effusions and septal lines are typically absent. The vascular pedicle is of normal width.

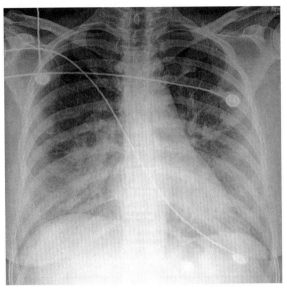

▲ **Figure 4-27.** Posteroanterior chest radiograph demonstrating airspace opacities predominantly in the lower lobes bilaterally. Septal thickening is not seen. Vascular pedicle width is normal.

Renal failure and volume overload may result in pulmonary edema, which may be chronic. When the degree of edema is small to moderate, patients are often reasonably well compensated and are able to carry out many activities of daily living.

EXERCISE 4-5. AIRWAY DISEASE

4-10. The most accurate description of this chest radiograph (Figure 4-28 A,B) is
   A. decreased lung volume.
   B. diffuse thickening of the bronchial walls.
   C. cardiomegaly.
   D. pleural effusion.
   E. mediastinal shift.

Radiologic Findings

4-10. In this case, the most prominent radiographic finding in Figure 4-28 A is coarse thickening of the bronchovascular bundles as they radiate from the hila. Thickened bronchial walls may be identified as tram-track lines, which refers to the appearance of the nearly parallel walls of bronchi oriented longitudinally. Careful inspection shows that these are present throughout both lungs and are located near the hila. Bronchial walls also project as ring-shaped opacities near the hila when

the bronchus is seen end-on. Both of these structures represent the thick walls of dilated bronchi (bronchiectasis). The hila themselves are slightly enlarged as a result of a combination of enlarged hilar lymph nodes and mild pulmonary arterial hypertension. The lung volume is increased. The anterior clear space (retrosternal area) is larger and more radiolucent than normal. (B is the correct answer to Question 4-10).

Discussion

The cause of this patient's bronchiectasis is cystic fibrosis. The mucus in patients with cystic fibrosis is thickened, and these patients do not have normal tracheobronchial clearance. This abnormal clearance may cause mucoid impaction, and atelectasis and pneumonia are frequent complications. Bronchiectasis can also occur as a result of pneumonia in patients without cystic fibrosis. In patients with pneumonia, the bronchiectasis is more likely to be confined to a single lobe, often a lower lobe. Bronchiectasis is divided into three groups: cylindrical, fusiform (or varicose), and saccular (or cystic). These three groups not only describe the appearance of the abnormal bronchi, but also give an indication as to its severity. Cylindrical bronchiectasis (Figure 4-29 A), the mildest form, is reversible and appears as thick-walled bronchi that fail to taper normally. The more severe forms, fusiform and saccular, are irreversible. Fusiform (Figure 4-29 B) bronchiectasis has a beaded appearance, whereas the bronchi in saccular (Figure 4-29 C) bronchiectasis end with clubbed, cystic areas. If the severe forms are localized, surgical resection may be curative. Medical therapy with bronchodilator and, when necessary, antibiotics is used when surgery is not indicated.

CT is the method of choice for determining the presence and extent of bronchiectasis. When the bronchus is perpendicular to the CT plane of section, bronchiectasis is identified as a ring shadow adjacent to an opaque circle. The ring represents the thickened dilated bronchial walls. The opaque circle represents the pulmonary artery adjacent to the dilated bronchus. This is called the "signet ring" sign (Figure 4-30). Bronchi and arteries travel together throughout the lung and are normally of the same caliber.

EXERCISE 4-6. SOLITARY PULMONARY NODULE

4-11. Characteristics suggesting that a nodule is benign are that
   A. the size of the nodule does not change over 2 months.
   B. it contains central calcification.
   C. CT attenuation values within the nodule are over 30 Hounsfield units.
   D. it is semisolid on CT.

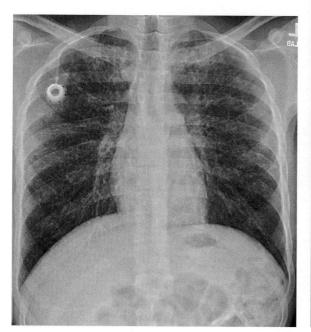

A

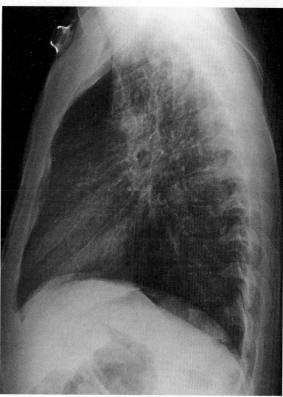

B

▲ **Figure 4-28.** **(A,B)** Case 4-10: 22-year-old man who has had chronic cough and copious mucus production since childhood.

Radiologic Findings

4-11. Frontal chest radiograph (Figure 4-31 A) shows a nodule in the left mid-lung that appears solid but is slightly lobulated. CT (Figure 4-31 B) of the chest demonstrates a popcorn pattern of calcification (arrow) (B is the correct answer to Question 4-11).

Discussion

In attempting to determine whether or not a nodule is benign, the characteristics to consider are the age of the patient, any history of previous malignancy, and the nodule's growth rate, density, shape, and edge characteristics. The most important of these are the growth rate and density. If a solid nodule has had no growth over a 2-year period and has calcification of the types associated with benign causes, then the nodule is almost certainly benign. Because of the importance of time in assessing growth, comparison with old images is the most important test and the least expensive method of determining whether a nodule is benign.

Doubling times of lung cancers are variable, but an increase in diameter of the tumor would be expected in a 2-year period. The absence of growth of a solid nodule over a 2-year period is evidence that the nodule is stable is size and must, therefore, be benign. If radiographs demonstrate growth over this 2-year interval, then the nodule should be assumed to be malignant.

If a solid nodule is diffusely and completely calcified (Figure 4-32 A), if it is calcified centrally (Figure 4-32 B), or if it has a laminated pattern (Figure 4-32 C), then the nodule may be assumed to be benign. A popcorn pattern of calcification, also benign (Figures 4-31 B, 4-32 D), can be seen in a hamartoma. Calcification may not be apparent on the initial radiograph because the most commonly used technique for chest radiography obscures subtle calcification. Demonstration of calcification may require fluoroscopy or repeated chest radiography with a lower kVp technique to enhance its depiction. When it is not clear from these studies whether calcification is present, CT should be used to identify it. CT has an extended range of tissue discrimination

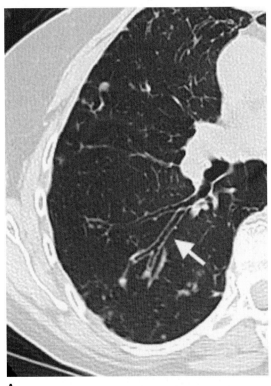

A

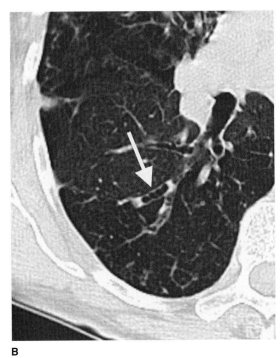

B

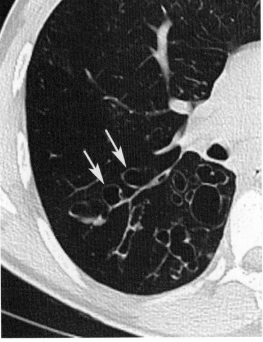

C

▲ **Figure 4-29.** Cylindrical (**A**), fusiform (**B**), and saccular (**C**) bronchiectasis (arrow) on axial CT.

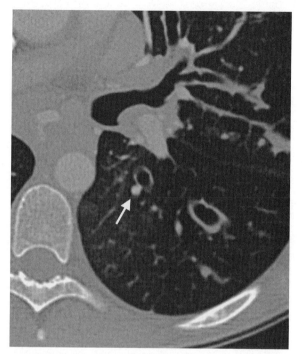

▲ **Figure 4-30.** Axial CT image demonstrates the "signet ring" sign (arrow) of bronchiectasis created by the dilated bronchus (the ring) and adjacent artery.

compared to conventional radiographs. The presence of calcification within a pulmonary nodule can be determined by evaluating the attenuation values within a region of interest (ROI) centered over the nodule (Figure 4-33 A–C). Air within the lung measures –800 Hounsfield units, noncalcified nodules measure 30 to 100 HU, and calcified nodules measure over 200 HU. Nodules with attenuation values between 0 and 200 are not necessarily malignant; they just do not have enough calcification to be categorized unequivocally as benign.

If a nodule is not calcified or if it has shown growth over a 2-year period, it should be considered as a possible malignancy, and further assessment should be dictated by the clinical circumstances. Most patients will need evaluation for possible tissue biopsy and surgical resection to determine the cause.

Nodules that are larger than 1 cm in diameter are generally evaluated with PET-CT. Smaller nodules are generally considered below the threshold of resolution for this technique. Nodules considered hypermetabolic on PET-CT (increased radiotracer uptake relative to background) are considered potentially malignant. Generally, these nodules then undergo percutaneous or surgical biopsy. However, whereas most cancers are hypermetabolic, bronchoalveolar cell carcinoma (BAC) and carcinoid may not be hypermetabolic (Figure 4-34). If these cancers are suspected on CT, a negative PET-CT examination could be a false-negative and should not preclude biopsy.

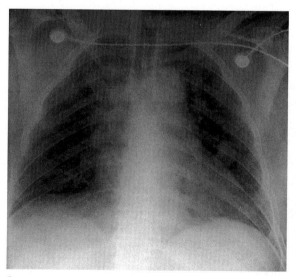

A

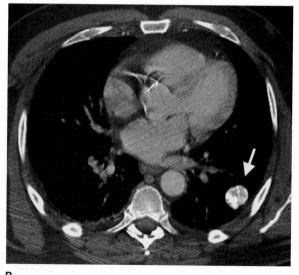

B

▲ **Figure 4-31.** Case 4-11: Preoperative chest radiograph (**A**) with subsequent CT of the chest (**B**) of a 53-year-old man who is scheduled for coronary artery bypass grafting.

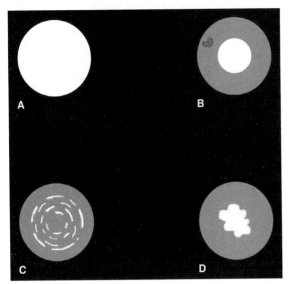

▲ **Figure 4-32.** Benign patterns of calcification on chest CT: (**A**) diffusely and completely calcified, (**B**) central calcification, (**C**) laminated pattern of calcification, (**D**) popcorn pattern of calcification.

Nodules can also be ground glass in appearance (Figure 4-35). However, this appearance is nonspecific and can be seen in multiple etiologies including infection as well as bronchoalveolar cell carcinoma. BAC can present as a ground-glass nodule that may not demonstrate any significant growth over a 2-year period. Therefore, ground-glass nodules require more extended monitoring than solid nodules do.

Nodules that are part solid and part ground glass can also be seen. These semisolid nodules behave more like solid nodules. Although they can be seen in an infectious or inflammatory process, semisolid nodules are more concerning for neoplasm. Semisolid nodules are particularly worrisome for bronchoalveolar cell carcinoma and warrant close follow-up with a low threshold for biopsy.

Bronchogenic carcinoma, particularly adenocarcinoma, frequently presents as a solitary pulmonary nodule in the periphery of the lung. A new solitary pulmonary nodule or nodule of indeterminate age, therefore, should be considered a possible malignancy. The most common cause of a solitary pulmonary nodule is a granuloma, typically the result of prior granulomatous infection, such as histoplasmosis or tuberculosis. These can frequently be identified as granulomata because of characteristic patterns of calcification.

Note that the margins of the lesion, whether smooth or spiculated, are of no value in determining the benignity or malignant potential of a lesion. Only uniform or central calcification, absence of growth over a 2-year period, or CT attenuation values over 200 HU throughout the nodule are reliable noninvasive indicators of benignity.

EXERCISE 4-7. PULMONARY NEOPLASM

4-12. The best description of the chest radiograph in Figure 4-36 A,B is
   A. mass in the left upper lobe.
   B. left upper lobe collapse.
   C. mediastinal mass.
   D. consolidation of the left upper lobe.
   E. enlargement of the left pulmonary artery.

Radiologic Findings

4-12. In this case, the chest radiographs show a smoothly marginated opacity projecting over the left upper lobe. Both hila are normal in size. The opacity seen on the PA view is smaller than the volume of the left upper lobe, and no air bronchograms are present; this excludes consolidation of the lung as an answer. The posterior margin of the opacity is not a long straight or gently curving line, as is the major fissure, and therefore left upper lobe atelectasis is not the correct answer. The one best description of the radiographic findings is mass in the left upper lobe (A is the correct answer to Question 4-12). In a patient with cough, weight loss, and a history of tobacco use, bronchogenic carcinoma should be the primary consideration. A CT examination in this patient (Figure 4-37 A) shows the mass in the left upper lobe, completely surrounded by aerated lung. PET-CT fusion imaging (Figure 4-37 B) demonstrates the expected hypermetabolic activity in the left upper lobe mass. A CT-guided percutaneous biopsy of this mass yielded a diagnosis of adenocarcinoma.

Discussion

There are more than 220,000 new cases of lung cancer, or bronchogenic carcinoma, and 160,000 deaths from lung cancer in the United States each year. Bronchogenic carcinoma is the more appropriate term, as most of them arise from the epithelium of the airways and not the lung per se. Because early recognition and surgical resection offer the patient the best chance for cure, it is important to be familiar with the variety of radiographic appearances of lung cancer. Four major cell types account for almost 90% of all lung cancers. The major cell types are squamous cell, adenocarcinoma,

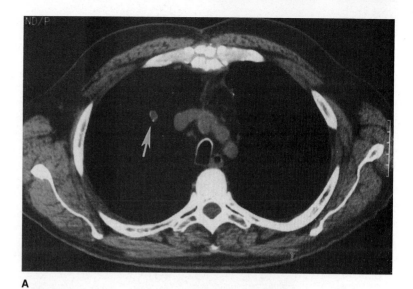

A

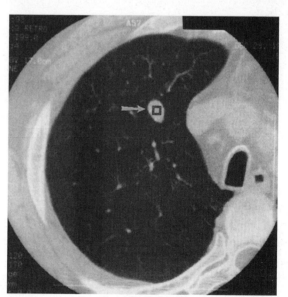

B

▲ Figure 4-33. (A) CT scan just above the aortic arch shows a nodule in the right upper lobe (arrow) with at least two eccentric regions of calcification. (B) A region of interest has been drawn on the nodule (arrow).

large cell, and small cell. For therapeutic purposes, lung cancer is divided into small-cell and non-small-cell lung cancer (NSCLC). This distinction is necessary because small-cell bronchogenic carcinoma is almost always widespread at the time of diagnosis and is best treated by chemotherapy and radiation therapy. Non-small-cell bronchogenic carcinoma, on the other hand, is best treated by surgical resection when the tumor is confined to one lung and regional lymph nodes. The typical radiographic appearance of small-cell carcinoma

is bulky hilar and/or mediastinal lymph nodes; the primary tumor sometimes is visible as a nodule within the lung (Figure 4-38).

Non-small-cell bronchogenic carcinoma includes adenocarcinoma, squamous-cell carcinoma, and large-cell carcinoma. Adenocarcinoma, the most common cell type, typically appears as a solitary pulmonary nodule in the periphery of the lung. Bronchioalveolar cell carcinoma is a subtype of adenocarcinoma that may present either as lobar

Report #1

Series: 3
Image: 17

	306	307	308	309	310	311	312	313	314	315	316
164	−10	14	85	87	53	61	54	22	16	26	−3
165	−7	19	75	78	69	113	112	37	−1	11	12
166	−9	3	17	45	113	205	220	114	17	−9	−2
167	23	0	12	89	232	374	370	225	77	−23	−40
168	4	−7	61	207	410	529	437	248	68	−56	−63
169	−21	22	130	301	504	557	363	131	9	−57	−46
170	13	41	187	331	440	424	219	31	−18	−17	−41
171	39	42	164	289	312	239	80	−34	−22	5	−48
172	38	25	122	235	227	102	−17	−74	−33	−6	−68
173	53	47	78	150	139	54	−34	−26	5	−10	−121
174	26	26	29	76	79	28	14	49	26	−68	−228

▲ **Figure 4-33.** *(Continued)* **(C)** The Hounsfield units in each pixel in the region of interest are demonstrated. Note the very high numbers in the central portion of the lesion, indicating calcification within those pixels.

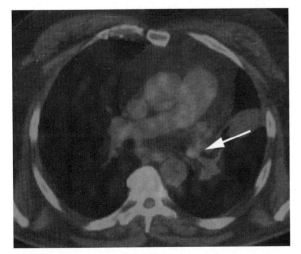

▲ **Figure 4-34.** Axial PET-CT fusion image demonstrates an endobronchial lesion with minimal hypermetabolic activity above the background level. This was biopsy-proven carcinoid, which may not be hypermetabolic on PET imaging.

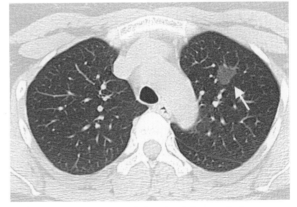

▲ **Figure 4-35.** CT scan of the chest demonstrates a ground-glass nodule in the left upper lobe. This was biopsy-proven bronchoalveolar cell carcinoma.

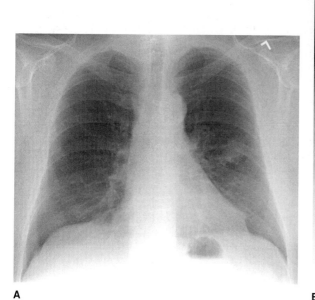
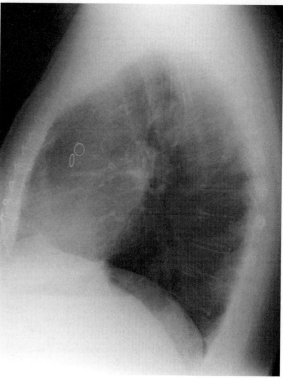

A   B

▲ **Figure 4-36.** **(A,B)** Case 4-12: 64-year-old man with cough and weight loss and a 50-pack-year history of tobacco use.

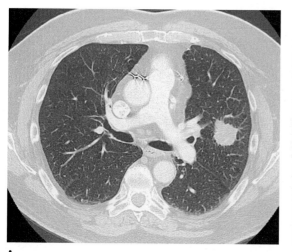
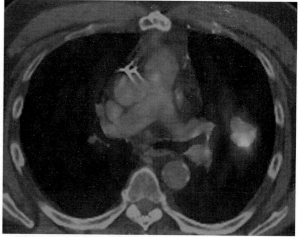

A   B

▲ **Figure 4-37.** **(A)** Axial CT image demonstrates a mass in the left upper lobe surrounded by aerated lung. This mass results in the opacity seen on chest radiograph. **(B)** PET-CT fusion image demonstrating hypermetabolic activity within the mass, consistent with malignancy in this case.

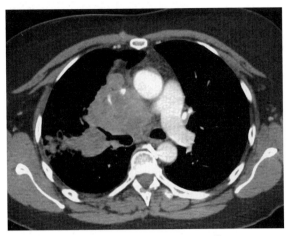

▲ **Figure 4-38.** Small-cell carcinoma typically presents with bulky mediastinal or hilar adenopathy.

airspace disease (Figure 4-39 A) or as diffuse, ill-defined pulmonary nodules (Figure 4-39 B). Bronchioalveolar cell carcinoma may also present as a solitary pulmonary nodule, usually a ground-glass nodule (see Figure 4-35). The second most common cell type, squamous-cell carcinoma, is associated with cigarette smoking and most often is found as an endobronchial tumor resulting in lobar collapse (Figures 4-13

and 4-18). The endobronchial tumor is visible bronchoscopically, and sputum cytology may be diagnostic in this tumor. Squamous-cell carcinoma can also appear radiographically as a solitary cavitary mass (Figure 4-39 C) or noncavitary mass. Large-cell carcinoma is the least frequent cell type. Its appearance is that of a bulky lesion within the lung.

When non-small-cell lung cancer is diagnosed, the patient undergoes a series of clinical and radiologic studies to determine the stage of the tumor. In the TNM staging system (Table 4-6), the categories of disease are stage IA, IB, IIA, IIB, IIIA, IIIB, or IV (Table 4-7). Stages I, II, and IIIA are surgically resectable. Patients with either stage IIIB or stage IV disease are not surgical candidates, but are treated with chemotherapy, radiation therapy, or both. In addition to helping define which treatment the patient should receive, the stage of the tumor helps provide prognosis. Patients with stage I disease have a 56% 5-year relative survival rate. Patients with stage IV disease have a 2% 5-year survival rate.

EXERCISE 4-8. MULTIPLE PULMONARY NODULES

4-13. The most likely cause of the multiple pulmonary nodules in Case 4-13 (Figure 4-40) is
   A. metastasis.
   B. herpes simplex pneumonia.

Table 4-6. Lung Cancer TNM Staging System

Tumor	Node	Metastasis
Tis Carcinoma in situ	N0 No lymph-node metastases	M0 No distant metastases
T1 A tumor 3 cm or less in greatest diameter, limited to the lung, and without invasion proximal to a lobar bronchus T1a Tumor 2 cm in greatest dimension or less T1b Tumor greater than 2 cm but less than 3 cm	N1 Metastases to ipsilateral intrapulmonary, hilar, or peribronchial lymph nodes	M1 Distant metastases
T2 A tumor larger than 3 cm but less than 7 cm; a tumor that invades the visceral pleura or produces collapse or consolidation of less than an entire lung; the tumor must be more than 2 cm distal to the carina T2a Tumor greater than 3 cm, but less than 5 cm T2b Tumor greater than 5 cm, but less than 7 cm	N2 Metastases to ipsilateral mediastinal or subcarinal lymph nodes	M1a Separate tumor nodule(s) in a contralateral lobe; tumor with pleural nodules or malignant pleural or pericardial effusion
T3 A tumor greater than 7 cm invading parietal pleura, chest wall, diaphragm, or mediastinal pleura or pericardium; a tumor less than 2 cm from the carina; or producing collapse or consolidation of an entire lung; or with separate nodule(s) in the same lobe	N3 Metastases to contralateral hilar or mediastinal lymph nodes; or scalene or supraclavicular lymph nodes	M1b Distant metastases
T4 A tumor of any size with invasion of the mediastinum or involving heart, great vessels, trachea, recurrent laryngeal nerve, esophagus, vertebral body, or carina; or separate tumor nodule(s) in a different ipsilateral lobe		

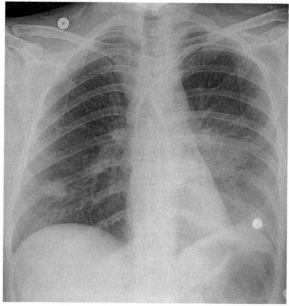

A

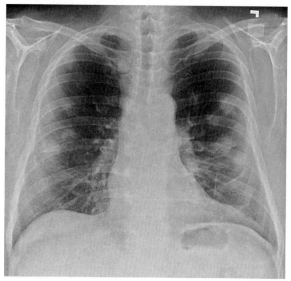

B

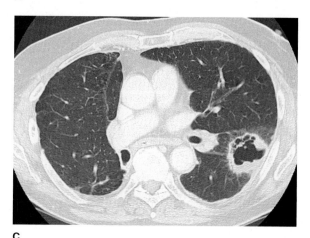

C

▲ **Figure 4-39.** (**A–C**) Forms of non-small-cell carcinoma. Presentations of bronchoalveolar cell carcinoma (a subtype of adenocarcinoma) on chest radiograph includes lobar airspace disease (**A**) and diffuse ill-defined pulmonary nodules (**B**). Air-fluid levels are present within a thick-walled cavitary mass in the left lower lobe, which was biopsy-proven squamous-cell carcinoma (**C**).

C. histoplasmosis.
D. Wegener's granulomatosis.
E. arteriovenous malformations.

Radiologic Findings

4-13.   In this case, the chest radiograph shows multiple, smoothly marginated, solid nodules in both lungs. These nodules are distributed diffusely and have various diameters (A is the correct answer to Question 4-13). The heart is normal in size and shape.

Discussion

The radiographic pattern of multiple pulmonary nodules is frequently encountered (Table 4-8). The clinical setting has considerable influence on the differential diagnosis in such cases and should always be taken into account when assessing patients with this pattern. However, the differential diagnosis may be narrowed by assessing the absolute size of the nodules, the uniformity of their size, their marginal characteristics, whether or not they are calcified, and whether or not they are cavitary. In adults the most common causes of

Table 4-7. Lung Cancer Staging Classifications

Stage 0	Stage IA	Stage IB	Stage IIA	Stage IIB	Stage IIIA	Stage IIIB	Stage IV
Tis N0 M0	T1a,b N0 M0	T2a N0 M0	T1a,b N1 M0 T2a N1 M0 T2b N0 M0	T2b N1 M0 T3 N0 M0	T1-2 N2 M0 T3 N1-2 M0 T4 N0,1 M0	T4 N2 M0 Any T N3 M0	Any T Any N M1a,b

multiple nodules are metastatic neoplasm and infectious disease. Metastatic neoplasm may result from carcinoma, sarcoma, or lymphoma. Pulmonary metastases may be of any size and number. In contrast to inflammatory nodules, nodular pulmonary metastases are often of various diameters. Metastases are usually of soft-tissue density similar to muscle or blood (Figure 4-41). Metastases may rarely be calcified if the patient has a sarcoma that makes bone or cartilage (eg, osteosarcoma). Differentiation is most commonly made by the clinical setting or review of old studies, but determination of the correct diagnosis may require tissue biopsy for confirmation.

Multiple pulmonary nodules may also be due to infectious disease, most commonly fungal or mycobacterial infections. In the United States, the most common fungus is histoplasmosis (Figure 4-42), although there are regional variations. Calcified nodules that are all of similar size suggest a previous infection with either histoplasmosis or tuberculosis. Nodules seen in acute infection are often not as sharply defined as metastases. This is especially true if the nodules represent acinar shadows. In these instances, the nodule is approximately 5 to 10 mm in diameter and is ill defined or fuzzy on its margin. Acinar nodules develop in patients with viral pneumonias such as herpes pneumonia or chicken pox (varicella) pneumonia.

Multiple pulmonary nodules may also develop in a wide variety of other disorders, including Wegener's granulomatosis and arteriovenous malformations, but would not be as numerous as in this case.

EXERCISE 4-9. CAVITARY DISEASE

4-14. The chest radiographic findings (Figure 4-43 A, B) in Case 4-14 could be best explained as
 A. multiple lung abscesses due to *Staphylococcus aureus*.
 B. pneumatoceles due to *Pneumocystis jiroveci* pneumonia.
 C. Wegener's granulomatosis.
 D. multiple cavities due to *Mycobacterium avium-intracellulare*.
 E. metastases from Kaposi's sarcoma.

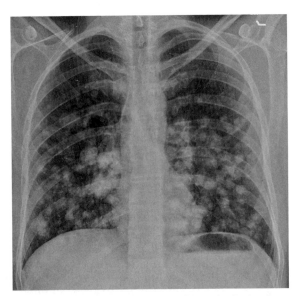

▲ **Figure 4-40.** Case 4-13: Chest radiograph obtained as part of a routine follow-up examination in a 43-year-old male with malignant melanoma of the right thigh treated with wide resection 3 years previously.

Table 4-8. Patterns of Multiple Pulmonary Nodules

Disease process	Nodule description	Nodule location
Metastases	Various sizes	Peripheral, hematogenous
Granulomas	Similar sizes, calcified	Diffuse
Septic emboli	Varying stages of cavitation	Peripheral
Wegener's granulomatosis	Generally larger, cavitary, hemorrhagic	Diffuse
Rheumatoid arthritis	Various sizes, cavitary, thick-walled	Peripheral

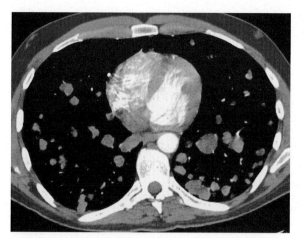

▲ **Figure 4-41.** Axial CT image from the same patient (Figure 4-40) demonstrating multiple soft tissue attenuation nodules throughout the lungs consistent with metastatic disease.

Radiologic Findings

4-14.   PA and lateral chest radiographs (Figures 4-43 A,B) and CT images (Figure 4-43 C,D) show at least two thick-walled cavitary lesions in the right lung (C is the correct answer to Question 4-14). There is no hilar or mediastinal lymph node enlargement. The heart and skeleton are normal.

Discussion

Inflammatory lesions are the most common cause of lung cavities (Table 4-9). The number of cavities may range from one to many. A wide variety of infecting organisms may result in cavitation, and the radiograph is nonspecific as to etiology. There is considerable overlap in appearances from the various organisms, so that culture or histologic evaluation is the only satisfactory means of identifying the etiology. If the lesion is single, a cavitating pneumonia should be the first

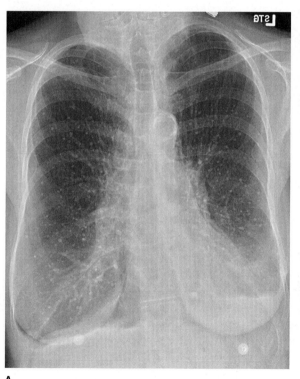

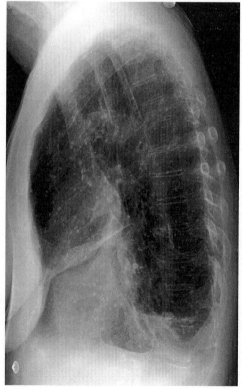

A   B

▲ **Figure 4-42.** Frontal (**A**) and lateral (**B**) chest radiographs show multiple small, dense nodules scattered throughout both lungs; these calcified nodules are the residua of prior histoplasmosis infection. Tuberculosis can also produce calcified granulomata. This patient also has small bilateral pleural effusions.

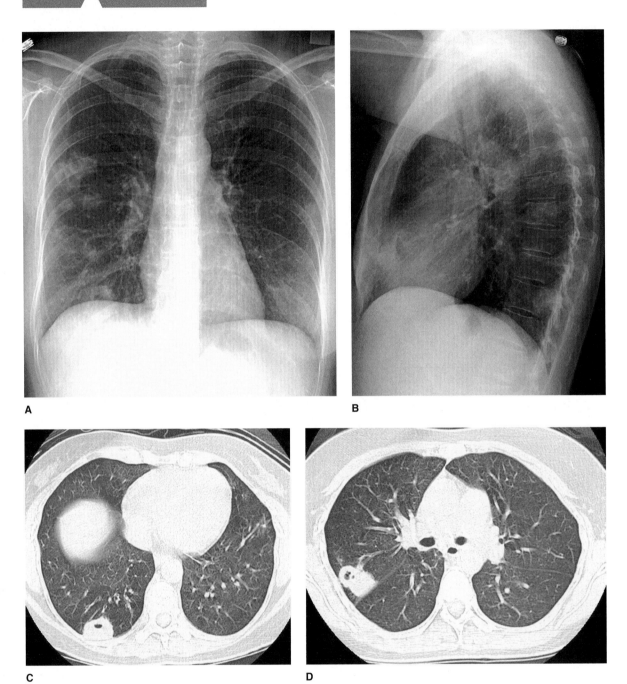

A

B

C

D

▲ **Figure 4-43.** (**A–D**) Case 4-14: 39-year-old female with a history of renal disease.

Table 4-9. Cavitary Lesion Differential Diagnoses (Partial List)

Solitary cavitary lesion	Multiple cavitary lesions
Lung abscess, including tuberculosis	Wegener's granulomatosis
Bronchogenic carcinoma	Metastases
Septic embolus	Septic emboli
Pneumatocele (trauma, *Pneumocystis* pneumonia)	Rheumatoid arthritis

consideration, especially if the patient is febrile. If multiple cavities are present (Figure 4-44), the infection is likely due to hematogenous dissemination, and a source for this dissemination should be sought. The source could be right-sided endocarditis or infected venous thrombi. *Staphylococcus aureus* pneumonias are frequently seen in intravenous drug users and usually appear as multiple cavities. These usually have thin walls (2 to 4 mm) that are slightly indistinct on their outer borders.

As the acquired immunodeficiency syndrome (AIDS) epidemic has progressed, it has been recognized that patients with *Pneumocystis jiroveci* may develop cavitary lesions in the lungs (Figure 4-45). These cavities may be reversible and result from pneumatoceles, or they may be due to a slowly progressive granulomatous reaction. The cavities are usually in the upper lobes and are thin walled. Pneumothorax can result when a peripheral cavity ruptures through the visceral pleura, into the pleural space.

Neoplasia, either primary or secondarily involving the lung, may also cavitate (see Figure 4-39 C). Cavities may re-

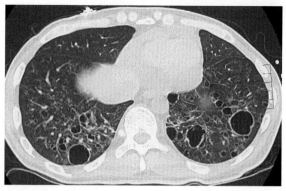

▲ **Figure 4-45.** CT scan of the chest in a patient with human immunodeficiency virus (HIV) demonstrates multiple thin-walled cysts consistent with pneumatoceles related to *Pneumocystis* pneumonia.

sult from pulmonary vasculitis, of which Wegener's granulomatosis is the prototype. Demonstrating the importance of clinical history, the supplied history of renal disease points toward Wegener's granulomatosis.

EXERCISE 4-10. OCCUPATIONAL DISORDERS

4-15. The most likely diagnosis in Figure 4-46 A,B is
  A. progressive massive fibrosis, due to silicosis.
  B. pneumonia in a patient with chronic interstitial lung disease.
  C. lung cancer in a patient with asbestosis.
  D. rounded atelectasis in a patient with asbestosis.
  E. calcified plaques in a patient with asbestos exposure.

4-16. The most likely diagnosis in Figure 4-47 A,B is
  A. progressive massive fibrosis, due to silicosis.
  B. pneumonia in a patient with chronic interstitial lung disease.
  C. lung cancer in a patient with asbestosis.
  D. rounded atelectasis in a patient with asbestosis.
  E. calcified plaques in a patient with asbestos exposure.

Radiologic Findings

4-15. The dense radiopaque lines projecting adjacent to both diaphragmatic surfaces on the PA and lateral radiographs represent calcified pleural plaques. These are better seen on the CT (Figure 4-48 A). When the pleural plaques are seen en face on the PA radiograph, they produce irregular opacities over the lung. These opacities have been described

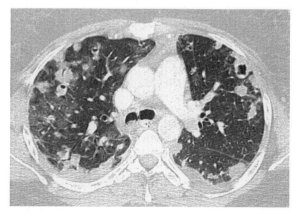

▲ **Figure 4-44.** Axial CT scan in a patient with positive blood cultures demonstrates multiple cavitary nodules. This patient has septic emboli.

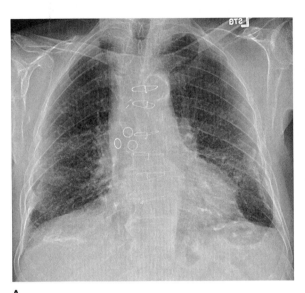

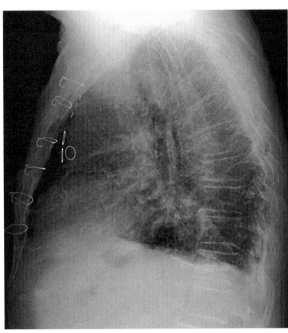

A   **B**

▲ **Figure 4-46. (A,B)** Case 4-15: 64-year-old man who previously worked in a naval shipyard.

as having a holly leaf appearance. At the lung bases, a network of fine lines is superimposed over the normal vascular shadows. These subpleural reticular markings represent interstitial pulmonary fibrosis, which almost certainly represents asbestosis (Figure 4-48 B). (E is the correct answer to Question 4-15.)

4-16.   The patient in Figures 4-47 A,B has two large opacities projecting over the upper lung zones bilaterally. Bilateral upper lobe volume loss is indicated by upward displacement of the hila. Nodular diseases that have an upper-lobe preponderance include silicosis, sarcoidosis, and eosinophilic granuloma. In this case, the nodules have coalesced into large masses, an entity known as progressive massive fibrosis. In this patient with a history of working in coal mines, the most likely of these diseases is silicosis, or coal worker's pneumoconiosis (A is the correct answer to Question 4-16).

Discussion

The two most commonly encountered occupational lung diseases in the United States are asbestosis and silicosis. Development of these diseases is dose dependent, and there is a latent period of many years between exposure and disease. Asbestos-related diseases occur after exposure to asbestos particles, which are found in many types of insulation, fireproofing materials, concrete, and brake linings. The patient with asbestos exposure is at an increased risk of developing lung cancer. If the patient also smokes, there is an additive risk, and these patients may be as much as 100 times more likely to develop lung cancer than the nonsmoking individual with no asbestos exposure.

The term *asbestosis* is used to refer to the pulmonary fibrosis that may be incited by the presence of the mineral and is not used in reference to the pleural disease. The pulmonary fibrosis is predominantly distributed in the lung bases. When severe, it is detected with conventional chest radiography. When it is more subtle, CT is required for its demonstration (see Figure 4-48 B). When the abnormalities are confined to the pleura, the process is called asbestos-related pleural disease. There are five manifestations of asbestos-related pleural disease: asbestos-related pleural effusion, diffuse pleural thickening, pleural plaques, rounded atelectasis, and malignant mesothelioma. Asbestos-related pleural effusion occurs from 7 to 15 years after exposure. It is self-limited and may resolve without sequelae or result in diffuse pleural thickening. Pleural plaques are fibrous plaques that occur predominately on

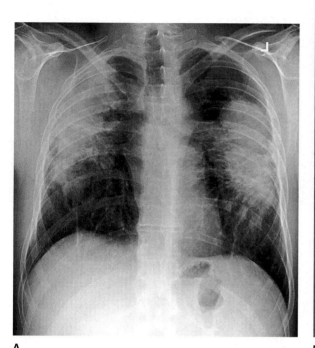
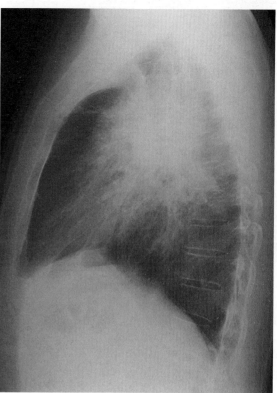

▲ **Figure 4-47.** (**A,B**) Case 4-16: 55-year-old man who worked as a coal miner for 30 years.

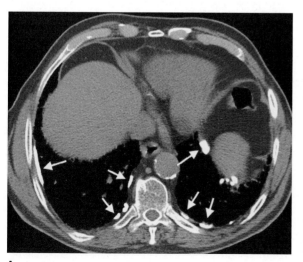
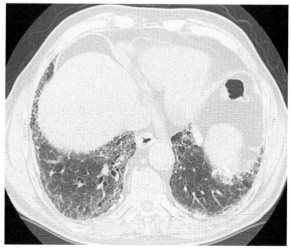

▲ **Figure 4-48.** (**A**) Axial CT image with mediastinal windows shows multiple peripheral calcified pleural plaques (arrows) consistent with asbestos exposure. (**B**) Axial CT image with lung windows shows subpleural reticulation in the lung bases. This is consistent with asbestosis in a patient with a history of asbestos exposure.

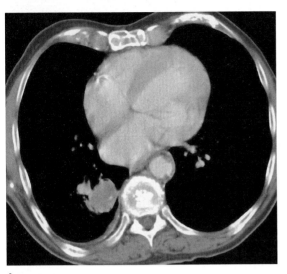
A

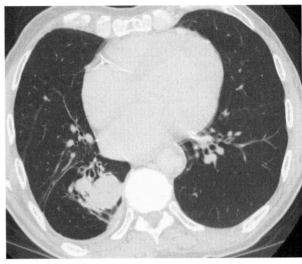
B

▲ **Figure 4-49.** Axial CT images in soft tissue (**A**) and lung (**B**) windows demonstrates a mass in the right lower lobe consistent with rounded atelectasis. Note the spiraling vessels into the mass, volume loss in the affected lobe, and adjacent pleural thickening.

the parietal pleural surfaces of the lower thoracic wall and diaphragmatic surfaces. Pleural plaques may be up to 8 to 10 mm thick, but are not easily visualized when seen en face. Oblique radiographs may show plaques that are projected en face on the PA chest radiograph. The plaques usually occur 10 years or more after exposure. Early in the development of pleural disease, the plaques are not calcified, but with time, the incidence of calcification increases. CT is the most sensitive method of identifying pleural plaques (see Figure 4-48 A). Diffuse pleural thickening may result from the scarring of a previous benign asbestos-related pleural effusion, or it sometimes is due to confluent pleural plaques. Rounded atelectasis (Figures 4-49 A,B) is a piece of folded lung tissue that appears as a mass adjacent to the chest wall. The parietal pleura adheres to an area of lung, usually in the posterior lower lobes, and gradually produces a spiraling folded area of lung, which mimics lung cancer. The comet-tail appearance of bronchi and vessels spiraling into the mass may suggest the correct diagnosis, but because there is such a great increase in the risk of lung cancer in the asbestos-exposed individual, the mass should be closely followed. PET scans and biopsy may be necessary to distinguish the mass of rounded atelectasis from lung cancer. The final asbestos-related disease of the pleura is malignant mesothelioma. This is a malignant tumor of the pleura that usually presents as pleural nodules or pleural effusion (Figure 4-50 A,B).

Silicosis is another form of pulmonary fibrosis that occurs after prolonged exposure to silica. Historically, it has

most often developed in coal miners. Because of improved ventilation standards and the increased automation of coal mining, silicosis is less commonly encountered today. There is an increased incidence of tuberculosis in coal miners, but no increased risk of lung cancer has been reported. Because of particle deposition, silicosis is predominantly an upper-lobe process. It first appears as small pulmonary nodules, and as the fibrosis progresses the hila are retracted upward over a period of years. The small granulomatous nodules of simple silicosis coalesce to form larger conglomerate masses. When these reach at least 1 cm in diameter, the disease is called complicated silicosis, and as they become larger still, it is designated progressive massive fibrosis. Very early disease may be seen only on CT, although in the later stages of the process, the small nodules and conglomerate masses are readily seen on either conventional radiographs or CT images (see Figure 4-47 A,B). Hilar and mediastinal lymph nodes may calcify in the periphery of the lymph node, a type of calcification known as eggshell calcification (Figure 4-51 A,B). An acute form of silicosis can occur in sandblasters who inhale a massive amount of sand. This type of silicosis radiographically resembles pulmonary edema. Coal worker's pneumoconiosis is a similar process that results from inhalation of coal of a relatively pure carbon content. This dust is relatively more inert than silica and incites less fibrosis. The nodules are less well defined on their periphery, and there is a lesser tendency to develop progressive massive fibrosis. These distinctions are rather artificial, as rock dust is usually not

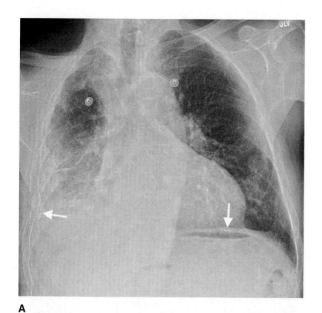

A

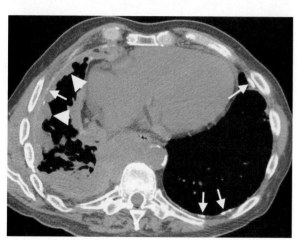

B

▲ **Figure 4-50.** (**A**) Frontal chest radiograph of a 56-year-old man with right-sided chest pain shows pleural opacity on the right. The patient was exposed to asbestos 20 years earlier. (**B**) CT scan through the midthorax show loss of volume in the right hemithorax, with nodular pleural thickening encasing the lung (arrowheads), representing malignant mesothelioma. Calcified pleural plaques are also present (arrows).

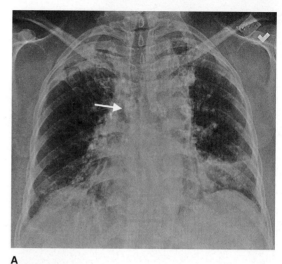

A

B

▲ **Figure 4-51.** Frontal (**A**) and lateral (**B**) radiographs of the chest in a 49-year-old man who shoveled sand in a glass factory with silica exposure demonstrate hilar and mediastinal adenopathy with an eggshell pattern of peripheral calcification (arrows) classically seen in silicosis or sarcoidosis.

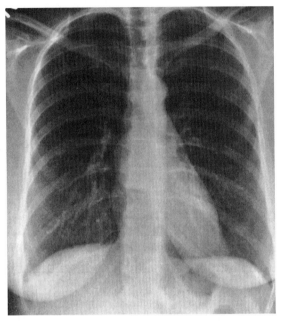
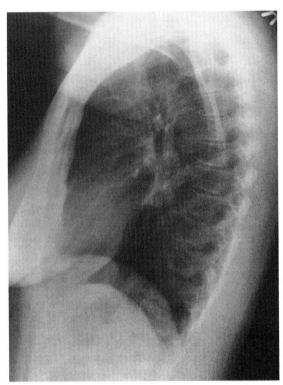

A **B**

▲ **Figure 4-52. (A,B)** Case 4-17: A routine chest radiograph in an asymptomatic 37-year-old woman.

very pure and contains a mixture of silica, carbon, and other minerals.

EXERCISE 4-11. MEDIASTINAL MASSES AND COMPARTMENTS

4-17. The chest radiograph in Figure 4-52 shows
 A. an anterior mediastinal mass.
 B. a middle mediastinal mass.
 C. a posterior mediastinal mass.
 D. a superior mediastinal mass.

4-18. The chest radiograph in Figure 4-53 shows
 A. an anterior mediastinal mass.
 B. a middle mediastinal mass.
 C. a posterior mediastinal mass.
 D. a superior mediastinal mass.

4-19. The chest radiograph in Figure 4-54 shows
 A. an anterior mediastinal mass.
 B. a middle mediastinal mass.
 C. a posterior mediastinal mass.
 D. a superior mediastinal mass.

Radiologic Findings

4-17. A spherical mass 4 cm in diameter is present in the subcarinal region on the frontal radiograph (Figure 4-52 A), and superimposed on the hilar region on the lateral radiograph (Figure 4-52 B). CT (Figure 4-55) shows that the lesion is of fluid attenuation (greater attenuation than the subcutaneous fat, but less attenuation than muscle). This mass is in the middle mediastinum. (B is the correct answer to Question 4-17.) In an asymptomatic individual, this most likely represents a congenital bronchogenic cyst. These masses can grow to sufficient size to cause symptoms such as dyspnea or dysphagia owing to compression of the trachea or esophagus. Bronchogenic cysts may also occur within the lungs and are often surgically resected because of the likelihood of pulmonary infection. The differential diagnosis of a middle mediastinal mass can be seen in Table 4-10.

4-18. The frontal radiograph (Figure 4-53) shows a lobulated mass to the right of the lower thoracic vertebrae. Note that the right heart border remains visible, suggesting that this mass is either anterior or posterior to

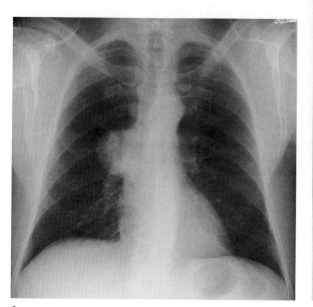

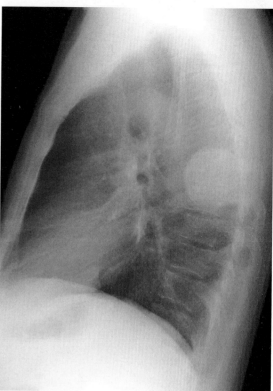

A   **B**

▲ **Figure 4-53.** (**A,B**) Case 4-18: 55-year-old man with multiple subcutaneous nodules.

the heart. On the lateral radiograph, the mass projects over the vertebral column consistent with a posterior mediastinal location. The coronal MR image in Figure 4-56 shows that the mass is paraspinal in location and associated with the neural foramen. Neurogenic tumors are the most common cause of posterior mediastinal masses. In this patient with multiple sub-

cutaneous nodules, this mass is most likely a neurofibroma (C is the correct answer to Question 4-18).

4-19.   In Figure 4-54, the frontal chest radiograph (Figures 4-54 A and 4-57 A) shows a mass projecting over the left hilum without obscuration of the interlobar pulmonary artery (arrowhead). Because the mass does not obliterate the margins of the vessel, it must be either anterior or

Table 4-10. Differential Diagnosis by Mediastinal Compartment (Partial List)

Superior	Anterior	Middle	Posterior
Thyroid goiter, carcinoma	Thymoma	Adenopathy	Neurogenic tumor
Cystic hygroma	Teratoma	Vascular abnormalities	Nerve root tumors
Adenopathy	Thyroid goiter, carcinoma	Bronchogenic cyst	Meningocele
Vascular abnormalities	Lymphoma	Pericardial cyst	Vascular abnormalities
Bronchogenic cyst		Esophageal duplication cyst Esophageal mass Hiatal hernia	Extramedullary hematopoiesis Diaphragmatic hernia Bone tumor

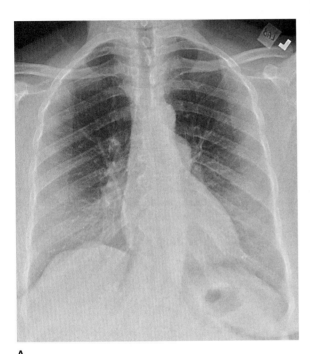

A

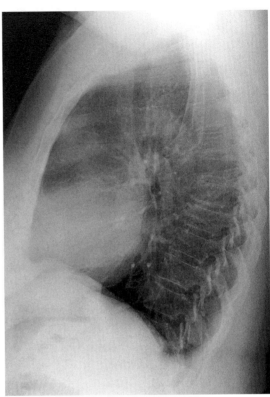

B

▲ **Figure 4-54.** (**A,B**) Case 4-19: 25-year-old woman with a nonproductive cough.

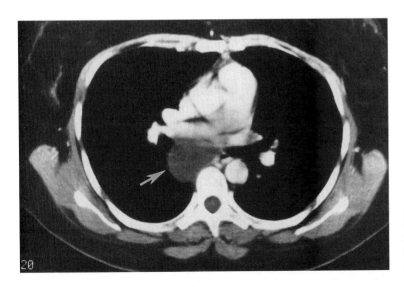

▲ **Figure 4-55.** Axial CT image of the same patient in Figure 4-52 shows a round mass (arrow) of fluid attenuation in the subcarinal position. This is a typical appearance of a bronchogenic cyst.

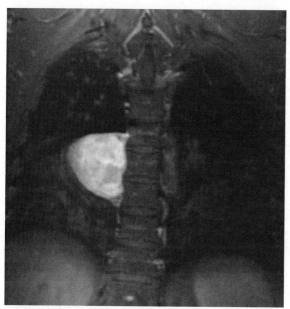

▲ **Figure 4-56.** Coronal MRI image of the same patient in Figure 4-53 demonstrates a right paraspinal mass.

posterior to the hilum. On the lateral view (Figure 4-57 B), the anterior clear space is somewhat opaque, and there is a suggestion of the margins of the mass. The CT scan (Figure 4-57 C) shows the mass, surrounded by fat, in the anterior mediastinum. The mass is solid and contains a few calcifications (arrow). (A is the correct answer to Question 4-19.)

Discussion

Two methods of dividing the mediastinum for radiographic purposes are in common use. The radiographic divisions are arbitrary and are intended to provide the most appropriate differential diagnosis for abnormalities that occur in these locations. Neither of the divisions follows the divisions used by anatomists. In the older system, the mediastinum is divided into three compartments. The anterior mediastinum is that portion of the mediastinum that is anterior to the anterior margin of the trachea and along the posterior margin of the pericardium and inferior vena cava. The posterior mediastinum lies behind a plane that extends the length of the thorax behind a line drawn 1 cm posteriorly to the anterior margin of the vertebral column. The middle mediastinum is the region between these two boundaries. This system has been superseded by a four-compartment model, which designates a superior mediastinal compartment as the space that lies above a plane

extending from the sternomanubrial junction to the lower border of the fourth thoracic vertebra. The anterior mediastinum is just caudad to the superior compartment and is anterior to a plane extending along the anterior aspect of the tracheal air column and along the anterior pericardium. Note that the heart shifts from the anterior to the middle mediastinum with the four-compartment system. The middle mediastinum occupies the area from the anterior pericardium backward to a plane 1 cm posterior to the anterior margin of the vertebral column. The addition of the fourth compartment occurred when CT was developed and it became easier to identify structures in each compartment.

The differential diagnosis of lesions occurring in each compartment is in part dependent on the structures that exist there (see Table 4-10). Note that there are vascular structures and lymph nodes in each of the compartments. Therefore, abnormalities of the blood vessels (eg, aneurysms) and lymph node diseases (eg, lymphoma) would have to be included in the differential diagnosis of diseases occurring there. The differential diagnosis lists include the most common disorders occurring in each region. The most common mass to occur in the superior mediastinum is an enlarged substernal thyroid, which may become large enough to extend into the anterior or middle mediastinum (Figure 4-58 A,B).

EXERCISE 4-12. PLEURAL ABNORMALITIES

4-20.   The most likely diagnosis in Case 4-20 (Figure 4-59 A,B) is
   A. pulmonary embolism.
   B. overinflation associated with asthma.
   C. pneumothorax.
   D. normal chest, with a skin fold projected over the right hemithorax.
   E. left lower lobe atelectasis.

Radiologic Findings

4-10.   In Figure 4-59, there is increased radiolucency in the periphery of the right hemithorax. On the close-up of the right lung (Figure 4-60 A), there is a thin white line (arrows) paralleling, but displaced from, the right lateral chest wall. The thin line represents the visceral pleura. There is air-filled lung medial to this thin white line, and there is air within the pleural space lateral to this line. Note the absence of pulmonary vessels lateral to the pleural line (C is the correct answer to Question 4-20).

Discussion

Pneumothorax is the presence of air in the pleural space. The lung collapses away from the chest wall because of its normal

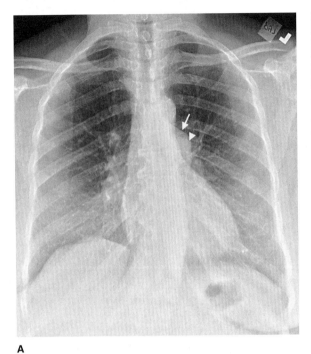

A

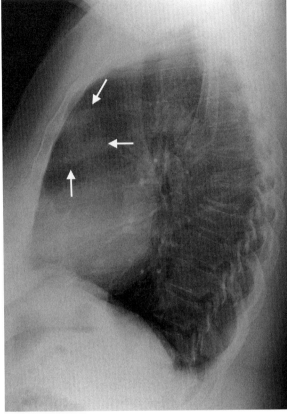

B

C

▲ **Figure 4-57.** Anterior mediastinal mass (arrow) of the same patient in Figure 4-54 is demonstrated on frontal (**A**) and lateral (**B**) radiographs of the chest. A single axial CT image from the same patient (**C**) reveals a mass anterior to the pulmonary artery with punctuate areas of calcification (arrow) as seen in a thymoma.

elastic recoil. In some instances, a ball valve mechanism is present, and air continues to enter the pleural space and further collapses the lung and displaces the mediastinum away from the side of the pneumothorax. The relationship of the air in the pleural space to the lung and chest wall can be clearly seen on the CT scan of a patient with a right pneumothorax (Figure 4-60 B). Note that air rises to the

highest point in the thorax, the anterior thorax in a supine patient and the lung apex in an upright patient. The visceral pleura covering the lung is visible as a thin white line on both chest radiographs and CT scans. No pulmonary vessels may be seen extending beyond the pleural line, and the air in the pleural space appears more radiolucent than the adjacent lung.

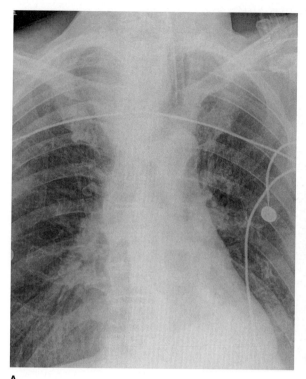

A

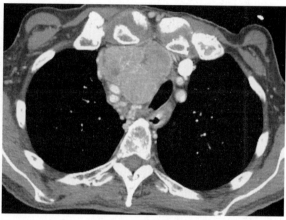

B

▲ **Figure 4-58.** (**A**) Close-up view of the superior mediastinum on a frontal radiograph shows an opacity resulting in shift of the trachea and endotracheal tube toward the left. (**B**) Axial CT of the chest in this patient reveals a heterogeneous superior mediastinal mass originating from the thyroid gland. This patient had biopsy-proven thyroid carcinoma.

The most common mimic of a pneumothorax, particularly in a supine patient, is a skin fold. The image receptor for portable AP chest radiographs is placed behind the patient's back. Skin folds may be pressed between the patient's back and the receptor. Radiographically, a skin fold produces an interface, or an edge of thick tissue outlined by the greater radiolucency of the superimposed lung (Figure 4-61). If you can distinguish an edge from a line, then you can distinguish a skin fold from a pneumothorax. The absence of pulmonary markings beyond the pleural line is supporting evidence for a pneumothorax. Because the vessels taper as they approach the lung periphery, the vessels in the extreme periphery of the lung may be too tiny to see.

Pneumothorax is considered spontaneous if it occurs in the absence of trauma (including barotrauma). Spontaneous pneumothorax may be primary and occur in the absence of significant other lung disease, or it may occur secondarily because of lung disease. Apical blebs are present in a high percentage of patients with primary spontaneous pneumothorax, and their rupture is thought to be the most frequent cause of spontaneous pneumothorax. For unknown reasons, it occurs most frequently in tall young men. Secondary spontaneous pneumothorax may occur in association with any cavitary lesion that lies in the periphery of the lung, as well as in emphysema, in bullous disease, and in pulmonary fibrosis of a variety of etiologies.

EXERCISE 4-13. PLEURAL EFFUSION

4-21. Which of the following radiographic signs generally does not suggest the presence of pleural effusion?
   A. Meniscus-shaped opacity in a posterior costophrenic angle on the lateral projection
   B. Biconvex lens-shaped opacity projecting in the midthorax on the lateral projection

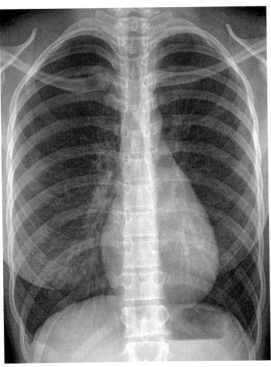
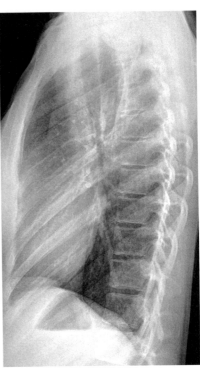

A   B

▲ **Figure 4-59.** **(A,B)** Case 4-20: Tall, 21-year-old female who noted the sudden onset of dyspnea and right-sided pleuritic chest pain.

C. Fluid levels that have the same lengths on the PA and lateral views in a hemithorax

D. Homogenous increased density in a hemithorax with preservation of the vascular shadows in the lungs

E. Separation of the gastric air bubble from the inferior lung margin by more than 2 cm

Radiologic Findings

The frontal chest radiograph (Figure 4-62 A) shows opacity at the lower hemithorax bilaterally, which has a concave border curving upward laterally adjacent to the chest wall. The overall lung volume is low in both the right and left lungs. There is separation of the gastric bubble from the inferior margin of the lung by several centimeters. On the lateral examination (Figure 4-62 B), the opacities obscure the posterior heart margin and have a margin curving slightly upward to the posterior chest wall. Neither hemidiaphragm can be followed posteriorly to the chest wall. The findings are those of bilateral pleural effusions (C is the correct answer to Question 4-21).

Discussion

The visceral pleura is the outer lining of the lung, and the parietal pleura is the lining of the chest cavity. Normally, these surfaces are smooth and are separated by a minimal amount of pleural fluid. This provides a nearly friction-free environment for movement of the lung within the thorax. The pleural space, therefore, is a potential space that, in the normal individual, contains no more than 3 to 5 mL of pleural fluid. Fluid may accumulate within the pleural space as a result of conditions that (1) increase pulmonary capillary pressure, (2) alter thoracic vascular or lymphatic pathways, (3) alter pleural capillary or lymphatic permeability, or (4) affect diaphragmatic peritoneal and pleural surfaces.

Pleural effusions are usually approached clinically according to whether the effusion develops because of alterations of the Starling equation, which controls fluid flow and maintenance in body compartments, or whether the pleura is affected primarily by a disease process. Processes resulting from alterations of the Starling equation include congestive heart failure, hypoproteinemia, fluid overload, liver failure, and nephrosis. These effusions are usually

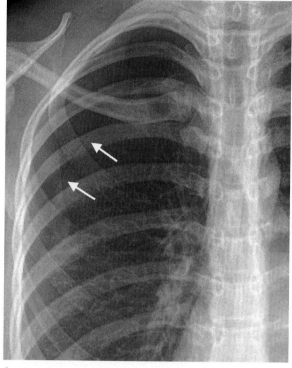

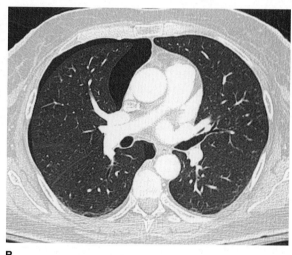

A

B

▲ **Figure 4-60.** **(A)** Close-up frontal view of the chest of the same patient in Figure 4-59 shows a thin white line (arrows), corresponding to the visceral pleura. Lucency on either side represents air in the pleural space laterally and normally aerated lung medially. This is the hallmark of pneumothorax. **(B)** Axial CT image (lung window settings) shows air in the right pleural space. Note that the pneumothorax in this supine patient rises to the nondependent area of the thorax.

transudates (clear or pale yellow, odorless fluid without elevation of the ratios of pleural fluid to serum protein and lactate dehydrogenase [LDH]). Processes that alter pleural capillary or lymphatic permeability include infection, inflammation, pulmonary embolism, and neoplasms. These effusions are usually exudates (clear, pale yellow or turbid, bloody, brownish fluid; pleural fluid protein: serum protein greater than 0.5; and pleural fluid LDH:serum LDH greater than 0.6). Enlarged lymph nodes or masses within the hila or mediastinum may obstruct lymphatic fluid flow and cause pleural exudates. Abdominal conditions that may produce pleural effusions include pancreatitis, subphrenic abscesses, liver abscesses, ovarian tumors, peritonitis, and ascites.

The most common radiographic sign of pleural effusion is pleural meniscus. The volume of fluid necessary to produce a pleural meniscus within a costophrenic angle varies from individual to individual. Approximately 100 mL of pleural fluid will cause appreciable blunting of the posterior costophrenic angle on the lateral view (Figure 4-63 A), and

200 mL will cause blunting of the lateral costophrenic angle on the PA projection in an upright patient (Figure 4-63 B). A lateral decubitus chest radiograph, with the side containing the pleural effusion placed down (dependent), will demonstrate even smaller amounts of free-flowing pleural effusions (Figure 4-63 C). Each millimeter of thickness of pleural fluid in the lateral decubitus projection corresponds to approximately 20 mL of pleural fluid. Large pleural effusions may usually be aspirated without guidance other than the chest radiograph. Small effusions are more difficult to aspirate and, if thoracentesis is planned, additional imaging guidance with ultrasonography or CT may be used. The effusion may simply be marked and aspirated by the clinical physician, or the effusion may be aspirated by a radiologist. If thoracentesis is attempted and fails for a large pleural effusion, it may be loculated and further imaging guidance is usually helpful.

When pleural adhesions develop, fluid in the pleural space becomes loculated (Figure 4-64 A–C) and may be trapped in nondependent areas of the thorax. The appearance of pleural

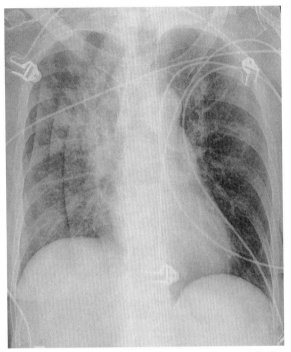

▲ **Figure 4-61.** Frontal chest radiograph shows multiple skin folds visualized as edges, or interfaces, projecting over the right hemithorax.

fluid may change and, rather than taking a meniscus shape, may assume the shape of a convex margin away from the chest wall. If air is introduced in the pleural space by penetration of the chest wall, or if fluid is trapped in the fissures, it will assume a biconvex lens shape (Figure 4-65). If a bronchopleural fistula develops, the patient will have a hydropneumothorax that may be recognized by air-fluid levels of different lengths on the PA and lateral chest radiographs (Figure 4-66). When cavities develop in the lung, the fluid levels are usually of the same length (Figure 4-67).

EXERCISE 4-14. PULMONARY VASCULAR DISEASE

4-22. The most likely cause for this patient's dyspnea and pleuritic chest pain (Figure 4-68 A–D) is
A. multifocal pneumonia.
B. malignant pleural effusion.
C. pulmonary embolism.
D. septic emboli.
E. drug-related pneumonitis.

Radiologic Findings

4-22. The chest x-ray shows a wedge-shaped opacity in the periphery of the right lung base. There is blunting of the right lateral costophrenic angle on the PA view of

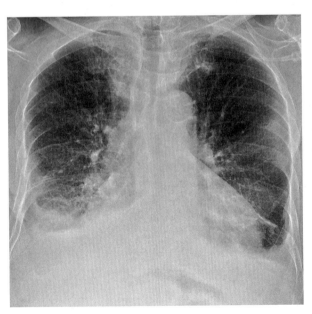

A

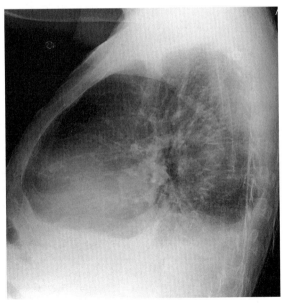

B

▲ **Figure 4-62.** (**A,B**) Case 4-21: 65-year-old man with increasing dyspnea of 1-week duration.

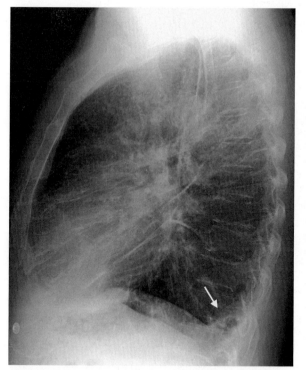

A

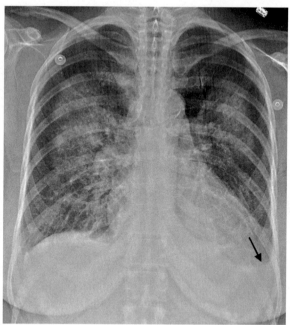

B

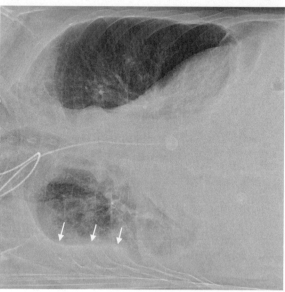

C

▲ **Figure 4-63.** Frontal (**A**) and lateral (**B**) views of the chest show blunting of both lateral costophrenic angles (arrow) as well as the posterior costophrenic angles (arrow) caused by small bilateral pleural effusions. Note the batwing appearance of pulmonary edema. (**C**) Right lateral decubitus chest radiograph from a different patient shows displacement of the lateral margin of the right lung (arrows) from the chest wall by free-flowing pleural effusion.

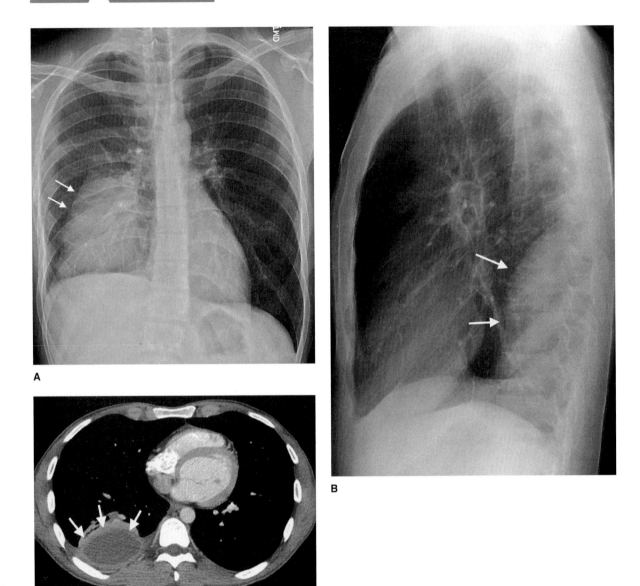

A

B

C

▲ **Figure 4-64.** **(A)** Posteroanterior radiograph shows an opacity (arrows) in the right lower hemithorax. The right pulmonary artery, right heart border, and right hemidiaphragm remain visible, suggesting that this opacity lies posteriorly. **(B)** Lateral chest radiograph demonstrates an opacity posteriorly contiguous with the pleural surface but with a well-defined anterior margin (arrows). Note the obtuse angle that the opacity makes with the posterior chest wall. **(C)** Axial contrasted CT image demonstrates the loculated pleural fluid seen on chest radiograph. The lung is displaced anteriorly. The pleura (arrows) is enhancing, suggesting an exudative process.

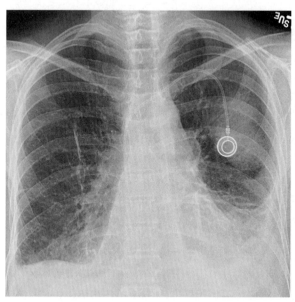

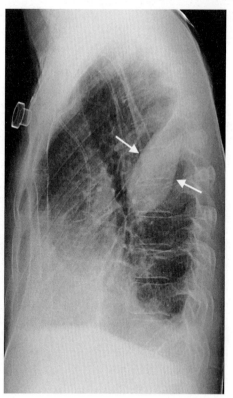

A   B

▲ **Figure 4-65.** **(A)** Posteroanterior radiograph shows an opacity in the left hemithorax behind the patient's central venous access device. This opacity is ill-defined on its superior and lateral margins. **(B)** Lateral chest radiograph demonstrates a well-defined lens-shaped opacity (arrows). This is characteristic of "pseudotumor" or fluid loculated in the fissure, in this case, the left major fissure.

the chest. The opacity could represent a Hampton's hump in the clinical setting of pulmonary embolus. Alternatively, pneumonia could have a similar presentation. The CT scan demonstrates filling defects within the pulmonary arteries bilaterally. At the levels shown, thromboemboli are visible within the right main pulmonary artery extending into the right upper lobe pulmonary artery (Figure 4-68 C) and within the basilar segmental arteries bilaterally (Figure 4-68 D). (C is the correct answer to Question 4-22.) The lung windows (Figure 4-68 E) show a peripheral area of increased attenuation, consistent with an area of reperfusion edema and/or pulmonary infarction.

Discussion

Pulmonary thromboembolism can occur as a result of deep venous thrombosis, typically from the veins of the pelvis and lower extremities. These thrombi dislodge (embolize) and travel via the inferior vena cava and right heart chambers to become trapped in the tapering branches of the pulmonary arterial system. Because pulmonary embolism often occurs without pulmonary infarction, the appearance of the chest radiograph is usually normal. The areas of lung deprived of pulmonary arterial flow are perfused by bronchial arterial collateral vessels. The chest radiograph may demonstrate subtle signs of volume loss or a small pleural effusion. Pulmonary opacities develop because of microatelectasis within the region of lung that has had an embolus, from edema as the blood flow is restored via the bronchial circulation, or from hemorrhage within a pulmonary infarction. Pulmonary infarction may occur if the pulmonary venous pressure is elevated or the bronchial arterial supply to a region is deficient for some reason. The cone-shaped area of pulmonary infarction has been called a Hampton's hump (Figure 4-68 A) and is

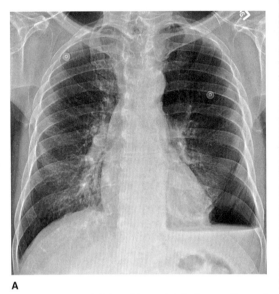
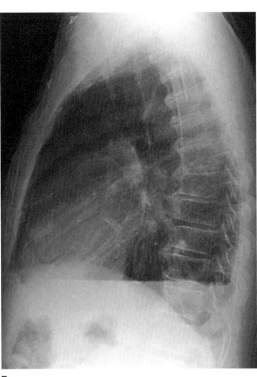

A   B

▲ **Figure 4-66.** Frontal (**A**) and lateral (**B**) chest radiographs demonstrate an air-fluid level in the left hemithorax. Note that the interface between the air and fluid in this patient's hydropneumothorax is of different length on the two views. This is characteristic of an air-fluid level in the pleural space.

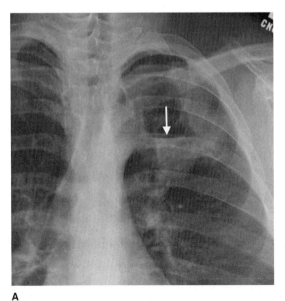
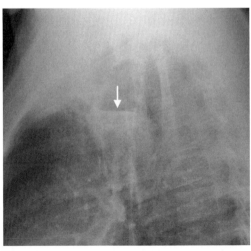

A   B

▲ **Figure 4-67.** Close-up frontal (**A**) and lateral (**B**) chest radiographs of the left upper lobe demonstrate an air-fluid level (arrow). In this patient, the line separating the air and fluid is the same length on both views, suggesting that the cavitary lesion is spherical in shape. This is characteristic of an air-fluid level in the lung parenchyma, in this case, a lung abscess.

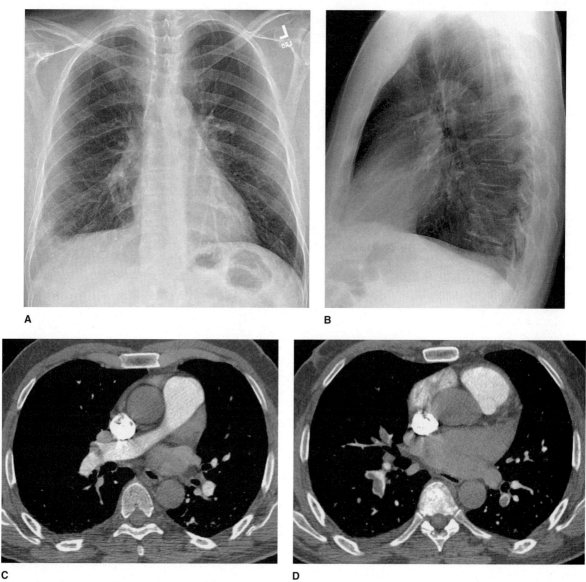

▲ **Figure 4-68.** Case 4-22: PA and lateral chest radiograph (**A, B**) and a CT scan with intravenous contrast (**C, D**) in a 57-year-old male who presents with worsening shortness of breath and pleuritic chest pain after a transatlantic flight 1 week prior.

named after the person who originally described it. An area of radiolucency, corresponding to diminished pulmonary vascularity distal to a pulmonary embolism, is occasionally seen and is called the Westermark sign. There may also be an increase in the size of the pulmonary artery proximal to a large central pulmonary embolus (Fleischner sign).

Two imaging modalities are widely used in the evaluation of a patient with suspected pulmonary embolism: radionuclide perfusion scan and chest CTA. The radionuclide perfusion scan may be the more appropriate examination in the patient with a normal chest radiograph and no preexisting cardiac or pulmonary disease. In the patient with an abnormal chest radiograph, or preexisting

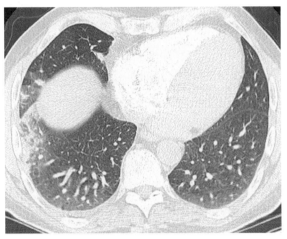

E

▲ **Figure 4-68.** *(Continued)* The lung windows (**E**) show a peripheral area of increased attenuation, consistent with an area of reperfusion edema and/or pulmonary infarction.

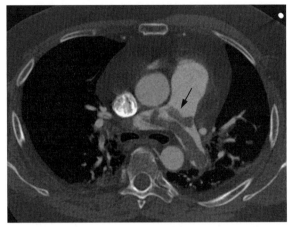

▲ **Figure 4-69.** Axial contrasted CT image from a CTA of the chest demonstrates tubular filling defects in the pulmonary trunk and extending from the right main pulmonary artery into the left main pulmonary artery. This is consistent with a "saddle embolus" that straddles the bifurcation of the pulmonary arteries (arrow).

cardiopulmonary disease, the V/Q scan is more likely to be interpreted as "indeterminate" and a chest CT becomes the preferred imaging modality. The chest CT also has the advantage of demonstrating unsuspected abnormalities, such as pericardial effusion, emphysema, esophagitis, or aortic dissection, which could be responsible for the patient's chest pain or dyspnea.

On chest CTA, thromboemboli are visible as filling defects within the contrast-filled pulmonary arteries. These are typically several centimeters long and often are seen draped across the bifurcation of an artery (saddle emboli) (Figure 4-69). In patients with acute pulmonary embolism, the filling defects are seen within the center of the arterial lumen, although they may also completely occlude the artery. In patients with chronic pulmonary embolism, the filling defects are more likely to be found against the wall of the artery. Calcification within the thrombus also confirms the chronic nature of the thrombus.

There will be some patients in whom the diagnosis of pulmonary embolism remains uncertain after either a V/Q scan or a chest CTA. These examinations can be inadequate for a number of both technical and clinical reasons. The chest CTA can be difficult to interpret unless the patient is able to suspend respiration for the duration of the scan. Fortunately, helical CT scans are able to scan the entire thorax in under 20 seconds. Many patients with severe dyspnea, however, are unable to achieve this. Pulmonary angiography can be obtained to further evaluate the pulmonary arterial circulation when either the V/Q scan or chest CTA is nondiagnostic.

EXERCISE 4-15. INTERSTITIAL LUNG DISEASE

4-23.   The most likely cause for this patient's dyspnea and pleuritic chest pain (Figure 4-70 A–C) is
A.   emphysema.
B.   empyema.
C.   pneumonia.
D.   pulmonary fibrosis.
E.   aspiration.

Radiologic Findings

4-23.   The chest x-ray (Figure 4-70 A,B) shows diffuse bilateral coarse interstitial opacities with slight basilar predominance. The hemidiaphragms are flattened on the lateral radiograph. The CT scan (Figure 4-70 C) demonstrates multiple small similar-sized cysts stacked along the lung periphery with some preservation of normal lung centrally, particularly on the right. There is traction bronchiectasis present as well (D is the correct answer to Question 4-23).

Discussion

The list of interstitial lung diseases is long, and the differentiation can be complex. However, pulmonary fibrosis can be readily identified. Fibrosis can be subtle, with visible linear markings in the lung periphery on CT, or as obvious as the cystic change seen in this patient. End-stage pulmonary fibrosis is most readily recognized as stacks of air-filled

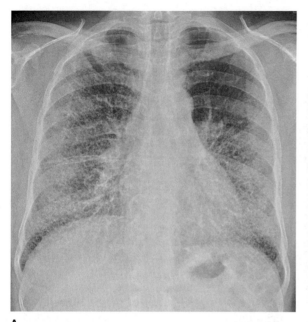

A

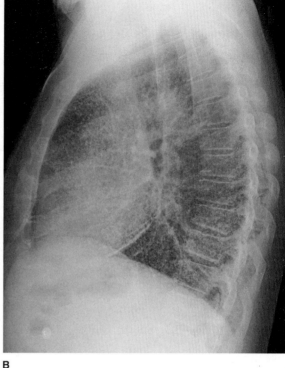

B

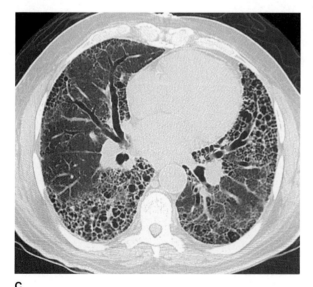

C

▲ **Figure 4-70. (A–C)** Case 4-23. A 66-year-old male on 2 liters oxygen per nasal cannula at home presents with dyspnea.

lucencies in the lung periphery in a pattern called "honey-combing" (Figure 4-70 C). This is often seen as the end stage of multiple interstitial lung diseases, most frequently in usual interstitial pneumonitis (UIP). These patients are almost certainly symptomatic, many requiring supplemental oxygen.

Lucencies in the lung can result from many causes. A lucency with a discernible wall is called a cavity. As described in previous exercises, infectious or neoplastic etiology can result in a cavity or air-filled lucency within the lung. However, these are rarely small and stacked as in this case. Empyema, or an infected pleural fluid collection, can also result in a cavity of air seen on chest radiograph. This cavity is generally larger and unilateral. Therefore, A, B, and E are incorrect.

In emphysema, the air-filled lucencies lack a discernable wall. (Figure 4-71 A). These lucencies are called bullae and, in centrilobular emphysema, have an upper lobe preponderance.

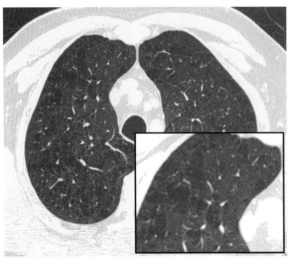

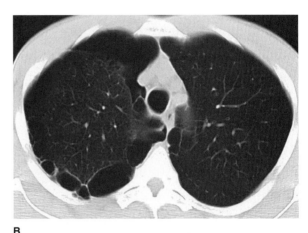

A   **B**

▲ **Figure 4-71. (A)** Axial CT image from a patient with centrilobular emphysema demonstrates multiple areas of lucency with barely perceptible walls in the lung parenchyma. Note that the vessels run through the lucencies rather than around them. **(B)** Axial CT image from a patient with paraseptal emphysema demonstrates a single layer of peripheral thin-walled cysts in the right upper lung.

These lucencies are not cysts, because a true lung cyst is lined with epithelium. Emphysema is a common cause of dyspnea and is most often smoking-related. In these patients, the lung volumes are often larger than normal, and the lungs appear more radiolucent. The bullous lesions of centrilobular emphysema are more easily recognized on CT than on chest radiographs. Unlike other cystic lung diseases, a vessel can generally be seen coursing through the bulla rather than around the lucency. Another form of emphysema is paraseptal emphysema, in which the bullae occur along the lung periphery (Figure 4-71 B).

GLOSSARY OF TERMS IN CHEST ROENTGENOLOGY

Acinar pattern (synonyms: alveolar pattern, airspace disease, consolidation): A collection of round or elliptic, ill-defined, discrete or partly confluent opacities in the lung, each

Adapted from Hansell DM, Bankier AA, MacMahon H, McLoud TC, Müller NL, Remy J. Fleischner Society: glossary of terms for thoracic imaging. *Radiology.* 2008;246:697-722, and Terms used in chest radiology. In Fraser RS, Muller NL, Colman N, Pare PD, editors. *Fraser and Pare's Diagnosis of Diseases of the Chest.* 4th ed. Philadelphia: WB. Saunders Co; 1999:xvii-xxxi.

measuring 4 to 8 mm in diameter and together producing an extended, inhomogeneous shadow.

Air bronchogram: A branching lucency that represents the roentgenographic shadow of an air-containing bronchus peripheral to the hilum and surrounded by airless lung (whether by virtue of absorption of air, replacement of air, or both), a finding generally regarded as evidence of the patency of the more proximal airway.

Air-fluid level: A local collection of gas and liquid that, when traversed by a horizontal x-ray beam, creates a shadow characterized by a sharp horizontal interface between a gas density above and liquid density below.

Air space: The gas-containing portion of lung parenchyma, including the acini and excluding the interstitium and purely conductive portions of the lung.

Anterior junction line: A vertically oriented linear opacity approximately 1 to 2 mm wide, produced by the shadows of the right and left pleural surfaces in intimate contact between the aerated lungs anterior to the great vessels. It is usually obliquely oriented, projected over the tracheal air column, below the level of the clavicles.

Aortopulmonary window: A zone of relative lucency seen on both the PA and lateral chest radiographs bounded medially by the left side of the trachea, superiorly by the inferior surface of the aortic arch, and inferiorly by the left pulmonary artery. The pleural surface of the aortopulmonary (AP) window is normally concave; convexity of the AP window suggests lymphadenopathy.

Atelectasis: Less than normal inflation of all or a portion of lung with corresponding diminution in volume. Qualifiers are often used to indicate extent and distribution (linear or platelike, subsegmental, segmental, lobar), as well as mechanism (resorption, relaxation, compressive, passive, cicatricial, adhesive).

Azygoesophageal recess: On the frontal chest radiograph, a vertically oriented interface between air in the right lower lobe, and the adjacent mediastinum containing the azygos vein and esophagus. It projects in the middle of the heart and spine on the frontal view.

Bleb: A thin-walled lucency within or contiguous to the visceral pleura.

Bulla: A sharply demarcated area of avascularity (lucency) within the lung measuring 1 cm or more in diameter and possessing a wall less than 1 mm in thickness.

Carina: The bifurcation of the trachea into right and left main bronchi.

Cavity: A gas-containing space within the lung surrounded by a wall whose thickness is greater than 1 mm and often irregular in contour.

Fissure: The infolding of visceral pleura that separates one lobe, or a portion of a lobe, from another. Radiographically visible as a linear opacity normally 1 mm or less in width. Qualifiers: minor (horizontal), major, accessory, azygos, anomalous.

Ground-glass pattern: A finely granular pattern of pulmonary opacity such that pulmonary vessels remain visible. The degree of opacity is not sufficient to result in air bronchograms.

Hilum (plural: hila): Anatomically, the depression or pit in that part of an organ where the vessels and nerves enter. On chest radiographs, the term *hilum* represents the composite shadow of the bronchi, pulmonary arteries and veins, and lymph nodes on the medial aspect of each lung.

Honeycomb pattern: A number of ring shadows or cystic spaces within the lung representing airspaces 5 to 10 mm in diameter with walls 2 to 3 mm thick that resemble a true honeycomb. The finding implies interstitial fibrosis and "end-stage" lung disease.

Interface (synonyms: edge, border): The boundary between the shadows of structures of different opacity (eg, the lung and the heart).

Interstitium: A continuum of loose connective tissue throughout the lung consisting of three subdivisions: (a) bronchoarterial (axial), surrounding the bronchoarterial bundles; (b) parenchymal (acinar), between the alveolar and capillary basement membranes; and (c) subpleural, between the pleura and lung parenchyma and continuous with the interlobular septa and perivenous interstitial space.

Line: A longitudinal opacity no greater than 2 mm in width.

Lobe: One of the principal divisions of the lungs (usually three on the right, two on the left) enveloped by the visceral pleura except at the hilum. The lobes are separated in whole or in part by pleural fissures.

Lucency (synonym: radiolucency): The shadow of tissue that attenuates the x-ray beam less effectively than surrounding tissue. On a radiograph, the area that appears more nearly black, usually applied to areas of air density or fat density.

Lymphadenopathy (synonym: adenopathy): Enlargement or abnormality of lymph nodes.

Mass: Any pulmonary or pleural lesion greater than 3 cm in diameter.

Miliary pattern: A collection of tiny (1 to 2 mm in diameter) discrete opacities in the lungs, generally uniform in size and widespread in distribution.

Nodular pattern: A collection of innumerable small, discrete opacities (2 to 10 mm in diameter), generally widespread in distribution.

Nodule: A sharply defined, discrete, circular opacity up to 3 cm in diameter within the lung.

Opacity: The shadow of tissue that attenuates the x-ray beam more than surrounding tissue. On a radiograph, areas that are more white than the surrounding area are said to be more opaque.

Posterior junction line: A vertically oriented, linear opacity approximately 2 mm wide, produced by the shadows of the right and left pleurae in intimate contact between the aerated lungs, representing the plane of contact between the lungs posterior to the trachea and esophagus, and anterior to the spine; the line may project above and below the suprasternal notch.

Posterior tracheal stripe: A vertically oriented linear opacity 2 to 5 mm wide, extending from the thoracic inlet to the bifurcation of the trachea, visible on the lateral radiograph, representing the posterior tracheal wall and contiguous mediastinal tissue (anterior, and often posterior, walls of the esophagus).

Primary complex: The combination of a focus of pneumonia due to a primary infection (eg, tuberculosis or histoplasmosis), with granulomas in the draining hilar or mediastinal lymph nodes. (Synonym: Ranke complex. The term *Ghon focus* describes the pulmonary lesion that has calcified. *Ranke complex* is the term to describe the combination of the Ghon focus and calcified hilar lymph nodes.)

Reticular pattern: A collection of innumerable small, linear opacities that together produce the appearance of a net.

Reticulonodular pattern: A collection of innumerable small, linear and nodular opacities that together produce the appearance of a net and superimposed small nodules.

Right tracheal stripe: A vertically oriented linear opacity 2 to 3 mm wide, extending from the thoracic inlet to the right tracheobronchial angle. It represents the right tracheal wall and contiguous mediastinal tissue (visceral and parietal pleurae of the right lung).

Septal line (synonym: Kerley line): A linear opacity, usually 1 to 2 mm in width, produced by thickening of the interlobular septa and often due to either edema or cellular infiltration.

Silhouette sign: The effacement of an anatomic soft-tissue border by either a normal anatomic structure or a pathologic state, such as airlessness of adjacent lung or accumulation of fluid in the contiguous pleural space.

Stripe: A longitudinal opacity 2 to 5 mm in width.

Tramline shadow: Parallel or slightly convergent linear opacities that suggest the projection of tubular structures, generally representing thickened bronchial walls.

SUGGESTED READING

1. Reed JC. *Chest Radiology: Plain Film Patterns and Differential Diagnoses.* 5th ed. Philadelphia: Mosby; 2003.

2. Groskin SA. *Heitzman's The Lung: Radiologic-Pathologic Correlations.* 3rd ed. St. Louis: Mosby; 1993.

3. Freundlich IM, Bragg DG. *A Radiologic Approach to Diseases of the Chest.* 2nd ed. Baltimore: Williams & Wilkins; 1997.

4. Collins J, Stern EJ. *Chest Radiology: The Essentials.* 2nd ed. Philadelphia: Lippincott, Williams & Wilkins; 2008.

5. Hansell DM, Armstrong P, Lynch DA, McAdams HP. *Imaging of Diseases of the Chest.* 4th ed. London: Mosby; 2005.

6. McLoud TC. *Thoracic Radiology: The Requisites.* 2nd ed. St Louis: Mosby; 2009.

7. Webb WR, Higgins CB. *Thoracic Imaging: Pulmonary and Cardiovascular Radiology.* Philadelphia: Lippincott, Williams & Wilkins; 2005.

8. Hansell DM, Bankier AA, MacMahon H, McLoud TC, Müller NL, Remy J. Fleischner Society: glossary of terms for thoracic imaging. *Radiology.* 2008;246:697-722.

Radiology of the Breast

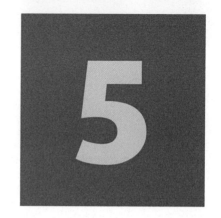

Rita I. Freimanis, MD
Joseph S. Ayoub, MD

Imaging of the breast is undertaken as part of a comprehensive evaluation of this organ, integrating the patient's history, clinical signs, and symptoms. Radiography of the breast is known as mammography, or radiomammography. When used periodically in asymptomatic patients, this is called screening mammography. When imaging is targeted to patients with signs or symptoms of breast cancer, it is referred to as diagnostic breast imaging and usually is a tailored evaluation consisting of some combination of mammography and other techniques described later. Using the integrated approach, it is often possible to make an accurate diagnosis nonoperatively, and treatment may be individualized according to each patient's needs. The primary purpose of breast imaging is to detect breast carcinoma. A secondary purpose is to evaluate benign disease, such as cyst formation, infection, implant complication, and trauma.

Before the 1980s, when breast imaging was much less widely used, the proportion of surgery for benign breast disease was higher, and treatment for breast carcinoma was initiated at later stages of the disease than at present. Breast imaging has increased the detection of tumors smaller than those found on clinical breast examination and has enabled patients to avoid unnecessary surgery.

The outcome of earlier diagnosis and treatment, however, is yet to be proven. Mortality from breast cancer has remained fairly stable for several decades in spite of the introduction and popularization of screening mammography. Debate continues as to the efficacy of routine breast screening in certain age groups. It is almost universally acknowledged that women over 50 years of age benefit from periodic screening mammography. Several large population studies have shown a decrease in mortality of around 30% in this group. However, controversy continues concerning the value of screening mammography for women under the age of 50 years. Because breast cancer has a lower prevalence in this age group, the impediment to mass screening is largely economic; that is, the number of lives saved relative to dollars spent must be justified. Another difference is that in younger women the breast parenchyma is more often dense and nodular. This condition decreases the sensitivity for detection for carcinoma and leads to more false-negative and false-positive results.

Besides a decrease in mortality, a second benefit of earlier diagnosis is that patients with breast carcinoma are afforded more treatment options; lumpectomy with radiation therapy is an option to mastectomy in many patients.

Mammography has been in common use since about 1980, and breast ultrasonography has been the most often used adjunctive technique during this time. The major contribution of ultrasonography has been its effectiveness in distinguishing cystic lesions from solid masses. Sonography has, therefore, helped to avoid unnecessary surgery, because asymptomatic simple cysts do not require intervention. Ultrasonography, together with mammography, is also used to help characterize solid lesions as benign, indeterminate, or suspicious.

Magnetic resonance (MR) imaging of the breast can be used in selected patients. Image-guided needle biopsy of the breast has become the first-line procedure for diagnosis of indeterminate lesions of the breast, with surgical biopsy being reserved for special cases. Nuclear medicine and contrast injection studies (ductography) are occasionally used under special circumstances with specific indications.

TECHNIQUE AND NORMAL ANATOMY

▶ Film-screen and Digital Radiography (Radiomammography)

The film-screen mammogram is created with x-rays, radiographic film, and intensifying screens adjacent to the film within the cassette; hence the term *film-screen mammography*. The digital mammogram is created using a similar system, but replacing the film and screen with a digital detector.

The routine examination consists of two views of each breast, the craniocaudal (C-C) view and the mediolateral oblique (MLO) view, with a total of four films. The C-C view can be considered the "top-down" view, and the MLO an angled view from the side (Figures 5-1, 5-2). The patient undresses from the waist up and stands for the examination, leaning slightly against the mammography unit. The technologist must mobilize, elevate, and pull the breast to place as much breast tissue as possible on the surface of the film cassette holder. A flat, plastic compression paddle is then gently

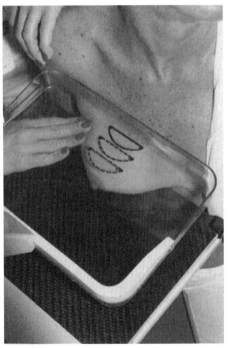

A

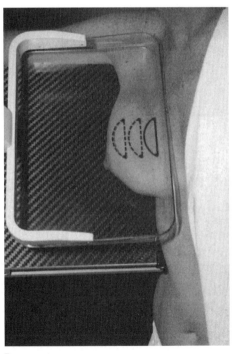

B

▲ **Figure 5-1. (A)** Positioning of the patient for the craniocaudal view of the mammogram. **(B)** Positioning of the patient for the mediolateral oblique view of the mammogram.

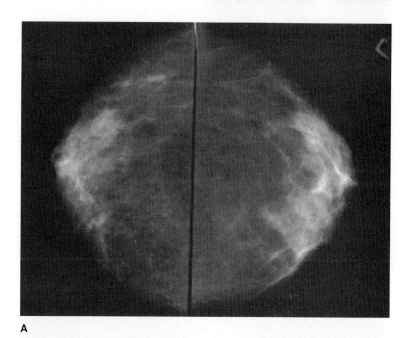

A

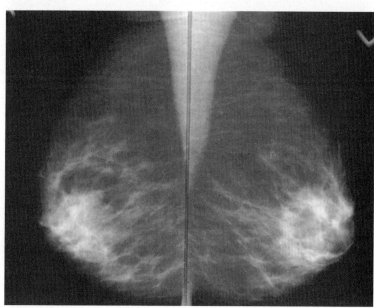

B

▲ Figure 5-2. (A) Normal bilateral cran-iocaudal views. (B) Normal bilateral mediolateral oblique views. This patient shows a moderate amount of residual fibroglandular density, having a mixed pattern of dense and fatty areas of the breast.

but firmly lowered onto the breast surface to compress the breast into as thin a layer as possible. This compression achieves both immobilization during exposure and dispersion of breast tissue shadows over a larger area, thereby permitting better visual separation of imaged structures. Compression may be uncomfortable, and may even be painful in a small proportion of patients. However, most patients accept this level of discomfort for the few seconds required for each exposure, particularly if they understand the need for compression and know what to expect during the examination. Mammography has proved to be more cost-effective, while maintaining resolution high enough to demonstrate early malignant lesions, than any other breast imaging technique. In its present state of evolution, however, the sensitivity of radiomammography ranges from 85% to 95%.

Limitations

Sensitivity is limited by three factors: (1) the nature of breast parenchyma, (2) the difficulty in positioning the organ for imaging, and (3) the nature of breast carcinoma.

The Nature of Breast Parenchyma

Very dense breast tissue may obscure masses lying within adjacent tissue. Masses are more easily detected in a fatty breast.

Positioning

A technologist performing mammography must include as much breast tissue as possible in the field of view for each image. The x-ray beam must pass through the breast tangentially to the thorax, and no other part of the body should intrude into the field of view, so as to not obscure any part of the breast. This requires both a cooperative patient and a skilled technologist. If a breast mass is located in a portion of the breast that is difficult to include in the image, mammography may fail to demonstrate the lesion. Also, because of these practical considerations, routine mammography is not performed in markedly debilitated patients.

The Nature of Breast Carcinoma

Some breast carcinomas are seen as well-defined rounded masses or as tiny, but bright, calcifications, and are easily detected. Others, however, may be poorly defined and irregular, mimicking normal breast tissue. Rarely, still others may have no radiographic signs at all.

   For these reasons, it must be remembered that mammography has significant limitations in detection of carcinoma. It cannot be overemphasized that any suspicious finding on breast physical examination should be evaluated further, even if the mammogram shows no abnormality. Occasionally, additional imaging may reveal an abnormality, but if not, short-term close clinical follow-up or biopsy is warranted.

Normal Structures

Normal breast is composed mainly of parenchyma (lobules and ducts), connective tissue, and fat. Lobules are drained by ducts, which arborize within lobes. There are about 15 to 20 lobes in the breast. The lobar ducts converge upon the nipple.

Parenchyma

The lobules are glandular units and are seen as ill-defined, splotchy opacities of medium density. Their size varies from 1 to several millimeters, and larger opacities result from conglomerates of lobules with little interspersed fat. The breast lobes are intertwined and are therefore not discretely identifiable. This parenchymal tissue is contained between the premammary and retromammary fascia.

   The amount and distribution of glandular tissue are highly variable. Younger women tend to have more glandular

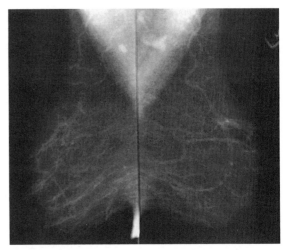

A

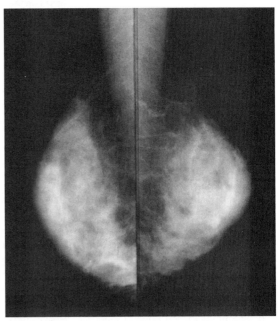

B

▲ **Figure 5-3.** (**A**) Normal mammograms of fatty breasts. (**B**) Normal mammograms of dense breasts. Note the extreme variation of the normal breast parenchymal pattern between patients. A small carcinoma would be much more difficult to detect in the patient with dense breasts than in the patient with fatty breasts.

tissue than do older women. Glandular atrophy begins inferomedially, and residual glandular density persists longer in the upper outer breast quadrants. However, any pattern can be seen at any adult age (Figure 5-3).

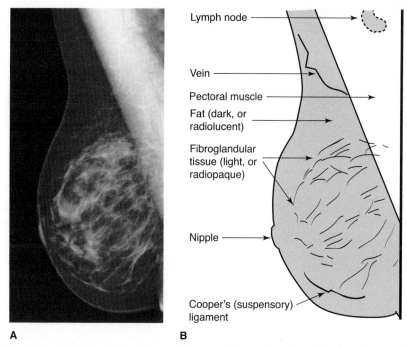

Lymph node

Vein

Pectoral muscle

Fat (dark, or radiolucent)

Fibroglandular tissue (light, or radiopaque)

Nipple

Cooper's (suspensory) ligament

A **B**

▲ **Figure 5-4. (A)** Mediolateral oblique view of normal breast. **(B)** Line drawing with identification of normal structures visible in part (A).

Along with glandular elements, the parenchyma consists of ductal tissue. Only major ducts are visualized mammographically, and these are seen in the subareolar region as thickened linear structures of medium density converging on the nipple.

Connective Tissue

Trabecular structures, which are condensations of connective tissue, appear as thin (<1 mm) linear opacities of medium to high density. Cooper's ligaments are the supporting trabeculae over the breast that give the organ its characteristic shape, and are thus seen as curved lines around fat lobules along the skin-parenchyma interface within any one breast (Figure 5-4).

Fat

The breast is composed of a large amount of fat, which is lucent, or almost black, on mammograms. Fat is distributed in the subcutaneous layer, in among the parenchymal elements centrally, and in the retromammary layer anterior to the pectoral muscle (Figure 5-4).

Lymph Nodes

Lymph nodes are seen in the axillae and occasionally in the breast itself (Figure 5-4).

Veins

Veins are seen traversing the breast as uniform, linear opacities, about 1 to 5 mm in diameter (Figure 5-4).

Arteries

Arteries appear as slightly thinner, uniform, linear densities and are best seen when calcified, as in patients with atherosclerosis, diabetes, or renal disease.

Skin

Skin lines are normally thin and are not easily seen without the aid of a bright light for film-screen mammograms. Various processing algorithms with digital mammography allow better visualization of the skin.

Screening Mammography

The standard mammogram (along with appropriate history-taking) makes up the entire screening mammogram. The indication for this examination is the search for occult carcinoma in an asymptomatic patient. Physical examination by the patient's physician, known as the clinical breast examination (CBE), is an indispensable element in complete breast screening. Although the American Cancer Society no longer recommends routine breast self-examination (BSE), particular attention should be paid to lumps identified by the patient as new or enlarging. Such patients should be referred for diagnostic mammography. Table 5-1 includes guidelines for frequency.

Diagnostic Mammography

The diagnostic mammogram begins with the two-view standard mammogram. Additional maneuvers are then used as

Table 5-1. American Cancer Society Recommendations for Breast Cancer Detection in Asymptomatic Women

Age group	Examination	Frequency
20 to 39	Breast self-examination Clinical breast examination	Optional Every 3 years
40 and older	Breast self-examination Clinical breast examination Mammography	Optional Annual Annual
High risk (>20% lifetime risk)	MRI	Annual
Moderate risk (15% to 20%)	MRI	Talk with doctor about possible annual examinations
Risk<15%	MRI	Not recommended

appropriate in each case, dictated by history, physical examination, and findings on initial mammography. Indications for diagnostic mammography are (1) a palpable mass or other symptom or sign (eg, skin dimpling, nipple retraction, or nipple discharge that is clear or bloody), and (2) a radiographic abnormality on a screening mammogram. Additionally, patients with a personal history of breast cancer may be considered in the diagnostic category.

Other projections, magnification, and spot compression may be used to further evaluate abnormalities. These techniques provide better detail and disperse overlapping breast tissue so that lesions are less obscured.

Implant Views

Patients with breast implants require specialized views to best image residual breast tissue because the implants obscure large areas of the breast tissue with routine mammography. These specialized views (Eklund, "push-back," or implant displacement view) displace the implants posteriorly while the breast tissue is pulled anteriorly as much as possible.

Computer-Aided Detection

Growing availability and affordability of computing power has led to the development of computer-aided detection (CAD). CAD utilizes complex algorithms to analyze the data from a mammogram for suspicious calcifications, masses, and architecture distortion. It then flags these areas so that the interpreting radiologist can give these areas special attention. Several studies show increased cancer detection when CAD is applied, and sensitivity and specificity continue to improve as these algorithms are refined.

▶ Ultrasonography

The indications for ultrasonography are (1) a mammographically detected mass, the nature of which is indeterminate, (2) a

palpable mass that is not seen on mammography, (3) a palpable mass in a patient below the age recommended for routine mammography, and (4) guidance for intervention. Ultrasonography is a highly reliable technique for differentiating cystic from solid masses. If criteria for a simple cyst are met, the diagnosis is over 99% accurate. Although certain features have been described as indicative of benign or malignant solid masses, this determination is more difficult to make and less accurate than the determination of the cystic nature of a mass.

A limitation of ultrasonography is that it is very operator-dependent. Also, it images only a small part of the breast at any one moment. Therefore, an overall inclusive survey is not possible in one image, and lesions may easily be missed.

Normal Structures

The skin, premammary and retromammary fasciae, trabeculae, walls of ducts and vessels, and pectoral fasciae are well seen as linear structures. The glandular and fat lobules are oval, of varying sizes, and hypoechoic relative to the surrounding connective tissue (Figure 5-5).

Simple cysts are anechoic (echo-free) and have thin, smooth walls. Increased echogenicity is seen deep to cysts (enhanced through-transmission). Most solid masses are hypoechoic relative to surrounding breast tissue.

▶ Magnetic Resonance Imaging

The role of MRI in mammography continues to expand, with common applications including (1) staging of and surgical planning for breast tumors, (2) searching for a primary tumor in patients who present with cancerous axillary lymph nodes, (3) evaluating tumor response to neoadjuvant chemotherapy, (4) differentiating tumor recurrence from posttreatment changes in patients with previous breast-conserving surgery and radiation, (5) screening of high-risk patients, (6) evaluating

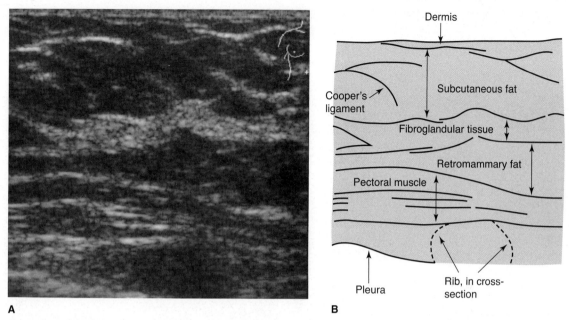

▲ **Figure 5-5. (A)** Ultrasonographic image of a portion of normal breast. **(B)** Line drawing identifying normal structures visible on the sonographic image.

implants, and (7) evaluating difficult (dense or fibrous) breasts. In addition, the technology for MR-guided breast biopsies is increasingly available.

The patient lies prone on the scanner table, and a specialized coil surrounds the breasts. Depending on the clinical question, a varying number of pulse sequences are performed to evaluate the breasts or the composition of a suspicious lesion. Scan times can range from 30 minutes to over an hour.

MRI can show whether a lesion is solid or contains fat or fluid. Dynamic scanning after administration of intravenous contrast shows whether structures enhance and at what rate. Cancers classically enhance rapidly with subsequent "washout." For instance, a lesion that enhances relatively rapidly on dynamic exam (think neovascularity) is more concerning for malignancy. If more than one suspicious lesion is identified, the relative proximity of these lesions can determine whether a patient would be a good candidate for lumpectomy rather than mastectomy. The wide field of view allows staging by evaluating the axillary and internal mammary nodes. Figure 5-6 shows an enhancing cancerous tumor.

Although MRI is quite sensitive (good for detecting disease), it is relatively nonspecific. This is due to the overlapping imaging characteristics of both benign and malignant processes. Like cancer, some benign breast structures show enhancement, although usually with a slower rate.

Because of the relatively low specificity, screening with MRI is best used in patients with a higher probability of

disease. The 2007 American Cancer Society recommendations include annual MRI breast screening of patients with a lifetime risk of 20% or greater.

Normal Structures

Tissues are differentiated by their pattern of change on different pulse sequences. The skin, nipple and areola, mammary fat, breast parenchyma, and connective tissue are normally seen, in addition to the anterior chest wall, including musculature, ribs and their cartilaginous portions, and portions of internal organs. Small calcifications are not visible, and small solid nodules may not be detected. Cystic structures are well seen. Normal implants appear as cystic structures with well-defined walls. Their location is deep to the breast parenchyma or subpectoral, depending on the surgical technique that was used to place the implants. Internal signal varies and depends on implant contents, either silicone or saline.

▶ Ductography

Ductography, or galactography, uses mammographic imaging with contrast injection into the breast ducts. The indication for use is a profuse, spontaneous, nonmilky nipple discharge from a single duct orifice. If these conditions are not present, the ductogram is likely to be of little help. The

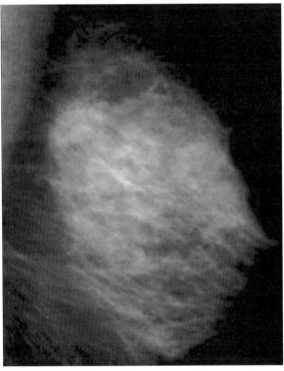

A

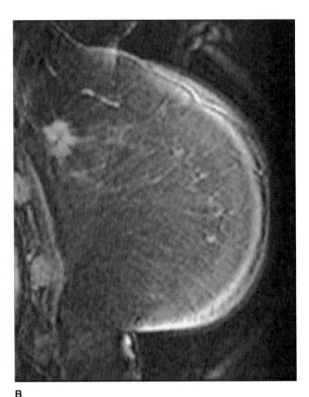

B

▲ **Figure 5-6. (A)** Mammogram showing dense breast tissue. **(B)** MRI of same breast showing enhancing cancer in otherwise minimally enhancing breast.

purpose is to reveal the location of the ductal system involved. The cause of the discharge is frequently not identified. Occasionally, an intraluminal abnormality is seen, but findings have low specificity.

The patient lies in supine position while the discharging duct is cannulated with a blunt-tipped needle or catheter under visual inspection and with the aid of a magnifying glass. A small amount of contrast material (usually not more than 1 mL) is injected gently by hand into the duct. Several mammographic images are then made. The procedure requires about 30 minutes and is not normally painful.

Normal Structures

Just deep to the opening of the duct on the nipple, the duct expands into the lactiferous sinus. After a few millimeters, the duct narrows again and then branches as it enters the lobe containing the glands drained by this ductal system. The normal caliber of the duct and its branches is highly variable, but normal duct walls should be smooth, without truncation or abrupt narrowing. With high-pressure injection, the lobules, as well as cystically dilated portions of ducts and lobules, may opacify.

▶ Image-Guided Needle Aspiration and Biopsy

The indications for needle aspiration and biopsy of breast lesions are varied and are variably interpreted by radiologists and referring physicians. Two categories are discussed here.

The first indication is aspiration of cystic lesions to confirm diagnosis, to relieve pain, or both. Nonpalpable cysts require either ultrasound or mammography to be seen. A fine needle (20- to 25-gauge) usually suffices to extract the fluid. The cystic fluid is not routinely sent for cytology unless it is bloody.

The second indication concerns solid lesions. Needle biopsy is used in this case (1) to confirm benignity of a lesion carrying a low suspicion of malignancy mammographically, (2) to confirm malignancy in a highly suspicious lesion prior to initiating further surgical planning and treatment, and (3) to evaluate any other relevant mammographic lesion for which either follow-up imaging or surgical excision is a less desirable option for further evaluation.

Guidance for needle biopsy can be accomplished with stereotactic mammography, ultrasound, and MR. Imaging modality for needle guidance is selected on the basis of lesion characteristics, availability of technology, and personal preference of the radiologist. Ultrasound and mammography are the most commonly used techniques.

Large core biopsy (typically 14-, 11-, or 8-gauge) has been shown to be more accurate for nonpalpable lesions than fine needle aspiration (20-gauge or smaller) and is often combined with vacuum assistance to further increase tissue yield.

Mammographic guidance is most easily and accurately performed with a stereotactic table unit. Lesions of only a few millimeters can be successfully biopsied. With stereotactic tables, the patient lies prone with the breast protruding through an opening in the table surface. A needle is mechanically guided to the proper location in the breast with computer assistance. The entire procedure requires 30 minutes to 1 hour.

▶ Image-Guided Needle Localization

When a nonpalpable breast lesion must be excised, imaging is used to guide placement of a needle into the breast, with the needle tip traversing or flanking the lesion. Either ultrasonographic or mammographic guidance can be used, and the choice again depends on lesion characteristics and personal preference. Once the needle is in the appropriate position, a hook wire is inserted through the needle to anchor the device in place. This prevents migration during patient transport and surgery. After needle placement, the patient is taken to the operating theater for excision of the lesion by the surgeon.

▶ Biopsy Specimen Radiography

When a lesion is excised from the breast, a surgical specimen can be radiographed to document that the mammographic abnormality was removed. This practice is routinely followed with needle-localized lesions, but palpable lesions excised may also be radiographed to confirm that the specimen contains an abnormality that may have been present on the mammogram.

TECHNIQUE SELECTION

As with other organ systems, the task of the referring physician with regard to breast imaging is to determine which patients may benefit from these studies and which are the appropriate studies to order. To do this, the physician first categorizes the patient as asymptomatic or symptomatic. (1) Asymptomatic patients: As a group, these patients will benefit from routine screening mammography performed according to published national guidelines. A particular patient may require an individualized program for specific reasons: for example, a 30-year-old asymptomatic woman whose mother died of breast cancer at age 35 may justifiably begin yearly screening mammography. (2) Symptomatic patients:

These are women who have any of the following signs or symptoms: a new or enlarging breast lump, skin changes (primarily dimpling), nipple retraction, eczematoid nipple changes, bloody or serous nipple discharge, and focal pain or tenderness. Diagnostic mammography is indicated in these patients. If the patient is under 35 years of age, the examinations may be differently tailored than for older patients. Consultation with the breast imager may be helpful in determining a suitable evaluation plan in any patient for whom the usual guidelines are not helpful.

If a diagnostic study is needed, a standard two-view mammogram is obtained first. The need for further studies will be determined by the results of the mammogram. Whether ultrasonography or another modality is needed is best decided by the person interpreting the films, provided that he or she has the necessary clinical information available. For example, it is imperative that the location and description of a suspected mass be made known to the radiologist so that a specific search can be made for a lesion.

Also, knowledge of prior surgery, inflammation, or trauma to the breast is a requirement for accurate image interpretation. The different disease processes may have overlapping appearances on breast images, and refining the differential diagnosis therefore depends on accurate breast physical examination and the patient's history.

When it has been determined that an abnormality is present, then the decision as to whether close follow-up, needle biopsy, or excision is warranted is best made by integrating the image-based diagnosis and clinical considerations. Good communication between the radiologist and the referring physician is needed to optimize management of breast lesions.

▶ Patient Preparation

For the mammogram, two-piece clothing is most convenient as the patient will need to undress from the waist up. Patients should not apply antiperspirant to the breast or axilla because it may cause artifacts.

Mammography is generally limited to ambulatory, cooperative patients because of the difficulties in proper positioning and because mammography units are not portable. If a debilitated patient has a palpable mass, then ultrasound would be a reasonable first step, followed by bedside needle aspiration or biopsy if the mass is solid. Screening mammography in markedly debilitated patients rarely has clinical utility.

Patients for whom stereotactic biopsy is being considered should be able to lie in prone position without moving for about 1 hour.

▶ Conflict with Other Procedures

Coordinating with other techniques is an infrequent problem with breast imaging. One situation that does occasionally cause difficulty occurs in the patient with a palpable mass that is aspirated with a needle prior to imaging. Aspiration of a simple cyst may cause bleeding into the lesion. Subsequent ultrasonography then shows a complex lesion with debris or some apparently solid elements, rather than a simple cyst. A complex lesion requires more aggressive management than does a simple cyst. Therefore, imaging is best performed prior to aspiration.

THE SYMPTOMATIC PATIENT

EXERCISE 5-1. THE PALPABLE MASS

(Please answer questions for this exercise before looking at the images, which are presented with the discussion.)

5-1.   In Case 5-1, a 34-year-old woman who noticed a new lump in her breast, which test should be ordered first?
A. Screening mammography
B. Excisional biopsy
C. Ultrasonography
D. Diagnostic mammography
E. Needle aspiration

5-2.   Case 5-2 is a 60-year-old woman who, on the insistence of her children, went for her first routine physical examination in many years. Her doctor found a mass in her breast. Which test should be ordered first?
A. Screening mammography
B. Excisional biopsy
C. Ultrasonography

D. Diagnostic mammography
E. Needle aspiration

5-3.   In Case 5-3, a 53-year-old woman thinks she feels a hard nodule deep in her breast. Her breasts have always been difficult to examine because of their dense nodular texture. What test should be ordered first?
A. Screening mammography
B. Excisional biopsy
C. Ultrasonography
D. Diagnostic mammography
E. Needle aspiration

5-4.   In Case 5-4, a 78-year-old woman with a soft, rounded mass discovered during physical examination, which one of the following statements is true?
A. A 78-year-old will not likely benefit from mammography.
B. Soft, rounded masses are benign and do not require biopsy.
C. This mass should initially be aspirated with a needle.
D. If this mass is carcinoma, the patient will probably die of this disease.
E. Her physical findings could easily be caused by a lipoma.

Radiologic Findings

5-1.   Ultrasonographic image of the patient in Figure 5-7. The anechoic, uniformly black area represents a simple

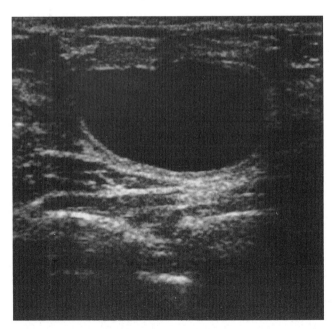

▲ **Figure 5-7.** Case 5-1. Ultrasonographic image of the patient. The anechoic, uniformly black area represents a simple cyst. Note that the walls of the cyst are sharp, and there is a brighter echo pattern deep to the cyst (enhanced through-transmission).

cyst. Note that the walls of the cyst are sharp, and there is a brighter echo pattern deep to the cyst (enhanced through-transmission) (C is the correct answer to Question 5-1). Figure 5-8 illustrates the mammographic features of a cyst. The shape is round or oval, and the margins are smooth and sharply delineated.

5-2. Detail of a mammogram (Figure 5-9) of the patient in Case 5-2. Note the spiculated mass in the upper outer quadrant of this otherwise fatty breast. Diagnosis: invasive ductal carcinoma (D is the correct answer to Question 5-2).

5-3. Detail of a mammogram (Figure 5-10 A) of the patient in Case 5-3. There is a dense nodular breast pattern with a vague, small, rounded opacity (arrow). Spot compression view (Figure 5-10 B) of the region of suspected abnormality in Figure 5-10 A. Note how much easier it is to see the lesion and the spiculation (around it) with spot compression. Note also the difficulty in detecting and evaluating this tumor within dense glandular tissue, compared with the fatty breast in Case 5-2 (D is the correct answer to Question 5-3).

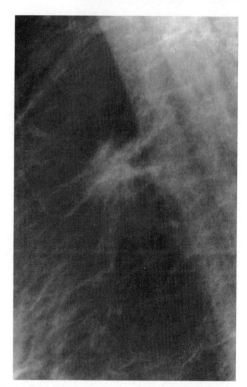

▲ **Figure 5-9.** Case 5-2. Detail of a mammogram of the patient. Note the spiculated mass in the upper outer quadrant of this otherwise fatty breast. Diagnosis: invasive ductal carcinoma.

5-4. The 78-year-old patient in Case 5-4 (Figure 5-11) has a soft mass in her breast and clearly needs a diagnostic mammogram because of her age and the palpable findings (E is the correct answer to Question 5-4).

Approach to the Palpable Lump

When a breast lump is found, several questions must be answered before proceeding with breast imaging. First, given that lumpy breasts are a normal variant, when is a lump significant? Experts in CBE advise palpation with the flat surface of two to three fingers, and not with the fingertips. With this technique, nonsignificant lumps will disperse into background breast density, but a significant lump will stand out as a dominant mass.

Second, is the lump new or enlarged? A new lump is more suspicious than a lump that has not changed over a few years.

Third, how big is the lump? Tiny pea-sized or smaller lumps, particularly in young women, are often observed closely with repeated CBE, because small breast nodules are extremely common, frequently resolve spontaneously, and

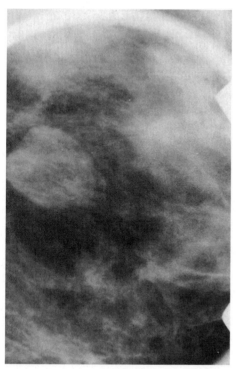

▲ **Figure 5-8.** Detail of a mammogram of a patient with a simple cyst. The smoothly circumscribed margin and the round-to-oval opacity, through which normal breast structures are visible, are characteristic of a simple cyst.

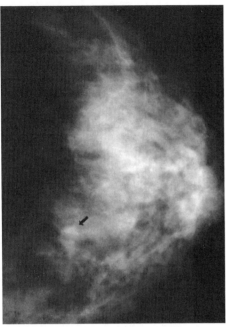
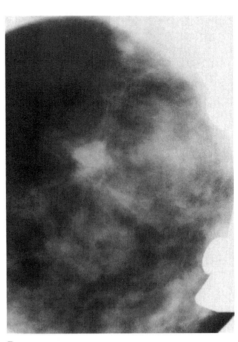

A   B

▲ **Figure 5-10.** Case 5-3. (**A**) Detail of a mammogram of the patient. There is a dense nodular breast pattern with a vague, small, rounded opacity (arrow). (**B**) Spot compression view of the region of suspected abnormality in Figure 5-10 A. Note how much easier it is to see the lesion and the spiculation (around it) with spot compression. Note also the difficulty in detecting and evaluating this tumor within dense glandular tissue, compared with the fatty breast in Case 5-2.

are usually benign. Repeating CBE in 6 weeks allows for interval menses, which frequently causes waning or resolution of the lump. If the lump persists, diagnostic mammography is indicated.

Fourth, how old is the patient? If the patient is less than 35 years of age, then radiation is avoided unless specifically indicated, because the younger breast is more sensitive to radiation. For patients over the age of 35 years, breast imaging begins with a diagnostic mammogram at the time a lump is deemed to be significant. The mammogram provides a view of the lump, as well as of the remainder of the involved breast and the opposite breast, where associated findings may aid in diagnosis and treatment planning.

If the patient is below 35 years of age, a significant lump is usually first examined with ultrasonography to determine whether a simple cyst is present. If there is no cyst, and the patient is below 30 years of age, the radiologist may choose to obtain a mammogram, but the density of the breast in such a young patient may limit the usefulness of radiomammography, so the mammogram may be limited to one breast or to a single view.

For women between the ages of 30 and 40 years, judgment is needed as to whether other imaging is indicated. Several factors should be weighed, including age, family history of breast carcinoma, reproductive history, and findings at CBE. If the primary care physician is uncertain of the significance of the findings of CBE, evaluation by a breast specialist may be helpful prior to requesting radiologic tests.

Discussion

The 34-year-old woman in Case 5-1 indeed has a dominant mass, 2 cm in diameter on CBE. She says it was definitely not present until recently. She has no risk factors for breast cancer. The mass most likely is a fibroadenoma or a cyst, but carcinoma cannot be excluded. The patient now needs breast ultrasonography.

Ultrasonography is best ordered before attempted needle aspiration because aspiration can alter the appearance of simple cysts, giving a misleading suspicious appearance. Therefore, answer E, needle aspiration, is incorrect.

Figure 5-7 shows an image from the ultrasound study that represents the area precisely in the location of the palpable mass. This area is echo-free, with sharply delineated walls and posterior acoustic enhancement (increased echogenicity deep to the anechoic area) consistent with a

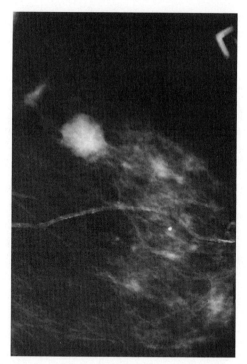

▲ **Figure 5-11.** Case 5-4. Detail of a mammogram of the patient.

simple cyst. If these three features are seen, the probability of a simple cyst is greater than 99% and no further treatment is indicated unless the patient has pain and needs cyst drainage for symptomatic relief. Therefore, option B, excisional biopsy, is inappropriate, because biopsy can be avoided by showing a simple cyst. No further imaging is needed. The patient is under the age of 40 years, not yet of screening age, and radiation should be avoided in young patients. Therefore, answers A and D, screening and diagnostic mammography, are not viable options until ultrasound is performed.

Simple cysts are very common in the premenopausal patient and in patients who are being treated with hormone replacement therapy. A complex cyst is one that has internal debris—blood, pus, or tumor. A complex cyst requires further evaluation, and a short-term follow-up (6 to 8 weeks) ultrasound may be sufficient. If the debris is due to attempted aspiration, it may clear on follow-up ultrasonography. Otherwise, excision or needle biopsy is indicated.

The 60-year-old woman in Case 5-2 has a 1.5-cm dominant mass on CBE. It is irregular and not freely mobile. The patient has never had a mammogram. Because she has a palpable mass, however, a screening mammogram is inappropriate, and option A is incorrect. Although the mass feels suspicious, she still needs a diagnostic mammogram prior to

biopsy (option B, excisional biopsy, is incorrect), to exclude other lesions such as multifocal carcinoma. The need for ultrasonography in a patient of this age is dictated by the mammographic appearance; therefore, option C, ultrasonography, is incorrect.

Her mammogram (Figure 5-9) shows a very fatty breast, making any abnormal findings readily apparent. There is a mass measuring 1 cm in the upper outer quadrant that corresponds to the area of the palpated mass. The mass is of high density, being white on the mammogram. There is abundant spiculation and stranding around the mass that is represented by the radiating linear densities around the periphery of the mass. There is also retraction of the linear patterns of the normal breast tissue; this retraction is known as architectural distortion. These findings represent the classical features of a malignant lesion on mammography, and this mass must be biopsied. A spiculated mass such as this is the most common appearance of invasive breast carcinoma. Less common signs are a circumscribed mass, asymmetric density, and architectural distortion alone. Intraductal (noninvasive) carcinoma is more commonly associated with calcifications.

Spiculation around an invasive carcinoma corresponds to fingers of tumor, as well as to a desmoplastic reaction of adjacent normal breast tissue responding to the presence of tumor. This patient has an invasive ductal carcinoma. About 90% of primary breast carcinomas are ductal carcinomas, and the other 10% are lobular carcinomas.

Besides carcinoma, the primary differential diagnosis for a spiculated mass includes postsurgical change, other trauma with hematoma, fat necrosis, infection, and radial scar (a complex, spontaneous benign lesion involving ductal proliferation, elastosis, and fibrosis).

There are no other lesions in our patient's breast, and the other breast appears normal. By mammographic criteria, then, the patient is a good candidate for treatment with lumpectomy and radiation therapy rather than mastectomy. Her tumor is solitary, localized to one quadrant, and her breast tissue is otherwise easy to evaluate mammographically. Recurrent tumor or additional lesions should, therefore, be readily seen on posttreatment follow-up mammograms.

For a mass that feels malignant and appears suspicious on a mammogram, fine-needle aspiration (FNA) at the bedside may provide a rapid cytological diagnosis of carcinoma. Because FNA best follows mammography, option E, needle aspiration, is incorrect. FNA may then be followed by definitive surgical treatment at a later date, after the patient has had time to consider the treatment options available. If FNA fails to disclose carcinoma, then excisional biopsy is required because of the suspicious findings on mammography and CBE. The occasional false-negative FNA occurs with tumors that do not shed cellular material readily.

Cytology of this palpable mass revealed ductal carcinoma, and this patient chose to have a lumpectomy.

The 53-year-old patient in Case 5-3 has an ill-defined 1.5-cm hardened nodular area in her breast. Results of screening mammography less than 1 year ago were normal. Her breast tissue is not fatty, as in Case 5-2, but she has quite dense, nodular, fibroglandular tissue, which may obscure small masses. The average doubling time of breast carcinoma makes it unlikely that she has a palpable carcinoma that is entirely new since her last mammogram. It is quite possible, however, that she has had a smaller cancer for a few years and that it has now grown large enough to be palpated. Breast tumors are typically not palpable unless they are at least 1 cm in diameter. Before this stage, in the preclinical phase, the tumor may be visible up to 2 or 3 years earlier on the mammogram if the breast is fatty. In dense breasts, as discussed previously, tumors may not be seen on the mammogram until later stages. For this reason, regular CBE is important. Mammography will miss some cancers, regardless of the situation, at a rate variably reported to be between 5% and 15%.

With a new area of abnormality on physical examination, being in a high-risk age group (over 50 years old), and having a dense parenchymal pattern, the patient needs another mammogram, this time a diagnostic mammogram of the involved breast only. Option A, screening mammogram, is incorrect, because it is too soon to repeat screening mammography at this time and the patient does have a palpable finding—a contraindication for a screening study.

Figure 5-10 A shows a vague, rounded opacity within dense fibroglandular tissue. This is in the area of the palpable mass, as indicated by a small BB placed on the skin over the abnormality. Detail is not adequate to make a judgment as to the possibility of malignancy here, or even to confirm that a real lesion is present. The appearance may merely be due to superimposed normal breast shadows. Compression spot films are needed to confirm the presence of a mass and to better define its borders.

Figure 5-10 B shows spot compression of the questioned opacity seen on initial images. This localized compression with a smaller paddle placed directly over the abnormality achieves two things. First, it separates the opacity from adjacent breast tissue, demonstrating this to be a discrete mass with high density and not merely superimposition of normal shadows. Second, it elicits clear spiculation and architectural distortion around the mass. These features are classic for breast carcinoma, and biopsy is therefore required. Biopsy of this lesion showed invasive ductal carcinoma.

The 78-year-old patient in Case 5-4 has a soft mass in her breast and clearly needs a diagnostic mammogram because of her age and the palpable findings. Soft, rounded masses on physical examination are often benign fibroadenomata or cysts, but carcinoma may also present this way (Statement B is false).

Other benign causes of these physical findings include hematoma, abscess, and lipoma (Statement E is true). Therefore, a mammogram may be beneficial for two reasons: (1) if a benign finding is revealed, biopsy may be avoided; and (2) if findings suggest malignancy, optimal treatment can be planned on the basis of extent of the lesion and presence or absence of additional lesions (Statement A is false).

Her mammogram (Figure 5-11) shows two findings. There is a rounded mass with multiple lobulations and circumscribed borders. The fact that the borders are not sharply outlined on all sides raises the suspicion level for this finding. Masses that are sharply delineated may be followed with serial mammograms at 6-month intervals if they are known not to be new, are nonpalpable, and show no other features of malignancy. This is not the case with the patient in Case 5-4. Note the fading margin along portions of the mass. This mass corresponds to the palpable finding. Ultrasonography would be useful to exclude a multiloculated cyst and show the lesion to be solid. Biopsy is indicated, but needle aspiration without imaging would have been inappropriate (Statement C is false).

A circumscribed mass representing carcinoma is seen less often than a spiculated mass. About 10% of invasive ductal carcinomas represent the better-differentiated subtypes, including medullary carcinoma, mucinous (colloid) carcinoma, and papillary carcinoma, all of which are frequently seen as circumscribed masses. They tend to have a better prognosis than the less well-differentiated garden-variety ductal carcinomas.

The differential diagnosis for the circumscribed mass on mammography includes carcinoma (primary as well as metastatic), fibroadenoma, and cysts; hematoma, abscess, and miscellaneous benign lesions are seen much less often. Correlation with clinical history and physical examination can help to narrow the differential diagnosis. When carcinoma cannot be excluded, either needle aspiration or excisional biopsy is required.

This patient had a needle biopsy. Because palpation alone could not reliably localize this lesion for needle biopsy because of its soft nature and the difficulty in fixing its position, stereotactic mammographic guidance was used in localizing the lesion for this procedure. The diagnosis of mucinous carcinoma was made by microscopic inspection of the specimen.

Now, were you astute enough to perceive the second lesion? Above and to the left of large mass is a smaller, dense spiculated mass. This was also biopsied and proved to be a carcinoma of the very well-differentiated tubular type. Even though the patient has two lesions now, both carry an excellent prognosis and they are unlikely to cause her death (Statement D is false). In fact, although mastectomy is certainly a reasonable treatment for her, local excision would also be an option with these nonaggressive lesions.

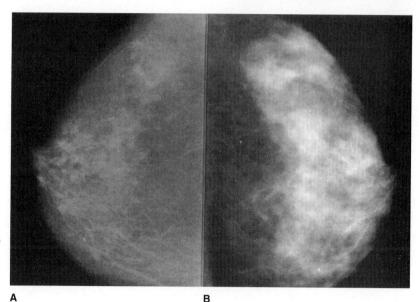

▲ **Figure 5-12.** (**A, B**) Case 5-5. The mammogram (**A** was taken 1 year before **B**) in a 82-year-old woman who complains of newly lumpy, painful breasts.

A   **B**

EXERCISE 5-2. LUMPINESS, NIPPLE DISCHARGE, AND PAIN

5-5. The most likely explanation for the patient's symptoms and mammographic change in Case 5-5 (Figure 5-12) is
   A. hormone effect.
   B. infectious mastitis.
   C. carcinoma.
   D. congestive heart failure.
   E. cystic disease.

5-6. With respect to ductography and the condition of the patient in Case 5-6 (Figure 5-13), which of the following statements is true?
   A. Ductography should be performed in all patients with nipple discharge.
   B. The cause for this patient's discharge is more likely to be malignant than benign.
   C. This ductogram shows an extraluminal filling defect.
   D. Ductography has a high specificity for malignant lesions.
   E. Ductography is helpful in guiding the surgeon's approach.

5-7. With respect to Case 5-7, which of the following statements is false (Figure 5-14)?
   A. There is diffuse abnormality on the left.
   B. Inflammatory carcinoma is high on the differential diagnostic list.

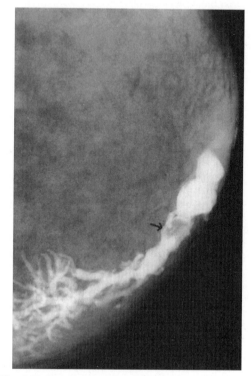

▲ **Figure 5-13.** Case 5-6. Ductography in a 45-year-old woman with a serous nipple discharge.

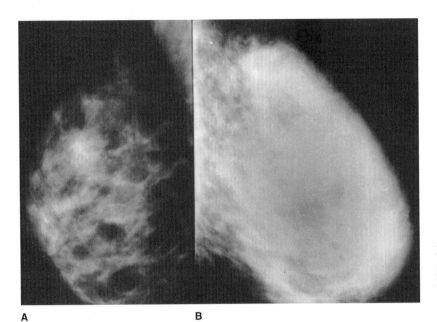

A   B

▲ **Figure 5-14. (A, B)** Case 5-7. The right (**A**) and left (**B**) breast in a 37-year-old woman who comes to the emergency department with a reddened, swollen, painful left breast.

C. Infectious mastitis is unlikely to be the cause in this nonlactating patient.
D. The mammographic appearance is nonspecific.
E. Follow-up imaging after a course of antibiotics would be appropriate.

5-8. With respect to Case 5-8, which one of the following statements is true (Figure 5-15)?
A. The soreness indicates a benign process.
B. The appearance is malignant, and biopsy is necessary.
C. Findings on physical examination and history may radically alter our management decision.
D. Bleeding, such as that due to anticoagulation therapy, would not have this appearance.
E. The most likely diagnosis is fibrocystic change.

Radiologic Findings

5-5. These mammograms show a diffuse marked increase in mammographic density with a nodular character (A is the correct answer to Question 5-5).
5-6. In this ductogram, contrast has been injected into a portion of a single ductal system with opacification of the lactiferous sinus and larger branching ducts. Most of the walls are smooth, as they should be. However, there is a filling defect in one of the major branches, as exhibited by the lucency outlined by contrast on all sides and indicated by the arrow (E is the correct answer to Question 5-6; Statement C is false).

5-7. Mammograms of the right and left breast show that the entire left breast (B) is abnormally dense (C is the correct answer to Question 5-7).
5-8. Mammogram shows a large band of high density with markedly spiculated margins in the upper part of the breast (C is the correct answer to Question 5-8).

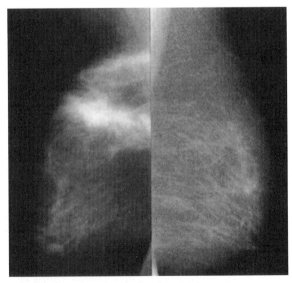

▲ **Figure 5-15.** Case 5-8. The mammogram in a 52-year-old woman with soreness in the right breast.

Discussion

Lumpy breasts are a variant of normal and, as such, require careful physical examination and mammography to avoid unnecessary surgery, as well as not to miss a carcinoma. Diffuse lumpiness is not a contraindication to screening mammography, but when a particular lump becomes dominant, a diagnostic study is indicated.

The two mammograms of the patient in Figure 5-12 were obtained 1 year apart. Between these two examinations, the patient began to exhibit menopause symptoms and was started on hormonal replacement therapy. The breasts, which were previously largely fatty (A), have become moderately dense and very lumpy on palpation 1 year later (B). This change can also be seen, although not usually as dramatically, in the perimenopausal time of estrogen flare.

Such changes can be seen asymmetrically or unilaterally, and it is useful to remember the estrogen effect when evaluating mammograms with interval changes. Correlation with clinical history is then needed.

Answer B, infectious mastitis, and Answer C, carcinoma, are incorrect as both of these entities are usually unilateral and focal. Option D, congestive heart failure (CHF), is incorrect because CHF causes bilateral changes that have a more linear pattern of trabecular thickening on mammography, rather than the patchy, ill-defined nodular pattern characteristic of glandular and cystic densities seen here. Answer E, cystic disease, is incorrect. Cysts are seen as a component of hormone-related breast changes, but spontaneous cystic disease alone is rare at this age.

In the patient in Case 5-6, there is a single intraluminal filling defect on ductography. However, we cannot determine from these findings alone whether the defect is due to a benign or a malignant nodule (Statement D is false), although approximately 90% of nipple discharges are due to benign causes (Statement B is false). The filling defect in this woman was a benign papilloma, the most common cause of bloody or serous discharge. Mammograms usually do not show these small, intraductal nodules.

Whether or not a filling defect is seen on a ductogram, biopsy is needed to rule out carcinoma, and the ductogram may be helpful in showing the surgeon which area of the breast harbors the cause of discharge (Statement E is true). However, many surgeons are able to identify the lobe(s) involved in the pathology by inspecting the nipple, noting the location of the discharging duct, and by palpation, observing which portion of the breast produces discharge when compressed. Usually, ductography is not easily performed and is of limited usefulness when discharge is not spontaneous, profuse, and confined to a single duct. Therefore, statement A is false; ductograms should not be performed on all patients with nipple discharge. Furthermore, only bloody or serous discharges are of concern. A large portion of patients with discharge have secretions typical of fibrocystic change (ie, a dark brownish or greenish fluid rather than a truly bloody or serous discharge). Milky discharge is normal.

In Case 5-7, the patient's entire left breast is abnormally dense (Statement A is true). There is skin thickening as well. This is a nonspecific appearance (Statement D is true); infection and inflammatory carcinoma are both high on the differential diagnosis list (B is true; C is false). Breast carcinoma may incite an inflammatory response in the breast, mimicking a benign infectious process both clinically and radiographically. The patient turns out to have an elevated white blood cell count and fever with marked pain. This information now makes infection more likely than tumor, and a course of antibiotics with follow-up imaging to monitor resolution is appropriate (Statement E is true).

Figure 5-16 shows the follow-up mammogram after significant clinical resolution. The mammographic findings have resolved, and the left breast now appears very similar to the right one.

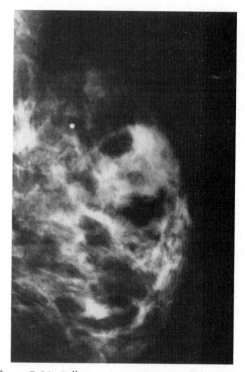

▲ **Figure 5-16.** Follow-up mammogram of the patient in Case 5-7 after a short course of antibiotics. Note the resolution of abnormal findings and the resultant symmetrical appearance compared with that of the opposite breast.

Infectious mastitis occurs more frequently in lactating women but is not uncommon in nonlactating women, particularly in diabetic patients. Imaging (mammography or ultrasound) is useful to exclude a drainable abscess collection and to provide a baseline for monitoring resolution to exclude carcinoma.

Case 5-8 illustrates the importance of correlation with history and physical examination. This patient has pain, as in the last case, but her mammographic abnormality is much more localized and appears more like a malignant mass, being a high-density opacity with excessive spiculation. However, this, too, is a benign process. The patient was in a motor vehicle accident 2 months earlier and sustained a severe injury to the right side of her chest. Physical examination shows a resolving laceration and contusion that extends in a linear fashion over the right breast (no wonder she is sore!). A CT scan performed at the time of trauma showed the acute injury precisely in the area shown on the mammogram. These mammographic features are consistent with a resolving hematoma from acute trauma. Therefore, no further action is warranted at this time, other than follow-up (Statement C is true). Although pain is not a prominent feature of carcinoma, patients with cancer may be symptomatic. Therefore, pain does not always indicate benignancy (Statement A is false).

The mammographic appearance would certainly be highly suspicious for invasive carcinoma in the absence of clinical information, but with careful correlation we are able to avoid biopsy in this case (Statement B is false).

Anticoagulation therapy with resultant bleeding could also have this appearance (Statement D is false).

Fibrocystic change, although very common, is an unlikely diagnosis. Fibrocystic change appears as increased cloudy densities, nodular densities, and occasionally some thickened linear densities, but rarely as a spiculated mass (Statement E is false).

THE ASYMPTOMATIC PATIENT

EXERCISE 5-3. THE FIRST MAMMOGRAM

5-9. According to the American Cancer Society, the best program of breast screening for this woman in Case 5-9 (Figure 5-17) includes all of the following except
  A. yearly MRI.
  B. yearly mammograms.
  C. cessation of routine mammograms at age 65.
  D. annual clinical breast examination.

5-10. The most likely diagnosis in Case 5-10 (Figure 5-18) is
  A. complex cyst.
  B. fibroadenolipoma.
  C. galactocele.
  D. ductal carcinoma.
  E. oil cyst.

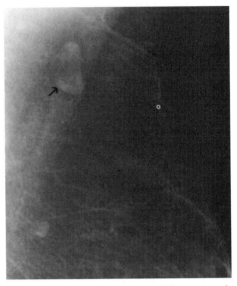

▲ **Figure 5-17.** Case 5-9. A 40-year-old woman whose mother died of breast carcinoma.

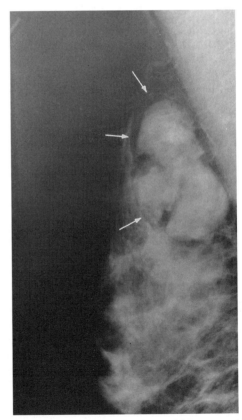

▲ **Figure 5-18.** Case 5-10. A 42-year-old woman with no risk factors for breast carcinoma. She has no symptoms.

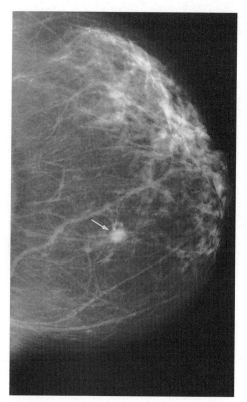

▲ **Figure 5-19.** Case 5-11. A 45-year-old woman, asymptomatic, with no risk factors.

5-11. The differential diagnosis in Case 5-11 (Figure 5-19) includes all of the following except
  A. invasive ductal carcinoma.
  B. cyst.
  C. intraductal comedocarcinoma.
  D. fibroadenoma.
  E. mucinous carcinoma.

Radiologic Findings

5-9. Detail of mammogram of the patient in this case shows a smoothly marginated small mass with a lucent center (arrow) (C is the correct answer to Question 5-9).

5-10. The mammogram in this case shows a circumscribed mass (arrows) with internal lucency as well as opacity (B is the correct answer to Question 5-10).

5-11. Mammogram of patient in this case shows a nodular density (arrow), with indistinct margins (C is the correct answer to Question 5-11).

Discussion

In Case 5-9, the 40-year-old woman has a strong family history of breast cancer, which puts her at high risk for develop-

ing the disease. As was stated in the introduction to this chapter, controversy exists concerning when mammographic screening should be initiated and the appropriate frequency of examinations in different groups. Most experts agree, however, that patients with a strong family history will benefit from screening beginning at age 40. The American Cancer Society (ACS) recommends annual screening from age 40 in all female patients; therefore, B is not the correct answer.

Although the upper age limit for mammographic screening has not been defined, we certainly cannot recommend cessation over age 65, because the prevalence of breast cancer is greatest in women in their 50s and 60s. Current ACS guidelines recommend yearly mammograms for all women over the age of 40 years. Appropriate age for termination of screening is best judged by the patient's physician, weighing life expectancy against potential benefits from screening.

ACS recommends annual screening MRI in women at high risk for breast cancer. ACS also recommends yearly physical examination by the physician to detect tumors missed by mammography, as well as those that become detectable between routine mammograms (interval cancers). Therefore, A and D are not correct answers to Question 5-9.

This patient's mammogram is normal and demonstrates a typical normal lymph node. The node is smoothly marginated and has a fatty hilum, indicated by the darker center.

In Case 5-10, there is a circumscribed mass in the axillary tail of this breast. The key to diagnosis is the mixture of densities within the lesion. There are medium-density opacities interspersed with lucencies within a smoothly marginated mass. This appearance is pathognomonic for a fibroadenolipoma, sometimes called by the misnomer hamartoma. Being composed of elements of normal breast (fatty, glandular, and fibrous tissues) organized within a thin capsule, a fibroadenolipoma forms a "breast within a breast." As such, it is benign and needs no further evaluation. It may be palpable as a soft mass.

The point to remember here is that fat-containing masses are always benign. Answer D, ductal carcinoma, is incorrect. The differential diagnosis of a fatty mass, besides fibroadenolipoma, includes lymph node, as in Case 5-9, galactocele, lipoma, and oil cyst. Galactoceles are usually smaller and are most commonly seen in lactating women (Answer C is incorrect).

Oil cysts result from fat necrosis and are usually smaller. Typically, they are entirely lucent, as they are filled with oil, except for a thin wall (Answer E is incorrect).

Option A, complex cyst, is incorrect because this entity would not contain fat. A cyst, whether it contains serous fluid, blood, or pus, is always opaque and of low to high density, not lucent.

In Case 5-11, an asymptomatic 45-year-old woman's first mammogram shows a 1-cm nodule centrally located in this breast. The differential diagnosis remains broad without further studies to help characterize this nodule. All choices except option C, intraductal comedocarcinoma, may have this

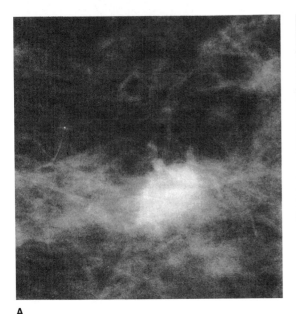 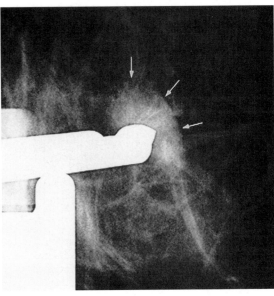

A   B

▲ **Figure 5-20.** (**A**) Spot compression of the nodule seen in Figure 5-19. The margins are indistinct and the shape is somewhat irregular. Biopsy is recommended. (**B**) Mammographic image obtained during stereotactic needle biopsy of the nodule in Case 5-11. The needle tip is about to pierce the nodule (arrows).

appearance. Intraductal carcinoma, when not mammographically occult, usually appears as microcalcifications. Because the margins are indistinct, however, the patient must be recalled for additional imaging to rule out carcinoma.

The sonographic image shows a solid lesion, ruling out a simple cyst. Spot compression is then used to evaluate the borders. If all margins were to appear smooth, one acceptable course of action would be serial 6-month follow-up mammograms for a period of 2 years to demonstrate stability. If any change occurs during this time, biopsy is indicated.

Spot compression (Figure 5-20 A) reveals that portions of the border are not smooth, raising the level of suspicion for malignancy. To exclude carcinoma, biopsy is needed.

Biopsy may be accomplished with excision or with needle biopsy. Excision would require needle localization of the nodule for the surgeon, because this is a nonpalpable lesion. Core needle biopsy, either stereotactic or ultrasound-guided, is preferable because it is minimally invasive, causes less morbidity to the patient, leaves no distortion in the breast or on the skin, and is often less expensive than surgical excision. Accurate needle biopsy devices, however, are expensive and are not universally available.

This nodule was diagnosed as a fibroadenoma with stereotactic core needle biopsy (Figure 5-20 B). Fibroadenomas are very common and are frequently the cause of benign breast biopsy. They occur in very young women (teenagers and women under 30 years of age) and persist undiscovered through the age at which the first mammogram is obtained, then, upon discovery, become a concern of both physician and patient. They may also become palpable or mammographically visible in older women after previously normal mammograms. They continue to be a management problem, because fibroadenoma and carcinoma have overlapping mammographic features and both are common lesions in middle-aged women. With age, fibroadenomas become involuted and heavily calcified, thereby revealing their true identity (Figure 5-21). Without this appearance, however, biopsy is often necessary.

A high index of suspicion and careful evaluation, together with either close follow-up or liberal use of needle biopsy, are needed to minimize both false-negative impressions and excessive breast surgery.

EXERCISE 5-4. ARCHITECTURAL DISTORTION AND ASYMMETRIC DENSITY

5-12. Concerning the architectural distortion in the right breast in Case 5-12 (Figure 5-22), which statement is false?

   A. Without history of biopsy, scarring is unlikely.

   B. Previous mammograms could be very helpful.

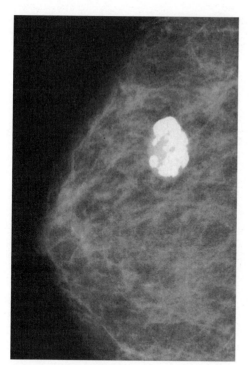

▲ Figure 5-21. Characteristic appearance of heavily calcified involuting fibroadenoma.

C. It is probably nonmalignant because the patient does not complain of a mass.
D. Invasive lobular carcinoma commonly has this appearance.
E. This is probably not an asymmetric response to hormone therapy.

5-13. The mammographic appearance in Case 5-13 (Figure 5-23) is least likely to be caused by
    A. normal breasts.
    B. postsurgical change.
    C. trauma.
    D. cystic disease.
    E. tumor.

Radiologic Findings

5-12. Bilateral craniocaudal views show architecture distortion in the right breast without a discrete dominant mass (C is the correct answer to Question 5-12).

5-13. Bilateral mediolateral oblique views of patient in this case show areas of asymmetric density in the left upper and right lower breast. The densities are interspersed with fat. Margins are generally concave, and there is no architectural distortion (D is the correct answer to Question 5-13).

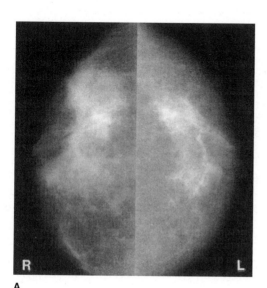

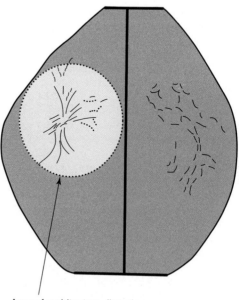

Area of architecture distortion, seen as retraction of parenchymal lines to a central point

A   B

▲ Figure 5-22. Case 5-12. A 51-year-old woman evaluated with screening mammography.

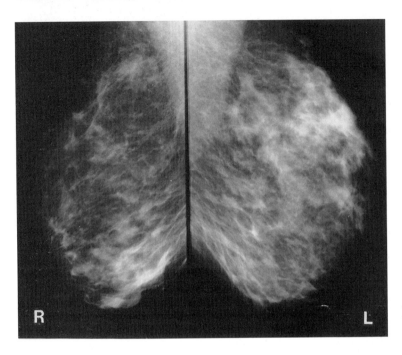

▲ **Figure 5-23.** Case 5-13. A 61-year-old woman evaluated with screening mammography.

Discussion

Although normal breast tissue is remarkably symmetric, it is never exactly the same on both sides. The challenge in mammography is to recognize normal variation and to be able to distinguish nonpathologic asymmetry from disease. This is not always possible, particularly in the asymptomatic group. A high index of suspicion is needed in evaluating the screening mammogram, just as in the baseline clinical breast examination. Once asymmetry is noted mammographically, a careful, focused breast examination is needed. If no suspicious areas are detected and if the radiographic features suggest fibroglandular tissue, then follow-up alone is adequate. Radiographically, we look for a homogeneous, nondistorted pattern of fat interspersed with lobular densities. Any dominant mass or architectural distortion should cause concern.

In Case 5-12, one area shows a different architectural pattern. The lines of tension appear to pull to a central focus. This is a classic appearance of invasive lobular carcinoma. Remember that 90% of the breast cancers are ductal in origin, and the other 10% are lobular, as in this case. This type of carcinoma shows a subtle infiltrating pattern much more often than does ductal carcinoma (Statement D is true).

One of the problems with this disease is that it is difficult to describe the extent of tumor mammographically. There is a large area of asymmetric architecture in this patient, but where the tumor ends is unclear. This patient had a carcinoma that measured 4 cm.

A correlated clinical examination often reveals abnormalities not detected without the guidance of mammographic findings (Statement C is false). Biopsy of any suspicious-feeling area is strongly recommended. Studies have shown that a high percentage of carcinomas "missed" at mammography appear as architecture distortion or asymmetric density. This patient did have a large area of thickening in the upper aspect of this breast, confirming the suspicious nature of the mammographic findings.

Previous mammograms are definitely useful in evaluating architecture distortion and asymmetric density. If the finding is unchanged over time, no further action may be needed. If the finding is new or is increasing, it is more easy to recognize (Statement B is true). Hormonal therapy may indeed have an asymmetric effect (Statement E is true), but it does not take the form of architecture distortion.

Surgical biopsy may result in such distortion of the architecture, but precise correlation with location and timing of the surgery is needed (Statement A is true).

Unlike the previous patient, the woman in Case 5-13 has multiple areas of breast asymmetric density. There is a large area in the upper part of the left breast and a smaller area in the lower part of the right breast. Both areas show fat interspersed with fibroglandular densities. There is no architectural distortion. Margins of the larger opacities are generally concave—a sign of benignity. There are no dominant or circumscribed masses, and cystic disease therefore would not be part of the differential diagnosis, because cysts are rounded masses. Having learned from the previous case that missed carcinoma often presents as asymmetric density, tumor must remain in the differential diagnosis, and answer E is incorrect.

Both trauma and postoperative change can lead to ill-defined asymmetric density. With trauma there may be bleeding, contusion, or actual deformity, if severe. With surgery, asymmetry results both from removal of normal tissues, leaving less density on the operated side, and from surgical trauma (hematoma and distortion), which causes increased localized densities. Therefore, options B and C are both incorrect. The most likely cause of this woman's mammographic appearance is normal breast tissue, and answer A is incorrect. The multiplicity and bilaterality of areas of asymmetry, the lack of signs or symptoms of breast cancer, and the fibroglandular characteristics of the densities all support this diagnosis.

EXERCISE 5-5. THE FOLLOW-UP MAMMOGRAM

5-14. Which of the following statements about Case 5-14 is false (Figure 5-24)?
   A. The abnormal finding is a spiculated mass.
   B. The rate of change is too slow for a breast cancer.
   C. A malpractice claim should not be encouraged.
   D. The lesion is probably not palpable.
   E. This change warrants biopsy.

5-15. With respect to the calcifications in Case 5-15 (Figure 5-25), which statement is false?
   A. They may be described as pleomorphic.
   B. The coarse nature of some of the calcifications suggests this is a benign process.
   C. They signal an aggressive malignancy.
   D. They are most likely due to necrosis in duct walls.
   E. Magnification should be performed to assess the extent of disease.

5-16. With respect to the calcifications in Case 5-16 (Figure 5-26), which statement is true?
   A. They may be described as granular.
   B. The regional distribution makes them highly suspicious.
   C. Follow-up alone would be inadequate.
   D. The new onset indicates a high probability of malignancy.
   E. They have a less than 20% chance of being malignant.

Radiologic Findings

5-14. This case shows back-to-back craniocaudal views of the right breast obtained 1 year apart. In the interval, a small spiculated mass has enlarged so as to become more apparent (arrow) (B is the correct answer to Question 5-14).

5-15. The mammogram of the patient in this case shows a cluster of microcalcifications posteriorly in the central aspect of the breast. Previous mammograms have been normal (B is the correct answer to Question 5-15).

5-16. Magnification view of a portion of the breast of the patient in this case shows coarse calcifications, some of which are rounded or ringlike (E is the correct answer to Question 5-16).

Discussion

Case 5-14 illustrates the concept of developing density. A developing density is any opacity that increases in size or density

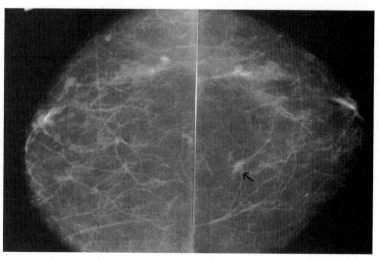

▲ **Figure 5-24. (A,B)** Case 5-14. The first mammogram **(A)** and the one obtained a year later **(B)** in a 70-year-woman who had two screening mammograms 1 year apart.

A   B

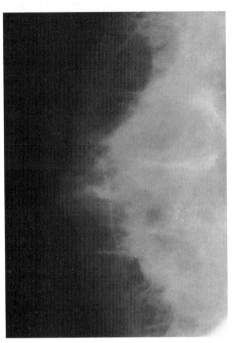

▲ **Figure 5-25.** Case 5-15. A 66-year-old woman with this screening mammogram after a previously normal mammogram.

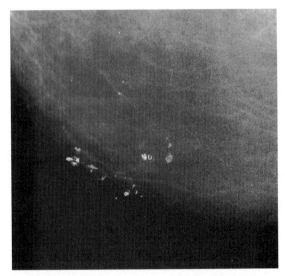

▲ **Figure 5-26.** Case 5-16. A 55-year-old woman who had a normal mammogram the previous year.

over time. All such opacities should be evaluated critically, as they can be signs of carcinoma. This concept is based on the natural behavior of breast cancer, which generally grows slowly. With periodic screening, the early tumor will be imaged but unrecognized on early images and may not be detected until 1, 2, 3, or more years later. Tumors 5 mm or smaller are very difficult to differentiate from normal breast tissue, but masses larger than 1 cm are more easily detected. The typical breast cancer has been present for several years by the time it is 1 cm in size. Therefore, breast cancers are routinely visible in retrospect on previous mammograms if the patient has had frequent screening. This does not mean, however, that malpractice has occurred. If the cancer is still small, no harm has been done and more harm could potentially be done by biopsying all such tiny densities, because most of them would be normal breast (Statement C is true). Being suspicious but judicious with any developing density, therefore, is necessary to detect breast cancer early without unnecessary biopsy.

This patient has a small (about 1 cm) spiculated mass in the central part of the breast (Statement A is true). It has increased slightly in size over 1 year, with a growth rate typical for breast carcinoma (Statement B is false and is the correct answer to Question 5-14). Being so small in a medium-sized breast, it is unlikely to be palpable (Statement D is true) and, therefore, would require imaging guidance for any biopsy. The spiculated margins, the rate of growth, and the patient's age group all make this a very suspicious lesion, and biopsy is warranted (Statement E is true). This lesion was an infiltrating ductal carcinoma.

Case 5-15 illustrates a new finding after a previous normal screening. There is a cluster of microcalcifications in the central area. Note that the calcifications are small and irregular, but we do not see their configuration exquisitely; nor can we be confident of the extent of disease, because there may be other smaller calcifications that we do not see. The patient, therefore, requires recall for magnification mammography (Figure 5-27) (Statement E is true). On magnification, we can appreciate that the calcifications are of many different sizes and shapes (ie, pleomorphic) (Statement A is true). Malignant microcalcifications are usually less than 0.5 mm in size, and the very coarse calcifications are classically benign. However, there is significant overlap, and configuration is generally a more helpful sign. Malignant calcifications are usually either granular or linear and branching.

These granular, linear, and branching calcifications are typical of intraductal carcinoma. The aggressive type of intraductal carcinoma, comedo or high-nuclear-grade carcinoma, causes necrosis in the cancerous mammary duct walls. Calcifications form in areas of necrosis, forming a "cast" of the duct. This process results in the linear and branching forms of calcification (Statements C and D are true). Pathologic analysis of this tissue showed intraductal carcinoma of the comedo type.

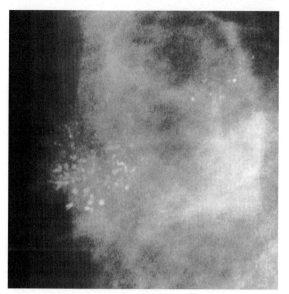

▲ **Figure 5-27.** Magnification view of microcalcifications seen on a screening mammogram of the patient in Case 5-15. Note the pleomorphism of the microcalcifications. The size varies from very fine to coarse, and shapes are bizarre. This appearance is typical of comedocarcinoma.

Lesser degrees of necrosis result in smaller, more granular calcifications, whereas extensive necrosis yields rather large rod-shaped or branched calcifications. Option B is false because, although large calcifications alone are usually benign, the mixture of tiny irregular calcifications with the coarse casting calcifications remains very suspicious for malignancy.

In Case 5-16, the mammogram detail shows typical benign calcifications. Benign calcifications take many forms, but if we see rings with lucent centers, as in this case, we can rest assured that they are benign. These rings are calcifying microcystic areas of fat necrosis. This is a very common benign finding. Punctate, or dotlike, calcifications are also usually benign if uniform and smooth. Granular calcifications are more angular, like broken needle tips, and would be more suspicious (Statement A is false).

Benign calcifying processes such as fibroadenoma, sclerosing adenosis, and fat necrosis can all be unifocal, or regional, as well as multifocal or diffuse; therefore, distribution alone does not make calcifications suspicious (Statement B is false).

Benign processes of many types do present in adulthood and therefore may appear de novo after a previously normal screening examination. Again, the configuration of calcifications is more helpful (Statement D is false).

For obviously benign calcifications such as these, routine follow-up alone is adequate (Statement C is false). Some calcifications are obviously malignant as in Case 5-15. A third group of calcifications is classified as indeterminate, and these require further evaluation, either close mammographic follow-up or some type of biopsy. Taken as a group, biopsied microcalcifications historically have had a rate of malignancy of only 20%. Therefore, Option E is true, because these ringlike calcifications have a better-than-average chance of being benign.

SUGGESTED READING

1. Kopans DB. *Breast Imaging.* 3rd ed. Philadelphia: Lippincott-Raven; 2007.
2. Soslow D, Boetes C, Burke W, et al. American Cancer Society guidelines for breast screening with MRI as an adjunct to mammography. *CA Cancer J Clin* 2007;57:75-89.
3. Cardenosa G. *Breast Imaging Companion.* 3rd ed. Philadelphia: Walters Kluwer, Lippincott Williams & Wilkins; 2008.
4. Ikeda DM. *Breast Imaging: The Requisites.* Philadelphia: Elsevier Mosby; 2004.

Musculoskeletal Imaging

Tamara Miner Haygood, MD, PhD
Mohamed M. H. Sayyouh, MD

When Wilhelm Conrad Roentgen discovered the x-ray in November 1895, he investigated it thoroughly, testing its ability to penetrate various inanimate objects and observing its effects on fluorescent screens and photographic film. He gazed in amazement at the image of the bones of his own hand as he allowed the new rays to penetrate his flesh. He made a photographic x-ray image of a hand (reportedly his wife's) and sent prints of it together with his paper describing the new phenomenon to a carefully selected list of scientific colleagues.

By mid-February 1896, Roentgen's paper had not only been published but also reprinted in other scientific journals including the American journal *Science*. Scientists everywhere repeated Roentgen's simple experiments and confirmed the truth of his discovery. Within a year, x-rays were in widespread use for medical purposes—chiefly for imaging of the skeleton.

Since Roentgen's time, many new imaging techniques have been developed that allow radiologists to see the muscles and other soft tissues of the musculoskeletal system as well as the bones and to evaluate the amount of metabolic activity in the bones and soft tissues. These techniques make skeletal imag-

ing an exciting area of radiology that can enhance patients' quality of life. The techniques can also be very expensive, however. This chapter is intended to introduce you to musculoskeletal imaging techniques and to suggest efficient ways to use them that will help you to make correct diagnoses without excessive cost. Naturally, the suggestions made in these pages must be tailored to the needs of individual patients.

TECHNIQUES

▶ Conventional Radiography

Conventional radiographs are the most frequently obtained imaging studies. They are chiefly useful for evaluation of the bones, but useful information about the adjacent soft tissues may also be obtained. Gas in the soft tissues may be a clue to an open wound, ulcer, or infection with a gas-producing organism. Calcifications in the soft tissues can indicate a tumor, myositis ossificans, or systemic disorders such as scleroderma or hyperparathyroidism.

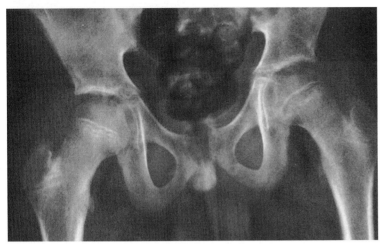

A

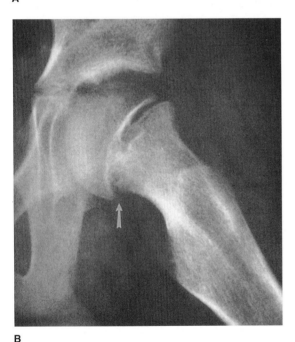

B

▲ **Figure 6-1. (A,B)** Slipped capital femoral epiphysis. **(A)** Anteroposterior (AP) radiograph of the pelvis. There are signs of a fracture through the physis of the left proximal femur: that femoral epiphysis is less well mineralized than the one on the right, the lucent line demarcating the physis is slightly widened, and the alignment of the edges of the epiphysis and metaphysis is abnormal. These signs are relatively subtle and could be easily missed. **(B)** Frog-leg lateral view of the left hip. This view, a lateral of the proximal femur, is much more obviously abnormal. Along the posterior edge of the femur, the cortices of the epiphysis and metaphysis should be flush but are instead offset by approximately 5 mm (arrow).

To get the most information possible from conventional radiographs, you should carefully choose the study to be ordered. At most hospitals and clinics, standardized sets of views have been developed that are routinely obtained together for evaluation of specific body areas in certain clinical settings. It is useful to know what will routinely be obtained when a certain set of films is ordered. Radiographs of the ankle, for example, usually include a straight frontal view of the ankle, a frontal view obtained with approximately 15 de-

grees internal rotation of the ankle (the mortise view), and a lateral view. There will be some variation among institutions, however. At a minimum, two views at right angles to one another should be obtained when a fracture or dislocation is suspected, because such injuries are notorious for being very subtle or even invisible in one projection, even when they are glaringly obvious in another view (Figure 6-1). Radiographs should be focused on the anatomic area being evaluated, free of overlapping, extraneous anatomy (Figure 6-2). If the knee

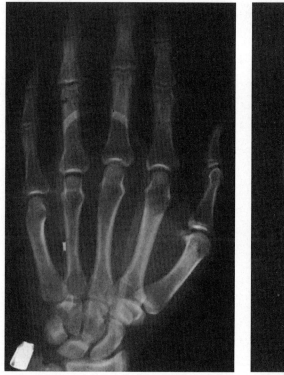 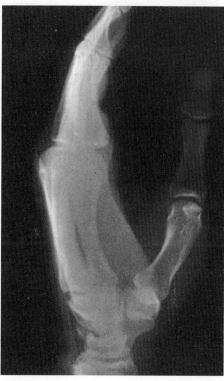

A   B

▲ Figure 6-2. (A,B) Phalangeal fracture. AP (A) and lateral (B) radiographs of the hand. This young man was first evaluated for trauma to the ring finger with frontal and lateral views of the whole hand. On the lateral view, all fingers other than the thumb are overlapped. No fracture was found.

is the site of trouble, do not order views of the entire tibia and fibula; you will be disappointed with the visualization of the knee. This principle must be abandoned more or less in young children and mentally impaired individuals who may not be able to localize their symptoms well, and also in trauma victims with so many injuries that the relatively minor ones may be overlooked.

In addition, when the radiographs will be studied by a consulting radiologist, it is helpful to provide a succinct yet accurate history pinpointing your clinical concerns. Simply indicating the site of injury will improve the likelihood that a subtle fracture will be discovered.

A conventional radiograph of a normal bone will show a smooth, homogenous cortex surrounding the medullary space. The cortex will be thicker along the shaft (diaphysis) of long bones and thinner in small, irregular bones such as the carpal and tarsal bones and at the ends of long bones (Figure 6-3). Exceptions are the normal roughening of the cortex at tendon and ligament insertion sites and the normal interruption of the cortex at the site of the nutrient arteries. Naturally

these occur at predictable places that differ from bone to bone. Within the medullary space of normal bone are trabeculae. These are visible in radiographs as thin, crisp white lines that are arranged not randomly but in predictable patterns that enhance the stress-bearing capability of the bone. It is beyond the scope of this chapter to address the appearance of each bone.

When questions arise concerning whether a particular appearance is normal or abnormal, several solutions are possible. Two books, Keats's *Normal Variants* and Kohler's *Borderlands*, are very useful in helping to distinguish the normal from the abnormal (see suggested reading). Correlation with the results of the history and physical examination may also be helpful. Finally, comparison with the patient's prior radiographs or with a radiograph of the opposite extremity may also help (Figure 6-4). Comparison views of the opposite extremity are especially helpful in children, in whom the open physes and accessory centers of ossification may vary considerably from individual to individual but tend to vary less from side to side than among different people.

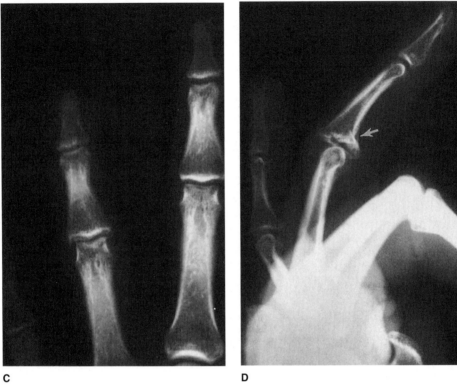

C   D

▲ **Figure 6-2.** *(Continued)* **(C,D)** AP and lateral radiographs of the finger. The patient returned 2½ months later, complaining that his finger still hurt. This time radiographs were coned more closely to the finger and care was taken on the lateral view to image the ring finger separately from the others. In that view the intra-articular fracture of the proximal aspect of the middle phalanx is quite obvious (arrow). It is far more subtle on the frontal view.

▶ Mammographic Techniques

Any soft-tissue area that can be pulled away from the skeleton and placed between the compression paddle and detector may be imaged with mammographic technique. In extremity imaging, mammographic technique is occasionally used to search for small calcifications or foreign bodies in the soft tissues.

▶ Fluoroscopy

Fluoroscopy plays an important role in evaluation of joint motion. It is often used by orthopedic surgeons to monitor placement of hardware. It may be of assistance in positioning patients for unusual or difficult conventional radiographic views.

▶ Computed Tomography

Tomography (either conventional complex-motion tomography or computed tomography [CT]) has two major uses in skeletal imaging. The first is evaluation of fracture fragment position. CT provides excellent delineation of fractures (Figure 6-5). Multislice scanners, which have become commonplace since about 2005, acquire data in blocks and can depict anatomy in any plane with the same resolution and accuracy that previously was possible only in the axial plane. In this way, a fracture may be evaluated in multiple planes of section, usually sagittal and coronal as well as axial. The decision to use CT for fracture evaluation should be based on whether the study will change treatment or will be of sufficient help in operative planning to justify the additional radiation and expense. Scapular fractures, for example, are often treated conservatively, but orthopedic surgeons differ on treatment of fractures that extend into the glenoid or involve the scapular spine. Some believe these benefit from internal fixation; others do not. Tomographic evaluation of these structures will be more useful to a surgeon who would use internal fixation selectively than to one who would use conservative therapy on all scapular fractures.

Three-dimensional reconstruction is available with many CT scanners. There is usually an extra charge. This may be justified if it helps the orthopedic surgeon to plan operative intervention and thus decrease the time required for surgery. Three-dimensional images are also useful for teaching

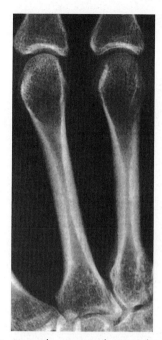

▲ **Figure 6-3.** Normal metacarpals. PA radiograph of the second and third metacarpals of a 36-year-old woman. The cortex is thick and homogenously white in the mid shaft of the metacarpal. It becomes progressively thinner as it approaches the ends of the bones. At the articular surfaces, the cortex has been reduced to a thin, yet distinct, white line.

purposes, as they can often be understood by less experienced individuals. They do not, however, contain information beyond that available in tomographic images.

The second major use of CT is in evaluation of bone tumors or tumor-like diseases. For this purpose, magnetic resonance (MR) imaging is the principal competing technique. CT is more sensitive than MRI in demonstrating small amounts of calcium and can show early periosteal new bone formation or small amounts of matrix calcification before they may be seen with conventional radiography. This finding can be helpful in narrowing the differential diagnosis of a tumor. MRI can easily obtain images in sagittal and coronal planes, which was once an advantage this technique had over CT. Multislice CT scanners have negated this advantage (Figure 6-6). Before MRI was developed, CT was also used widely for determining the extent of soft-tissue tumors, including osseous tumors that have spread into the soft tissues. MRI, however, is now more often used for staging. Its superior contrast resolution greatly eases the task of determining tumor extent within bone marrow and muscle or other soft tissues (Figure 6-7).

▶ Magnetic Resonance Imaging

The exquisite contrast of MRI makes it ideal for evaluation of soft tissues. Its most frequent use in skeletal imaging, therefore, is for diagnosis of injuries to muscles, tendons, or ligaments about joints. This superb contrast resolution also makes it very useful for evaluating disorders of the bone marrow including neoplasm, marrow-packing diseases such as

▲ **Figure 6-4. (A,B)** Nutrient canal. **(A)** PA radiographs of the small finger. The smooth white cortex of the radial side of the proximal phalanx of the small finger is interrupted by a thin, obliquely oriented dark line (arrow). The soft tissues are swollen, and there is tenderness in this area. How can you distinguish this nutrient canal from a fracture? It is in a typical location for a nutrient canal. Its borders are smooth and sclerotic, not jagged. For definitive proof, delve into the patient's film folder. **(B)** The same lucency was present 2½ years earlier. In this case, the soft-tissue swelling was due to cellulitis after a cat bite.

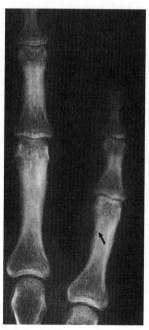 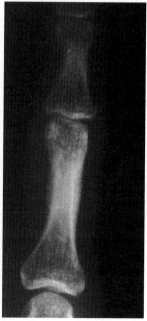

A   B

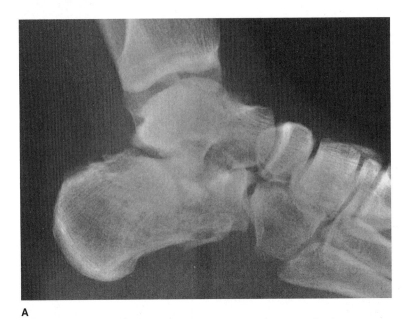

A

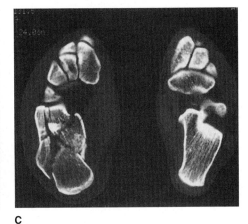

B   C

▲ **Figure 6-5.** Calcaneal fracture. (**A**) Lateral radiograph of the foot. The calcaneus of this 27-year-old man has a comminuted fracture that can easily be diagnosed with this conventional radiograph, but the degree of involvement of the articular surfaces is difficult to appreciate. (**B**) Direct coronal CT image through the posterior and middle subtalar joints demonstrates obliquely oriented fracture lines entering the posterior facet (arrows). There is a gap of approximately 8 mm between the fracture margins, and the lateral fragment has been rotated outward. (**C**) Axial CT image demonstrates a comminuted fracture of the inferior aspect of the calcaneocuboid joint.

Gaucher's disease, osteomyelitis, fractures that are occult on conventional radiographs, and avascular necrosis. Unfortunately, although MRI is very sensitive to these abnormalities, it is also very nonspecific. Many diseases of marrow cause similar signal alteration. One must then narrow the differential diagnosis based on the distribution of the abnormalities together, the radiographic appearance, and the clinical history. Diffusion-weighted MR imaging may be used to identify areas of an organ that have recently been damaged or injured. Diffusion-weighted MR imaging of the vertebral body may differentiate benign from malignant fracture, although its usefulness is still controversial.

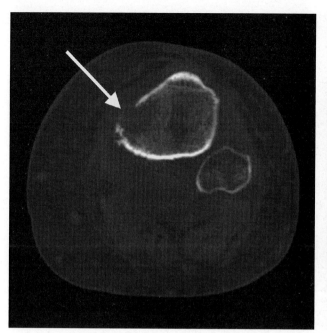

A

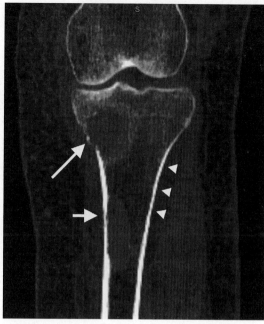

B

▲ **Figure 6-6.** **(A)** Axial coronal CT image of the left proximal tibia and fibula. The axial image demonstrates destruction of a portion of the medial cortex (arrow), due to an underlying intramedullary lesion of multiple myeloma. **(B)** Coronal CT image was obtained with a multislice scanner using helical technique. Reconstruction in the coronal plane clearly demonstrates the same area of cortical destruction (arrow). There is also a more distal area of abnormal cortex (short arrow) adjacent to an intramedullary lesion evident by replacement of the marrow fat by soft-tissue density similar to that of the muscles. The reconstruction is quite smooth, differing from the axial image primarily in the presence of tiny stair-step artifacts along curved edges (arrowheads).

▶ Nuclear Medicine

Several nuclear medicine studies are used for skeletal disease. The two most common are the technetium bone scan and fused positron emission tomography and computed tomography (PET-CT). One of several phosphate compounds of technetium-99m is selected for use in bone scan. Methylene diphosphonate (MDP) is used most frequently. If there is a specific anatomic area of interest, images may be acquired over that area at the time the radionuclide is injected, as well as 3 to 4 hours later. The immediate images reflect the amount of blood flow to the area; the delayed images reflect the amount of bone remodeling occurring there.

Bone scintigraphy is a sensitive but not very specific technique. Most osseous abnormalities of clinical significance will cause an increase in radionuclide accumulation. Exceptions are destructive lesions that incite little reparative reaction in the host bone or that destroy bone so quickly that it cannot remodel.

Because of their sensitivity and because they provide physiologic rather than anatomic information, bone scans can be used to find abnormalities before they are detectable

by conventional radiography. In particular, they are often used for screening for bone metastases in patients with known malignancy. Both multiple myeloma in adults and Langerhans cell histiocytosis in children, however, are notorious for causing no increased accumulation on bone scans. Therefore, in these diseases conventional radiographs or skeletal surveys are better than bone scans for screening for osseous involvement. MR imaging is sometimes also used for screening for myeloma or metastatic disease.

Fused positron emission tomography–computed tomography (PET/CT) combines in a single gantry system both PET scanner and CT scanner, so that images acquired from both techniques can be taken sequentially in the same session and combined into a single superimposed image. Thus, functional imaging obtained by PET, which depicts the spatial distribution of metabolic or biochemical activity in the body, can be more precisely aligned or correlated with anatomic imaging obtained by CT scanning. Other imaging studies may also be fused to combine metabolic information of a nuclear study with anatomic information. For example, a SPECT bone scan may be combined with CT or a PET scan may be combined with MRI.

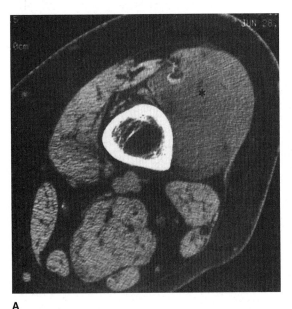

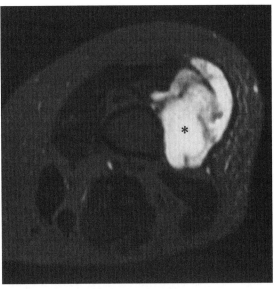

A   B

▲ **Figure 6-7.** (**A**) Axial CT image of the distal thigh. This 49-year-old woman complained of a palpable mass in her thigh. It had been present for a year and was painless. The internal architecture of the vastus lateralis muscle (*) is disrupted. The interdigitated fat and muscle tissues evident in the patient's other muscles have been replaced with a more homogenous mass of decreased attenuation. There is no apparent associated calcification. The mass closely approximates the femur but is not causing osseous destruction. (**B**) T2-weighted (2500/80) MR image of the thigh at approximately the same level. Although this tumor (*) could be seen on the CT scan, on the MR image it is far more obvious and more easily distinguished from normal tissue. The superiority of MR imaging in detecting soft-tissue neoplasms makes it excellent for determining the extent of primary soft-tissue tumors like this myxoid liposarcoma as well as for evaluating the spread of primary bone tumors into the adjacent soft tissues.

▶ Biopsy

When tumor or infection is suspected, it is often useful to obtain a tissue sample for cytologic or histologic analysis or for culture. This may be accomplished by means of an "open" procedure in the operating room or a percutaneous needle puncture of the lesion to obtain a cellular aspirate or slender core of tissue. Needle biopsies of palpable lesions do not necessarily need radiologic intervention. When the lesion is not palpable, however, biopsy may be accomplished under fluoroscopic, CT, ultrasound, or MRI guidance.

When skeletal lesions should be biopsied and by whom are important questions that can have a tremendous impact on the patient's outcome. For example, sarcomas have been reported to grow along the surgical or needle tracks after diagnostic biopsies. Therefore, when planning biopsies of suspected musculoskeletal sarcomas, care must be taken to approach the lesion through a track that can be resected en bloc with the tumor at the time of ultimate excision. These biopsies should always be carried out in close consultation with the surgeon who will be performing the definitive surgery.

When systemic disease such as metastatic carcinoma is the primary consideration, percutaneous needle biopsy is the most efficacious means of making a diagnosis if the lesion is amenable to this procedure. In this setting, the yield of needle biopsy is very good (90% or more of such biopsies yield a positive diagnosis when tumor is truly present) and a negative result is less likely to lead to open biopsy than it would in some suspected primary tumors. Nonetheless, biopsy should still be performed in consultation with the oncologist or other physician giving overall care.

TECHNIQUE SELECTION

In general, as in most other organ systems, the radiograph is the initial imaging test after history and physical examination. The selection of subsequent (often more expensive) imaging tests depends not only on medical need but also on a variety of other factors, including availability, expense, and the preferences of the radiologist, clinician, and patient.

▶ Trauma

Rely on conventional radiography. When a strongly suspected fracture is not identified, you may choose among repetition of conventional radiograph in 7 to 10 days, nuclear medicine bone scanning, and MRI. CT may be substituted for MRI if the latter is unavailable or there are contraindications to its use. If a fracture is noticed and more information is needed concerning the location of fragments, CT is useful.

▶ Bone or Soft-Tissue Tumors

For local staging of both bone and soft-tissue neoplasms, MRI is the best technique. When a bone tumor is suspected but is not discovered with conventional radiographs, MRI is a useful secondary screening tool.

▶ Metastatic Tumors

Symptomatic sites suspected of being involved by metastatic neoplasm are best evaluated initially with radiographs. An overall survey for osseous metastases may be performed by nuclear medicine bone scan or by MRI. Conventional radiography is then used to evaluate sites of possible tumor involvement. Suspected soft-tissue metastases are best evaluated by MRI. PET/CT scans are also useful in staging of many tumors.

▶ Infection

Conventional radiographs should be obtained first for suspected osteomyelitis. If these are normal or inconclusive, then MRI, nuclear medicine bone scan, or white blood cell scanning may be helpful. MRI is also useful for detecting the soft-tissue extent of infection and for finding complications including abscesses or necrotic tissue.

EXERCISE 6-1. TRAUMA

6-1. You are supposed to look at the radiographs for Case 6-1 (Figure 6-8) and call your colleagues in the

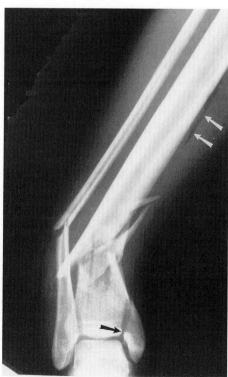
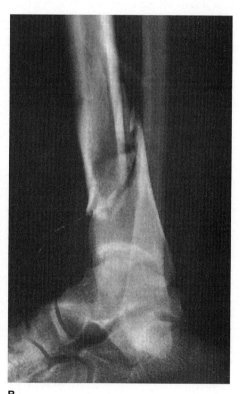

A   **B**

▲ **Figure 6-8.** Case 6-1. On the first day of your medical school rotation in orthopedic surgery, the resident and attending physician send you to the emergency department to see a 26-year-old man with a broken leg (AP and lateral views of the distal tibia and fibula).

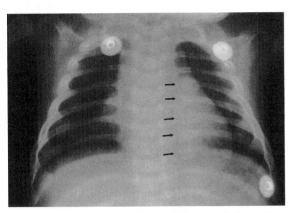

▲ **Figure 6-9.** Case 6-2. Infant with low-grade fever. You obtain a chest radiograph to evaluate for pneumonia (frontal view of the chest).

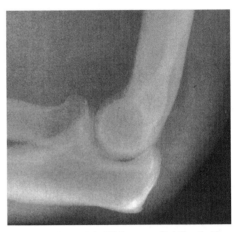

▲ **Figure 6-10.** Case 6-3. While moonlighting in the emergency department of a small community hospital, you examine a 25-year-old man who fell on an outstretched hand and now complains of elbow pain. You obtain an AP and lateral view of his elbow (lateral view of the elbow).

operating room to describe the fracture. Which of the following statements concerning the fracture would you wish to make?
A. The distal tibial fragment is displaced 1 cm anteriorly.
B. There is no comminution of the tibial fracture.
C. There is slight valgus angulation of the distal tibial fragment.
D. This is an open or compound fracture.

6-2. You interpret the chest radiograph for Case 6-2 (Figure 6-9) and render the following opinion:
A. Normal chest radiograph
B. Round pneumonia
C. Healing rib fractures
D. Pneumothorax

6-3. You first examine the lateral view of the elbow in Case 6-3 (Figure 6-10). You find
A. a lytic lesion in the distal humerus.
B. displacement of the fat pads of the elbow.
C. a fracture through the proximal ulna.
D. dislocation of the elbow.

6-4. You examine the radiographs for Case 6-4. Only the AP view is shown here (Figure 6-11). You tell the patient he has broken his ankle, but you want to get one more study:
A. Entire tibia and fibula, to exclude more proximal fractures
B. Ipsilateral foot, to exclude a fracture of the fifth metatarsal
C. Contralateral ankle, for comparison purposes
D. CT, for precise evaluation of the alignment of the fracture

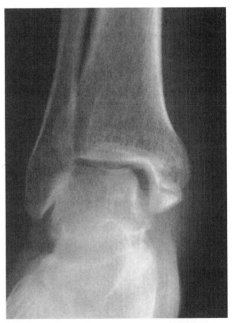

▲ **Figure 6-11.** Case 6-4. A week later you are once again moonlighting in the same small emergency department when a 29-year-old man is carried in complaining of ankle pain after a twisting injury. His ankle is swollen and ecchymotic, and he is tender to palpation along the medial malleolus. He has no other complaints. You order frontal, lateral, and oblique views of the ankle (AP view of the ankle).

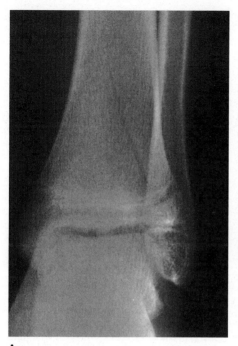 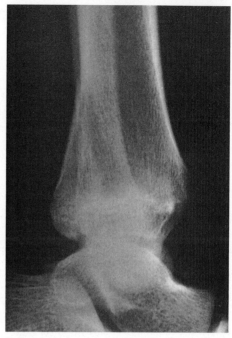

A   B

▲ **Figure 6-12.** Case 6-5. A 15-year-old boy complains of ankle pain after a fall (AP and lateral views of the ankle).

6-5. What is the abnormality in Case 6-5 (Figure 6-12)?
   A. Sprain of the lateral ligaments
   B. Fracture of the distal fibula
   C. Stress fracture of the talus
   D. Triplane fracture of the distal tibia

Radiologic Findings

6-1. Figure 6-8 shows comminuted fractures of the distal tibia and fibula with intra-articular extension of the tibial fracture (black arrow). The main distal fracture fragment is displaced posteriorly. As seen on the frontal view, the distal fragments are angulated so they are pointing medially. Gas density (white arrows) indicates that air has penetrated into the soft tissues through a skin wound, so this is an open fracture. A fracture line extends to the tibial articular surface (black arrow) (D is the correct answer to Question 6-1).

6-2. In Figure 6-9, a row of rounded opacities (arrows) in the left chest represents posterior healing rib fractures (C is the correct answer to Question 6-2).

6-3. This patient's anterior fat pad is pushed away from the bone, creating a small triangular "sail" (Figure 6-13, arrowheads). The posterior fat pad (arrow) is visible as a dark line behind the distal humerus, when it

should not normally be visible at all. There is no visible fracture or dislocation. (B is the correct answer to Question 6-3).

6-4. Figure 6-11 indicates a transverse fracture of the distal medial malleolus with widening of the medial

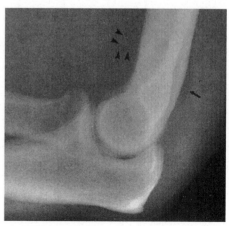

▲ **Figure 6-13.** Lateral view of the elbow with anterior (arrowheads) and posterior (arrow) fat pad signs.

aspect of the ankle joint. This type of fracture is often associated with a more proximal fibular fracture (A is the correct answer to Question 6-4).

6-5. Abnormal lucencies run vertically through the epiphysis on the frontal view (Figure 6-12) and obliquely through the metaphysis on both the frontal and the lateral views. The lateral aspect of the distal tibial physis or growth plate is widened (D is the correct answer to Question 6-5).

Discussion

Case 6-1: Your mission is to describe accurately and succinctly the features of this fracture that will affect treatment and outcome. You should discuss the alignment of the largest tibial and fibular fragments. Address both displacement and angulation. Displacement is always described in terms of the position of the distal fragment relative to that of the proximal fragment. The lateral view shows that the distal tibial fragment is displaced 1 cm posteriorly.

On the frontal view there is obvious angulation (Figure 6-8 A). Angulation may be described either in terms of the direction of shift of the distal fragment or in terms of the direction in which the apex of the angle points. In either case, it is better to give a measurement than to use subjective modifiers such as "slight" or "moderate." This angulation may correctly be described as "30 degrees of varus angulation of the distal fragment" or "30 degrees lateral apical angulation" (Figure 6-14).

Case 6-2: Rib fractures in a young child suggest child abuse. As most rib fractures in infants are caused by nonaccidental injury, you should reexamine the child for other stigmata of child abuse, such as bruises, welts, burns, or retinal hemorrhages, notify protective services, and obtain a skeletal survey. If you are unsure of your diagnosis or desire confirmation of the radiographic findings, you should obtain a radiology consult, as discharging the patient could place the child in serious danger. Figure 6-15 from the skeletal survey reveals the classic metaphyseal "corner" (large arrows) and "bucket handle"(small arrows) fractures virtually pathognomonic of infant abuse. The astute observer will also note a healing fracture of the superior pubic ramus. In summary, radiologic findings with moderate to high specificity for infant abuse include posterior rib fractures, metaphyseal fractures, multiple fractures, and fractures at different stages of healing.

Case 6-3: When examining a radiograph for a suspected fracture, it is important to evaluate not only the bones themselves but also the adjacent soft tissues. In a number of areas of the body there are normal deposits of fat, termed fat pads, which may be displaced by accumulation of blood or fluid in the underlying tissues. The fat pads of the elbow are particularly helpful. Displacement of the elbow fat pad is a nonspecific sign that indicates distension of the joint. Effusions due to rheumatoid arthritis, an infected joint, or

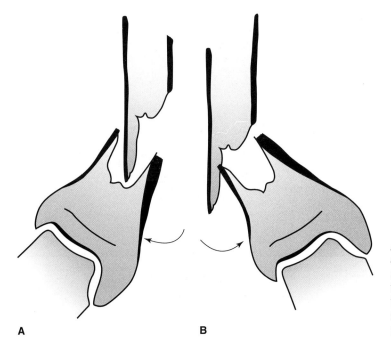

A　　　　　　　　**B**

▲ **Figure 6-14. (A,B)** Varus and valgus angulation. In **(A)** the distal tibial fragment has shifted laterally with respect to the proximal tibia. This is valgus angulation. In **(B)** the distal tibial fragment has shifted medially with respect to the proximal fragment. This is varus angulation.

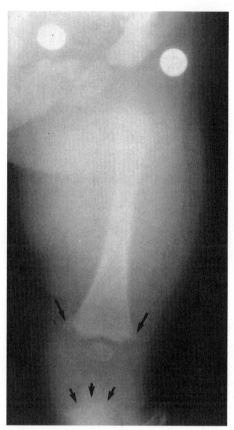

▲ **Figure 6-15.** AP view of the distal femur and proximal tibia. There are metaphyseal fractures of both the femur (arrows) and tibia (small arrows).

hemorrhage, especially in a patient with bleeding disorder, could all cause the "fat pad sign" seen in this patient. In an otherwise healthy person who has suffered trauma, however, a radial head fracture should be suspected because it is the most common elbow fracture in an adult. This patient's frontal view did actually demonstrate a small lucent fracture line in the radial head. Even without that, however, the most prudent course is to treat the patient as though he had a radial head fracture with immobilization and arrange for follow-up care with a physician accustomed to caring for fractures.

Case 6-4: Transverse medial malleolar fracture usually accompanies eversion of the ankle and is often associated with a fibular fracture. The fibular injury may occur at any level from the ankle to the knee. When there is no apparent distal fibular fracture on ankle views, the remainder of the bone should be imaged. In this case, there is, indeed, a fracture of

the proximal fibula (Figure 6-16). This fracture is also called the "Maisonneure" fracture, named for the surgeon Jules Germain Francois Maisonneure, and indicates rupture of the interosseous membrane all along its course from the ankle to the fibular fracture. This is an unstable injury that many orthopedic surgeons will treat with open reduction and internal fixation of the malleolar component and of the syndesmosis. Fractures of the proximal fifth metatarsal may accompany ankle inversion and may be difficult to distinguish clinically from other ankle injuries. Therefore, this part of the foot should always be included on at least one view of the ankle. If it is not, then it is prudent when possible to obtain one more view, but this should not ordinarily be considered a separate study or incur an additional charge. CT is not necessary in this situation.

Case 6-5: This adolescent patient has suffered a relatively common growth plate injury with a typical but somewhat complex fracture pattern. It is called a "triplane" fracture because it has components that run, more or less, in all three primary planes of section. It travels in the sagittal plane through the epiphysis, in the axial plane through the unfused portion of the physis or growth plate, and in the coronal plane through the metaphysis. It is a Salter-Harris type IV fracture (Figure 6-17). It can be diagnosed on the

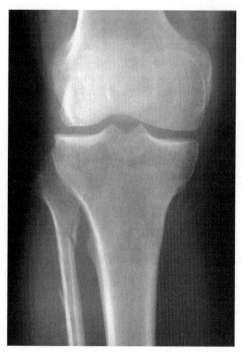

▲ **Figure 6-16.** AP view of the knee. The proximal fibula is fractured.

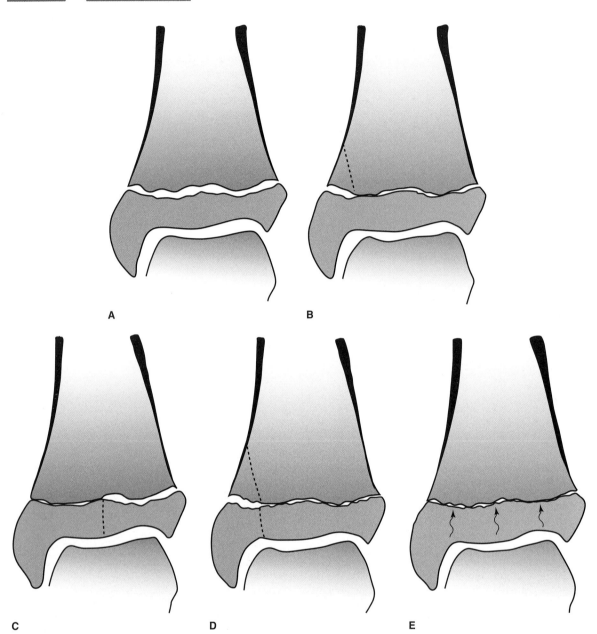

▲ **Figure 6-17.** Salter-Harris classification of physeal injuries. This is a commonly used method of describing fractures through the physis of skeletally immature individuals. Outcome worsens as the number describing the fracture increases. (**A**) Salter-Harris I fractures are through the physis or growth plate without involvement of the bone of the epiphysis or metaphysis. The slipped capital femoral epiphysis shown in Figure 6-1 is a type of Salter-Harris I fracture. (**B**) Salter-Harris II fractures involve part of the metaphysis (often only a small flake) and extend to the physis. (**C**) Salter-Harris III fractures involve the epiphysis and extend to the physis. The Salter-Harris III fracture illustrated here is similar to the epiphyseal and physeal components of the triplane fracture without extension to the metaphysis. It also is a fairly common injury pattern. (**D**) The Salter-Harris IV fracture involves both the metaphysis and epiphysis. (**E**) The Salter-Harris V injury involves only the physis and is a compressive injury secondary to axial loading forces.

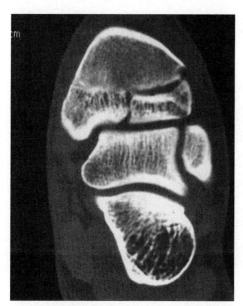

▲ **Figure 6-18.** Coronal CT scan of the ankle. This image demonstrates widening of the physis laterally and the sagittal split through the epiphysis.

conventional radiographs. Overlapping of several bones in the ankle region, together with the inferiorly concave shape of the articular surface of the distal tibia, the tibial plafond, complicates evaluation of fracture fragment position, and so a CT scan was obtained (Figure 6-18).

EXERCISE 6-2. LOCAL DISEASE

6-6. Based on the history, physical examination, and radiographs for Case 6-6 (Figure 6-19), which of the following choices is the best working diagnosis?
A. A bone tumor, most likely benign
B. A bone tumor, most likely malignant
C. An infection of the bone
D. A stress fracture of the proximal fibula

6-7. What is the most likely diagnosis for Case 6-7 (Figure 6-20)?
A. Osteomyelitis
B. A malignant bone tumor
C. A Salter-Harris IV fracture
D. Langerhans cell histiocytosis

6-8. What should you do about the calcified lump in the patient's arm in Case 6-8 (Figure 6-21)?
A. Needle biopsy
B. Open excisional biopsy

C. Reassure the patient
D. Bone scan

6-9. What is the lump in Case 6-9 (Figure 6-22)?
A. An osteosarcoma
B. An osteochondroma
C. A normal variant
D. A soft tissue sarcoma

Radiologic Findings

6-6. Focal lytic lesion in the proximal fibular metadiaphysis with an intact shell of new cortex and a well-defined, short zone of transition between itself and adjacent normal bone (A is the correct answer to Question 6-6).

6-7. There is a well-defined lytic lesion in the proximal tibia. Its edges are slightly sclerotic. It extends across the physis to involve portions of both the metaphysis and epiphysis (A is the correct answer to Question 6-7).

6-8. A well-defined ossified mass projects in the musculature of the posterolateral arm. It has a thin but distinct cortex (arrows) surrounding trabeculae (Figure 6-21) (C is the correct answer to Question 6-8).

6-9. Arising from the medial cortex of the femur is an ossified mass topped by a cauliflower-like thin shell of cortex (Figure 6-22). The cortex of the remainder of the femur is continuous with the cortex of the tumor (arrowheads), and the trabecular bone of the femoral metaphysis blends imperceptibly with that of the mass. The mass has grown away from its metaphyseal place of origin and points toward the diaphysis and away from the joint (B is the correct answer to Question 6-9).

Discussion

Case 6-6: The radiographs demonstrate a focal lytic lesion in the proximal fibular metadiaphysis. The cortex appears intact around the lesion, and the bone is widened. Cortex is not pliable; it will not stretch to accommodate a growing lesion. Instead it will slowly remodel by resorption of endosteal bone and deposition of periosteal new bone. The process takes time, so intact but extended cortex implies a slow growth rate for this lesion. Another indication of a slow growth rate is the sharp demarcation or short zone of transition between the lesion and adjacent normal bone.

In general, osteomyelitis will not cause apparent expansion of bone the way this lesion has. Stress fractures are usually linear lesions and usually are oriented transversely across the bone, though there are exceptions. Stress fractures may be lucent, if a gap in cortical bone is their primary manifestation, or sclerotic, either due to compression of trabeculae with resultant overlap or due to healing. The periosteal

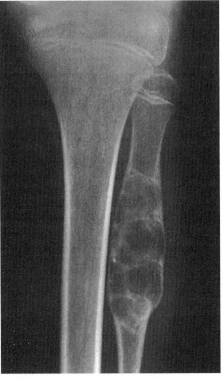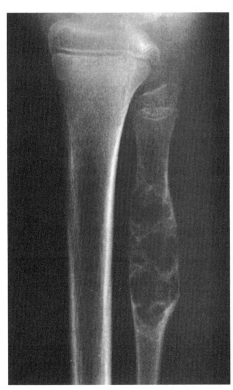

A   **B**

▲ **Figure 6-19.** Case 6-6. A 12-year-old girl comes to your pediatrics office complaining of 2 weeks of knee pain. There is no history of trauma. She is slightly swollen, tender, and erythematous over the proximal fibula. You obtain frontal and lateral views of the tibia and fibula (AP and lateral views of the proximal tibia and fibula).

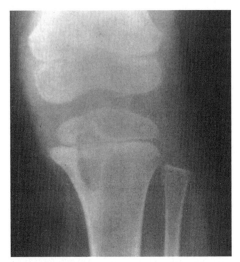

▲ **Figure 6-20.** Case 6-7. This 5-year-old girl has been limping off and on for 2 months. Her knee is warm and swollen (AP view of the knee).

reaction that they engender may cause them to be mistaken for bone tumors, but they will not look like this particular lesion (Figure 6-23).

Of the choices given in the question, the remaining ones are benign and malignant bone tumor. For the most part, malignant bone tumors in children have a rapid growth rate. This will cause them to have poorly defined borders. In addition, where they destroy cortex, the periosteum will be unable to contain them with solidly mineralized new bone, as has occurred here. There may be gaps in the cortex where tumor has broken through (Figure 6-24). The periosteal new bone may mineralize at 90-degree angles to the diaphysis or may be lamellated (like onion skin) or incomplete. The intact shell of periosteal new bone seen in this patient and the short zone of transition are more typical of a benign than a malignant tumor.

A primary bone tumor, no matter how benign its appearance, is most appropriately handled by an orthopedic oncologic surgeon experienced with tumors. As you have been stipulated to be a pediatrician, the patient should be sent to an orthopedic surgeon who specializes in the treatment of tumors.

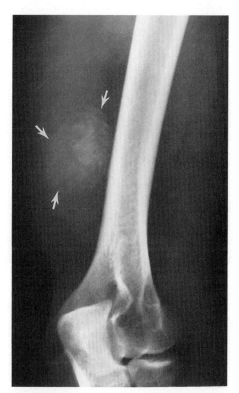

▲ **Figure 6-21.** Case 6-8. A 35-year-old man complains of a lump in the soft tissues of the right arm. He first noticed the lump 6 months ago after hurting his arm in a fall from a bicycle (AP view of the arm).

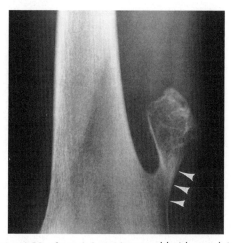

▲ **Figure 6-22.** Case 6-9. A 10-year-old girl complains of a lump on the inside of her thigh near the knee. It has been there as long as she can remember but has been annoying her since she recently took up horseback riding (AP view of the distal femur).

Performing a percutaneous needle biopsy has the potential to cause great harm if a poorly chosen route is taken. For example, if the needle passed close to the common peroneal nerve and then the lesion proved unexpectedly to be malignant, the nerve might have to be sacrificed in order to obtain a curative resection.

Obtaining additional imaging studies to evaluate this lesion further is not a bad idea. It is better, however, to allow the orthopedic surgeon to whom the patient will be referred (in consultation with the radiologist) to decide

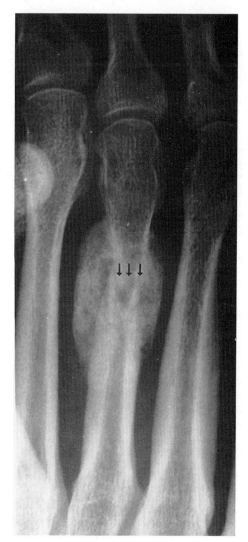

▲ **Figure 6-23.** Stress fracture. Oblique view of the third metatarsal. This typical healing stress fracture demonstrates both a transverse fracture oriented perpendicular to the shaft (arrows), and abundant callus formation.

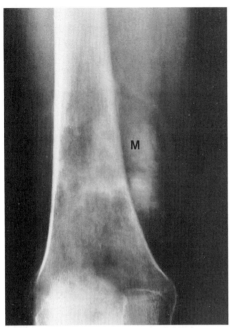

▲ **Figure 6-24.** AP view of the distal femur. Many of the radiographic features of this osteosarcoma mark it as a malignant tumor. The abnormal area of mottled lucent and sclerotic tumor in the metaphysis fades gradually into the shadows of surrounding normal bone. It is difficult to see where the tumor begins and ends; there is a large soft-tissue mass adjacent to the bone (M). The periosteum has been unable to maintain a shell of mineralized new bone around this mass. The sclerotic areas within the bone and the mineralized portions of the soft-tissue mass both have a relatively amorphous, smudged appearance that is seen with calcified osteoid matrix.

which imaging tests are most appropriate to evaluate the lesion more thoroughly rather than ordering additional tests before referral.

Case 6-7: The edges of malignant tumors are usually not as well defined as those of this lesion. Malignant tumors may extent across the growth plate, but it is uncommon for them to do so while they are still as small as this lesion.

Osteomyelitis, on the other hand, often breaches the growth plate. The most common organisms to cause osteomyelitis are species of *Staphylococcus* and *Streptococcus* (Figure 6-25). The relatively long history of limping, however, should suggest a more indolent organism. This case was due to *Mycobacterium tuberculosis*. Skeletal tuberculosis is uncommon and thus often is overlooked as a diagnostic possibility. Today, it is most commonly seen in the immunocompromised individual. Because it is curable yet

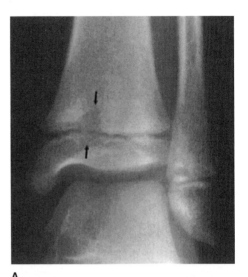

A

B

▲ **Figure 6-25.** **(A,B)** AP view **(A)** and sagittal tomogram **(B)** of the ankle. This focus of osteomyelitis (arrows), occurring in a 5-year-old boy, also crosses the growth plate. It is radiographically indistinguishable from the case of tuberculous osteomyelitis, yet it was due to *Staphylococcus*. The distinction between pyogenic and tuberculous osteomyelitis must be made on clinical grounds and sometimes must be proven by biopsy.

responds to very different drugs than would be used for pyogenic osteomyelitis, it is important to keep it in mind. It may occur at any site, but it is most common in the spine. In the extremities, it most often occurs in or near the hip and knee.

Langerhans cell histiocytosis (eosinophilic granuloma) is much less common than osteomyelitis and is thus not as likely a diagnosis. When it does occur, its favorite location is the skull.

Case 6-8: This ossified mass represents myositis ossificans, also known as heterotopic new bone formation. Though often associated with trauma, it may also be seen in patients without a distinct history of trauma. When it resembles mature bone as closely as in this patient, it is not a diagnostic dilemma, and you can reassure the patient that there is a benign cause for his lump.

Occasionally, myositis ossificans warrants excision on the basis of mechanical interference with the use of a muscle or joint. Recurrence is less likely if excision is performed after the lesion has matured. A bone scan may help to distinguish between mature and immature lesions. An immature lesion that is still undergoing ossification will exhibit marked radionuclide uptake. Once ossification is complete, radionuclide accumulation will resemble that of other bones.

Myositis ossificans may be diagnosed more confidently with radiography than with histology. An immature lesion will be full of immature, rapidly proliferating cells that may be mistaken for sarcoma by the pathologist. Radiologically, however, there is a distinct difference between the two. Myositis ossificans ossifies from the outside in. Sarcomas ossify from the inside out. See Figure 6-24 and notice that the central portion of the soft-tissue mass is denser (more ossified) than the outer portion. If it is not entirely clear from conventional radiographs where and how the ossification is occurring, a CT scan is the test of choice because of its ability to demonstrate calcium.

Case 6-9: This mass has the characteristic appearance of an osteochondroma, the most common of all benign, cartilaginous neoplasms. Osteochondromas may be very large or very small, pedunculated or sessile (Figure 6-26). They grow as the child grows and should cease growth by adulthood. Often asymptomatic, they may be an incidental finding. They may, however, cause a wide range of symptoms. The most common complaint is that they interfere with activities or with wearing certain clothes, such as tight blue jeans. They may be painful as a result of irritation of an overlying bursa (Figure 6-27). And they are subject to fracture. An uncommon (1% or less) but feared complication is malignant transformation, usually resulting in chondrosarcoma. Signs of such transformation include enlargement of the osteochondroma in an adult, thickening of the cartilaginous cap that covers the tumor, development of a soft-tissue mass, and destruction of bone.

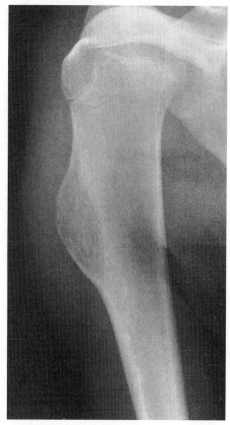

▲ **Figure 6-26.** AP view of the proximal humerus. There is a sessile osteochondroma on the lateral aspect of this child's humerus.

When further radiologic studies are needed, MR imaging or ultrasound are probably the most useful modalities. Both can demonstrate the cartilage cap and any associated soft tissue mass. When the diagnosis is not as obvious as in this case by conventional radiography, MRI can assist in confirming the identity of the tumor by demonstrating continuity between the cortices and medullary spaces of the tumor and the host bone.

EXERCISE 6-3. SYSTEMIC DISEASE

6-10.   For Case 6-10 (Figure 6-28), which of the following studies would be *least* useful today?
   A.   Chest CT
   B.   Left hip x-ray
   C.   Bone scan
   D.   Skeletal survey
   E.   Mammography

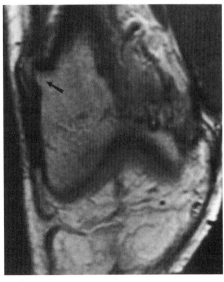
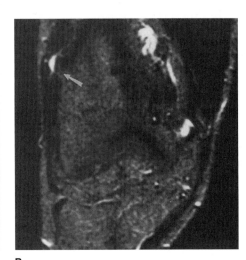

A   **B**

▲ **Figure 6-27. (A,B)** Proton-density **(A)** and T2-weighted **(B)** coronal MR images of the knee. A very tiny osteochondroma arises from the lateral metaphysis of the distal femur (arrow). Notice that the signal intensity (shade of gray) inside this diminutive tumor is the same as that of the adjoining marrow space. The bright area over the osteochondroma in Figure 6-27 B represents a small, fluid-filled bursa. This patient complained of a snapping sensation which most likely was due to movement of the iliotibial band back and forth over the osteochondroma.

6-11. For Case 6-11 (Figure 6-29), what is the next study you should order?
   A. Bone scan
   B. MRI of the knee
   C. Hand films
   D. Chest radiograph

6-12. For Case 6-12 (Figure 6-30), there is no evidence of pneumonia, but there are several abnormalities that are clues to the nature of this patient's chronic illness. Which finding is such a clue?
   A. The presence of a central venous line
   B. Enlargement of the pulmonary artery segment of the mediastinum
   C. Depression in the endplates of numerous vertebrae
   D. Asymmetry of the breast shadows

6-13. For Case 6-13 (Figure 6-31), which of the following imaging tests is most likely to help determine if this patient has progressive myeloma?
   A. PET-CT
   B. Bone Scan
   C. Chest x-ray
   D. CT of the spine

Radiologic Findings

6-10. D is the correct answer to Question 6-10.

6-11. A thin rim of calcium added to the bony contour of both sides of the right femoral metaphysis (Figure 6-29, arrows) is due to periosteal elevation. Similar findings were present on the left femur and both tibiae (D is the correct answer to Question 6-11).

6-12. Many vertebral bodies, as best appreciated in the lateral view, are shaped like the letter H (arrowheads), with central depressions in the superior and inferior end plates. (Figure 6-30) (C is the correct answer to Question 6-12).

6-13. A is the correct answer to Question 6-13.

Discussion

Case 6-10: Option E, mammography, is a reasonable screening examination. This would be a good test to order for this patient even without new symptoms. Indeed, mammography should be obtained in any woman of 45 years every year for screening purposes, irrespective of her history. Bone scans are also often ordered as screens for metastatic disease

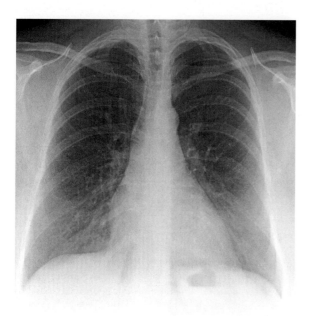

▲ **Figure 6-28.** Case 6-10. As a medical student on the oncology team, you see in clinic a 45-year-old woman with a history of breast cancer diagnosed 3 years previously. She underwent surgery and since that time has been free of disease. She has come for her routine follow-up appointment and complains only of vague, aching discomfort in her left hip. A chest x-ray shows no evidence of metastatic disease.

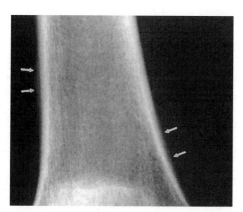

▲ **Figure 6-29.** Case 6-11. A 40-year-old man complains of knee pain and swelling of 3 weeks' duration. He has no other known disease. You order conventional radiographs of the knee. You notice some periosteal elevation on both femurs and tibiae (AP view of the right distal femur).

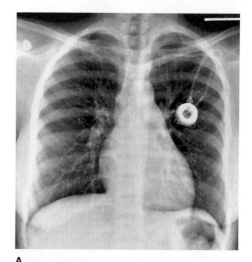

A

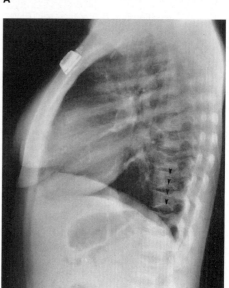

B

▲ **Figure 6-30.** Case 6-12. This chest radiograph was obtained to exclude pneumonia in a chronically ill 26-year-old woman (PA and lateral views of the chest).

in asymptomatic breast cancer patients, particularly for the first 2 to 3 years after diagnosis. Because this patient is complaining of skeletal pain, both a bone scan (Figure 6-32 A) and conventional radiographs of the affected area (Figure 6-32 B) are indicated. A chest CT can be helpful to find small pulmonary metastases that may not be apparent on a conventional chest radiograph. Whether to order it for this

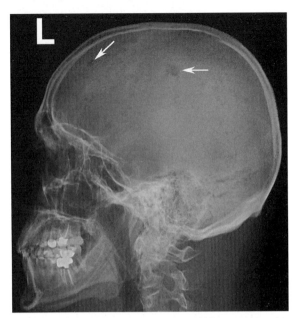

▲ **Figure 6-31.** Case 6-13. A 50-year-old man with multiple myeloma was treated successfully with chemotherapy and has been in remission for 2 years. Recent immunoelectrophoreses showed slight elevation of his paraproteins, which causes his oncologist to worry about progression of his myeloma. A bone survey showed well-defined lytic lesions in the skull, typical of myeloma, which had been stable since treatment began (arrows on two of the lesions).

woman may depend in part on the preferences of the attending oncologist and on risk factors such as the size of the original tumor and nodal status at the time of diagnosis. Option D, a skeletal survey, is inappropriate. Bone surveys are generally utilized in breast cancer only for follow-up of patients with widespread osseous metastatic disease.

In this patient's case, a bone scan revealed multiple areas of abnormally increased accumulation of radionuclide, including the left acetabulum (Figure 6-32 A,B). The multiplicity of lesions, together with the history of breast cancer (which often metastasizes to bone and may do so after a disease-free interval of many years), is very suggestive of metastatic disease. Some oncologists would choose to treat the patient for presumed metastatic disease on the basis of the bone scan, history, and current symptoms. Others would prefer a biopsy before proceeding to further treatment. This patient underwent a CT-guided needle aspiration of the acetabular lesion, which revealed metastatic tumor (Figure 6-32 C). To evaluate for possible impending pathologic fracture (Figure 6-33), most oncologists would also request conventional radiographs of areas demonstrating increased activity on the bone scan, particularly those in weight-bearing bones.

Case 6-11: Periosteal elevation is a nonspecific finding that occurs with local disorders such as fracture, bone tumors, and osteomyelitis and also with systemic or multifocal disorders such as bone infarction (Figure 6-34), venous stasis, and secondary hypertrophic osteoarthropathy. Because this finding is bilateral, it is more likely due to a systemic or multifocal disorder than to a local one.

Of all systemic disorders that may be associated with periosteal new bone formation, secondary hypertrophic osteoarthropathy is the most important to exclude. At one time it was called hypertrophic pulmonary osteoarthropathy because it is usually caused by pulmonary disease. The designation secondary hypertrophic osteoarthropathy reflects current understanding that this disorder may also be due to nonpulmonary diseases such as inflammatory bowel disease or congenital cardiac anomalies. Nonetheless, pulmonary disease, specifically lung cancer, remains the most common cause. This patient, in fact, had lung cancer (Figure 6-35).

A bone scan could be useful if you did not notice the periosteal new bone or were not sure of its presence. Hand films could demonstrate clubbing, which may be seen with some of the same disorders that cause hypertrophic osteoarthropathy, but simple physical inspection of the patient's hands would accomplish the same thing. MRI of the knees will not be helpful in this case.

Case 6-12: This patient (see Figure 6-30) has sickle cell disease. The peculiar shape of multiple vertebral bodies is very characteristic of sickle cell anemia, though it may occasionally be seen in other diseases affecting the marrow cavity, particularly Gaucher's disease. It may be caused by infarction of bone beneath the endplates, with remodeling of the cortex to produce the H-shape.

When red cells sickle, they clump together and may block blood vessels. In bone this leads to avascular necrosis, which may be widespread, involving many bones simultaneously. The mottled appearance of this patient's humeral heads is due to avascular necrosis and is a common finding in patients with sickle cell anemia.

Though they were not included among the possible answers to the question, there are other findings on this examination that are clues to the diagnosis. The gas-filled splenic flexure of the colon occupies too much of the left upper quadrant on the frontal view. There is no room for a spleen of normal size. In sickle cell patients, the spleen is often infarcted so that by any time they reach adulthood, it has shrunk to a small fraction of normal size. People with sickle cell disease are prone to early development of calcium bilirubinate gallstones (cholelithiasis).

Modest enlargement of the pulmonary artery, as seen in this patient, is so common in young women that it is considered normal in that population. The central line may be seen in many patients with a variety of disorders requiring chronic intravenous therapy.

Case 6-13: Multiple myeloma is a disease that can never really be considered cured. The goals of therapy are control of

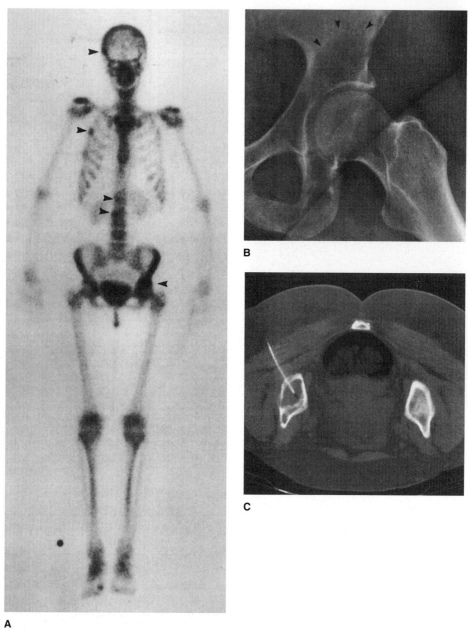

▲ **Figure 6-32. (A)** Anterior view from a ^{99m}Tc-MDP whole-body bone scan. In several areas more radionuclide has accumulated than in the remainder of the skeleton, and these areas appear darker: left acetabulum, two upper lumbar vertebrae, the lateral aspect of the right third rib, and the right side of the skull (arrowheads). Numerous foci of increased radioactivity, sprinkled somewhat haphazardly about the body but mostly involving the axial skeleton, are very typical of the appearance of metastatic cancer. **(B)** Frog-leg lateral view of the left hip. The ilium just above the acetabulum is too lucent, and a thin, irregular white line (arrowheads) demarcates the edge of the lucency. **(C)** Axial CT scan, obtained with the patient prone. The trabecular bone of the left ilium has been replaced by material of approximately the same density as the muscle. Using a percutaneous approach through the left buttock, a needle has been placed into the center of the lesion. Aspiration of cells yielded a diagnosis of metastatic breast carcinoma. The needle appears to be wholly embedded within the patient because it has traveled an oblique course. The rest of it would be apparent on adjacent sections.

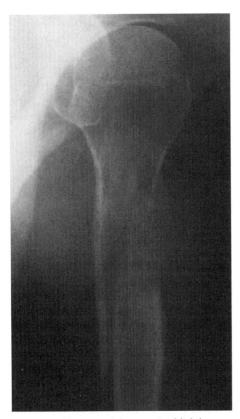

▲ **Figure 6-33.** AP view of the proximal left humerus. An acute fracture has occurred through an area of bone destruction caused by metastatic carcinoma. Conventional radiographs are used to identify bony metastases that have destroyed enough bone to make a pathologic fracture likely.

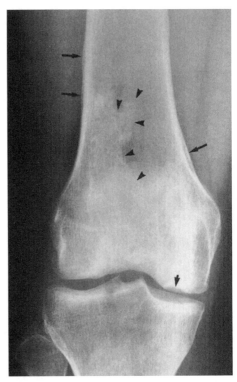

▲ **Figure 6-34.** AP view of the knee. This is an example of periosteal new bone formation (arrows) associated with bone infarction. The infarction is marked by an irregular sclerotic area in the metaphysis (arrowheads), as well as a small, rounded lucent defect in the articular surface of the medial femoral condyle (short arrow).

symptoms and, if possible, induction of remission. Remission may last months or even years, and during remission the patient is monitored for any signs that the disease has returned and is progressing. In this patient's case, the oncologists are looking for any imaging-based evidence of disease progression to back up a fairly weak clinical indicator.

A challenge is that the patient is already known to have lytic bone disease. Even though the myeloma has been in remission, the lytic lesions will not have gone away. Therefore, imaging studies that rely primarily on anatomy will only be helpful if they unequivocally show evidence of new lytic lesions. The bone survey has already been asserted to be unchanged, so no other conventional radiographs are likely to be helpful, either. Therefore, a chest x-ray will not be a good choice. CT scans are also anatomically based tests and can be expected to show lytic lesions without necessarily helping to

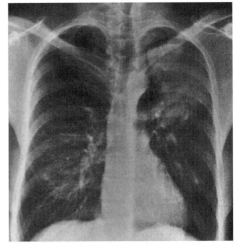

▲ **Figure 6-35.** PA view of the chest. A large mass in the left upper lobe represents primary lung carcinoma.

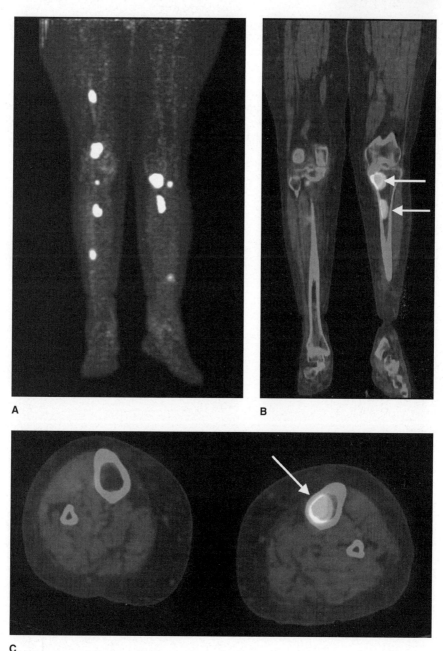

▲ **Figure 6-36.** A maximum intensity projection (MIP) image from a PET-CT. This is the same patient whose CT is presented in Figure 6-6. The bright white spots scattered in the bones of the lower extremities bilaterally represent areas of actively growing myeloma. (**B**) Coronal section of fused PET-CT at approximately the same level as the Figure 6-6. The two lesions in the left tibia (arrows) represent the lesions that are causing cortical destruction in Figure 6-6. A color image of this same section is located on the cover of the book. (**C**) Axial section of fused PET-CT at the level of the more distal of the two left tibial lesions confirms the location of the lesion inside the medullary cavity of the proximal left tibia (arrow).

determine if the lesions are old and quiescent or if they are actively growing.

What is needed is a test that will assess the metabolic activity of this patient's multiple myeloma, preferably with some associated anatomic information. MRI may be helpful in such situations. It is a good anatomic test, and if contrast is given, it also demonstrates areas of hyperemia. MRI, however, was not one of the answer choices. Bone scans are metabolic tests, but myeloma is a notorious source of false negative bone scans.

PET-CT may be quite useful for differentiating quiescent from metabolically active, growing lesions of myeloma (Figure 6-36).

Acknowledgment *Special thanks to Murray K. Dalinka, MD, for providing Figure 6-20 for use in this chapter.*

SUGGESTED READING

1. Schmidt H, Kohler A, Zimmer EA. *Borderlands of Normal and Early Pathologic Findings in Skeletal Radiography*. 4th ed. New York: Thieme Medical Publishers; 1993.
2. Keats TE, Anderson M. *Atlas of Normal Roentgen Variants That May Simulate Disease*. 7th ed. St. Louis: Mosby; 2001.
3. Berquist TH. *MRI of the Musculoskeletal System*. 5th ed. Philadelphia: Lippincott Williams & Williams; 2006.
4. Chew FS, Roberts CC. *Musculoskeletal Imaging: A Teaching File*. 2nd ed. Philadelphia: Lippincott Williams & Williams; 2006.

Imaging of Joints

Paul L. Wasserman, DO
Thomas L. Pope, MD

TECHNIQUES AND NORMAL ANATOMY

▶ Radiography

Conventional radiography is the most commonly used imaging technique to evaluate the joints of the musculoskeletal system. This technique should always be the first imaging study performed in a patient suspected of having joint problems. Radiography has the following important advantages: It is almost universally available, is relatively inexpensive compared to other imaging studies and delivers only a small radiation dose to the patient. When possible, orthogonal projections should be obtained, meaning two images of the joint that are perpendicular to each other (usually a frontal projection in either in the anteroposterior [AP] or posteroanterior [PA] directions and a lateral). In some instances oblique images may also be obtained, depending on the preferences of the referring physician or radiologist or the clinical situation. In certain instances it may also be important to obtain images of the joint proximal and distal to the injury. Examples of this include the forearm and lower leg (paired bones), as the joints proximal and distal are often injured. Because conventional radiography uses ionizing radiation, it should be used judiciously, especially in pediatric patients and pregnant women.

Historically, radiographic images were printed on film. However, with widespread adoption of PACS (picture archiving and communications system), images can be electronically processed and viewed on computer work screens. These images then can be transmitted anywhere electronically via the Internet.

▶ Conventional Tomography

Conventional tomography is mentioned mainly for historical interest. High radiation dose, relatively poor image resolution, and imaging that is only possible in one plane were its major disadvantages. The technique has been almost totally replaced by other imaging tests, especially computed tomographic (CT) and magnetic resonance (MR) imaging. Orthopantograms are one of the few remaining vestiges of this imaging technique.

▶ Arthrography

Arthrography is a technique in which contrast is injected into the joint using fluoroscopic guidance. The joint is then imaged using radiography, CT, or MR imaging or a combination of these techniques. The injected contrast may be an iodine-containing water-soluble compound (eg, Conray), subsequently imaged with radiography or CT (Figure 7-1). Alternatively, a paramagnetic compound (eg, gadolinium pentazocine) may be injected and imaged with MRI. MR arthrographic images of the joint may also be performed after intravenous injection of the paramagnetic contrast agent, although this technique does not distend the joint, and thereby is not used commonly today. MR arthrography is mainly used to evaluate the labrum of the hip or glenohumeral

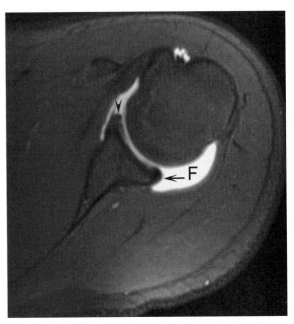

▲ **Figure 7-2.** Axial T1 weighted, fat-saturated MR arthrogram of the shoulder shows marked joint distention with contrast (F) and the normal glenoid labrum anteriorly (arrowhead) and posteriorly (arrow). MR arthrography is used mainly to evaluate the shoulder for tears of the labrum and symptoms of instability.

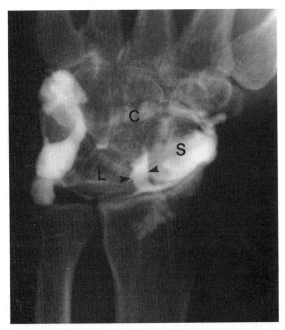

▲ **Figure 7-1.** Contrast arthrogram with plain radiograph: AP wrist arthrogram view obtained after injection of contrast material into the radiocarpal joint shows contrast material passing through the scaphoid (S) and lunate (L) space from the radiocarpal joint into the mid-carpal joint (arrowheads). This indicates a tear in the scapholunate ligament (C, capitate bone).

joint (Figure 7-2) but is also useful in the evaluation of the structures of the wrist and elbow joints. CT arthrography, and less commonly conventional arthrography can be useful in patients who cannot undergo, or have contraindications to, MR imaging (Figure 7-3).

▶ Computed Tomography

Computed tomography (CT), a technique that makes individual axial (transverse) slices of the patient, uses the same ionizing radiation as in conventional radiography. CT technique has been vastly improved in the past decade. The development of spiral or helical CT has major advantages over earlier CT technology. With the spiral CT technique, axial (transverse) images are acquired much more rapidly with dramatic decreases in radiation dose. For instance, a CT of the chest, abdomen, and pelvis can be performed in about 16 seconds. CT data is stored in three-dimensional packets that can then be reconstructed and displayed in almost any other plane. The most common images reconstructed from the axial plane are the sagittal and coronal planes (Figure 7-4).

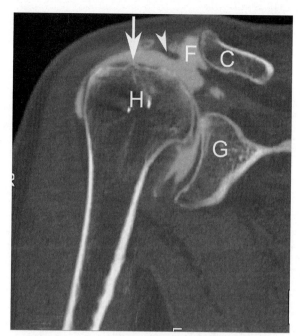

▲ **Figure 7-3.** CT arthrography. Coronal reformatted CT image of the shoulder after fluoroscopically guided, intraarticular contrast administration. CT arthrography is often used when the patient has contraindications to MR imaging. The image reveals a full-thickness rotator cuff tear with contrast in the subacromial-subdeltoid bursa (arrow) and contrast interposed between the acromioclavicular joint, the CT "geyser sign" (arrowhead). H, humeral head; G, glenoid; C, distal clavicle; F, contrast.

▶ Magnetic Resonance Imaging

MR imaging has revolutionized the imaging evaluation of almost all body areas, but particularly those of the central nervous system and musculoskeletal system. It has tremendous advantages over other imaging modalities in the evaluation of joints because of its excellent soft-tissue contrast, high resolution, and ability to image in every plane. This technique may show pathophysiologic events even before they are seen on conventional radiographs or CT, for example, revealing the early changes of avascular necrosis (Figure 7-5). Because of its exquisite soft-tissue contrast, MR imaging allows radiologists to visualize subtle differences in soft tissues that had never before been seen with other imaging modalities. For example, the subtle contrast between fat and muscle seen on a conventional radiographs or CT is dramatically highlighted with the use of MR imaging because of their very different chemical compositions (Figure 7-6). MR imaging can also depict subtle changes within the bone marrow cavity, an area difficult to evaluate with conventional radiography or CT. Therefore, MR imaging is a tremendous aid to preoperative evaluation of any patient who has unexplained joint pain or who has had joint trauma. One of the major disadvantages of MR imaging is that some patients with claustrophobia cannot tolerate the prolonged imaging time in the small bore of the magnet. In addition, patients with metallic foreign bodies or non-MR-compatible medical devices or hardware have contraindications to MR imaging. Concerns include motion of the objects, abnormal electrical arcs resulting in burns, and device malfunction.

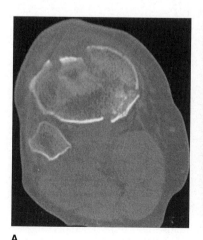
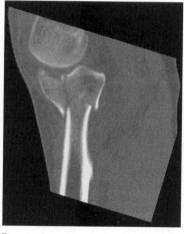
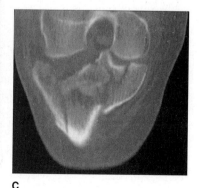

A   B   C

▲ **Figure 7-4.** (**A**) Axial CT scan showing a comminuted fracture of the proximal tibia. (**B**) Sagittal reconstruction of the axial data, again showing the comminuted tibial fracture. (**C**) Coronal reconstructed CT image showing the markedly comminuted fracture of the proximal tibia with extension into the joint. Current CT applications can be used to reconstruct data in multiple planes.

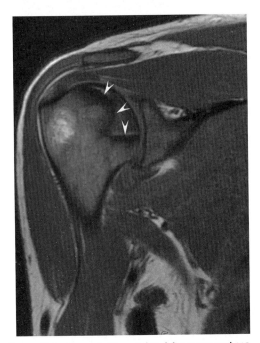

▲ **Figure 7-5.** Coronal, T2 weighted fat-saturated MR image of avascular necrosis of the humeral head. MR image of the shoulder reveals an area of bone infarct adjacent to the articular surface of the humeral head (arrowheads). MR imaging can show this abnormality much earlier than conventional radiography.

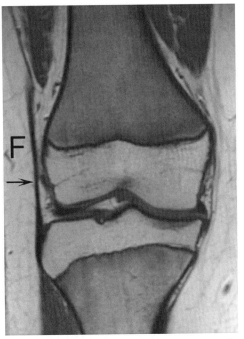

▲ **Figure 7-6.** Coronal T1 image of the knee reveals the significant difference of signal between the subcutaneous fat (F) and the iliotibial band (arrow). MR can accentuate the small differences in soft-tissue water content to produce remarkable images.

▶ Ultrasonography

Ultrasonography, first developed for use in World War II for detection of submarines, was adopted after the war for use in medical imaging. High-frequency transmission of sound can be used to evaluate the soft tissues, tendons, ligaments, and even the cartilage of the joint. The ultrasound waves cannot be transmitted through cortical bone, so the intramedullary cavity cannot be imaged with this technique. Ultrasound is used more extensively in Europe than in the United States; however, there is increasing interest in this modality within the United States. The main drawback of this modality is that it is highly user-dependent, relying heavily on the skill of the operator (Figure 7-7).

▶ Radionuclide Imaging (Nuclear Medicine Bone Scans)

Radionuclide imaging uses radioactive materials that are injected intravenously and then localize in regions of abnormally increased blood flow (hyperemia), increased osteoblastic activity, or heightened metabolic activity. The major uses of bone scanning are in patients suspected of

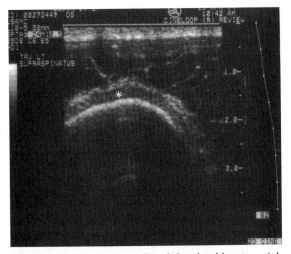

▲ **Figure 7-7.** Ultrasonography of the shoulder. An axial (transverse) ultrasonographic image of the shoulder shows an intact supraspinatus tendon (*), seen as a zone of hypoechogenicity (low-signal echoes) on the scan. This technique is very operator-dependent.

having metastatic disease or infection. This modality is very sensitive, but it has limited specificity, and often the findings must be correlated with other imaging modalities, especially radiography. Therefore, this technique is not usually used as a primary modality for the evaluation of joint disease.

Anatomy of the Normal Joint

The typical normal synovial joint consists of at least two articulating bones enclosed in a synovium-lined joint capsule. The apposing bony surfaces are covered by smooth articular cartilage (hyaline cartilage). On radiographs, the normal joint has a separation between the adjacent bones representing the region occupied by the hyaline or articular cartilage, menisci, and joint fluid (the so-called articular space) depending on which joint is imaged. Because of the limited soft-tissue contrast of the technique, these structures are not normally depicted on radiographs unless they are calcified (Figure 7-8). However, MR imaging exquisitely shows the components of the normal joint (Figure 7-9).

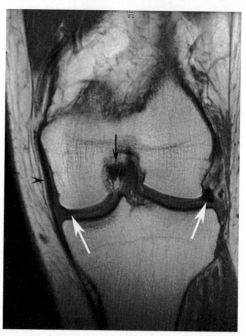

▲ **Figure 7-9.** Coronal T1 weighted MR image showing the normal components of the knee joint. Note the menisci (white arrows), the posterior cruciate ligament (black arrow), and the medial (tibial) collateral ligament (arrowhead).

Joint Disease

The clinical signs and symptoms of joint disease are manifestations of abnormal function such as reduced mobility, hypermobility, and pain. Altered function may be due to pain, discomfort, apprehension, or instability. The wide range of joint abnormalities is summarized below, and many of these processes are discussed in the exercises. Any of these signs may occur in isolation or in combination with any others.

Radiographically, joint disease may be diagnosed by any of the following:

1. Incongruity of the articulating bone as is seen with dislocations, for example, traumatic dislocation or dislocations caused by arthropathies such as lupus arthritis or rheumatoid arthritis.

2. Irregularity of articulating bone surfaces and margins, as in erosions (eg, in psoriasis or gout).

3. Increased density or sclerosis of articulating bone surface (also called "eburnation"), as in osteoarthritis.

4. Bony outgrowths (proliferation) at bone ends, known as osteophytes.

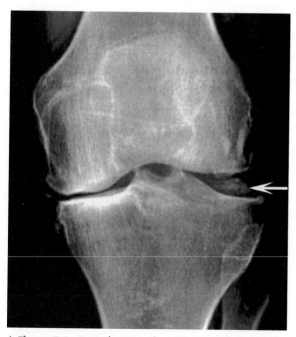

▲ **Figure 7-8.** Frontal views of an 82-year-old woman showing chondrocalcinosis represented by calcification within the menisci (chondrocalcinosis) (arrow). The menisci are not normally demonstrated on radiography unless they are calcified.

5. Diffuse decrease of bone density adjacent to articular surfaces, described as juxtaarticular or periarticular osteopenia (eg, rheumatoid arthritis, tuberculous arthritis).

6. Focal, well-defined, spherical lucencies within subchondral bone, known as subchondral cysts or geodes (eg, osteoarthritis, rheumatoid arthritis).

7. Loss of articular joint space from articular cartilage destruction (eg, septic arthritis, osteoarthritis).

8. Accumulation of excess joint fluid within the joint (joint effusion). Excess joint fluid is a common manifestation of joint disorders. The fluid may be synovial fluid, blood, or even pus, depending on the etiology of the joint disease.

9. Calcification of articular (hyaline) cartilage or fibrocartilage (chondrocalcinosis), or intraarticular soft-tissue calcification such as that seen in scleroderma or polymyositis or dermatomyositis.

10. Synovial proliferation or abnormal increase in the synovial lining, such as that seen with pigmented villonodular synovitis (PVNS).

TECHNIQUE SELECTION

Radiography should always be the initial imaging test to evaluate the joints and should be obtained after the patient has had a thorough history and physical examination and there is a clear indication to obtain the study. Various projections may be used depending on the clinical indication or the situation, but at least two orthogonal projections should be obtained. Often radiographs alone will confirm or refute the clinical diagnosis. In many instances, however, it may be necessary to use more sophisticated imaging techniques to clarify the radiographic findings or to further evaluate depending on the clinical scenario. The following paragraphs discuss the selection of the imaging techniques in a few common clinical scenarios.

▶ Congenital Diseases

Conventional radiographs should be the initial modality of choice when confronted with a possible congenital anomaly or pediatric joint abnormality, or in a child presenting with a limp.

Given that the joint structures are not well mineralized in children, further evaluation of the joint with ultrasonography or MR imaging is often required to make a definitive diagnosis, as these modalities have superior soft-tissue resolution. If MR imaging facilities are not available, congenital abnormalities can be investigated with a combination of conventional radiography, ultrasonography, and CT.

▶ Acute Trauma

In acute trauma, the conventional radiograph remains the mainstay of the initial imaging assessment. If fractures are identified, additional imaging will depend on the needs of the clinician or sub-specialist physician as dictated by the clinical situation. Generally, fractures that extend into the joint surface (intraarticular fractures) are treated with greater concern because of the importance of reestablishing the integrity of the joint. Intraarticular fractures are frequently treated by operative reduction and internal fixation, especially if the fracture fragments are severely displaced. CT examination of the injured limb and joints is used preoperatively for surgical planning and postoperatively to assess the results of surgical intervention. The advantages of CT are that it enables precise assessment of joint reconstitution and also identifies any intraarticular bone fragments or entrapped tendons that could interfere with proper reduction and healing (see Figure 7-4).

▶ Subacute and Remote Trauma

Conventional radiographs are used initially to determine the integrity of the joint. If the joint is normal and there is a persistent clinical suspicion of injury, MR imaging should be employed because of its superior soft-tissue contrast and resolution. It is, therefore, particularly suited for investigation of the intraarticular and periarticular soft-tissue structures and cartilage (see Figures 7-5, 7-6).

▶ Nontraumatic Cases

Likewise, if the initial conventional radiographs are normal, MR imaging is the next modality of choice in the patient with a painful joint. MR imaging may detect evidence of a small joint effusion, inflamed synovium, and subtle erosions that could suggest the diagnosis of an inflammatory arthropathy or a septic joint. Percutaneous joint aspiration of synovial fluid, often fluoroscopically guided, may result in confirmation of infection or yield abnormal crystal deposits within the joint, such as with gout.

EXERCISE 7-1. CONGENITAL JOINT DISORDERS

7-1. The most likely diagnosis in Case 7-1 (Figure 7-10) is
   A. bilateral developmental dysplasia of the hips (DDH).
   B. Legg-Calvé-Perthes disease.
   C. proximal focal femoral deficiency syndrome (PFFDS).
   D. neuropathic joint disease.

7-2. In Case 7-2 (Figure 7-11), the next best imaging test would be
   A. tomography of both hips.
   B. MR imaging of the hips.
   C. radionuclide bone scan of the pelvis.
   D. CT of the hips.

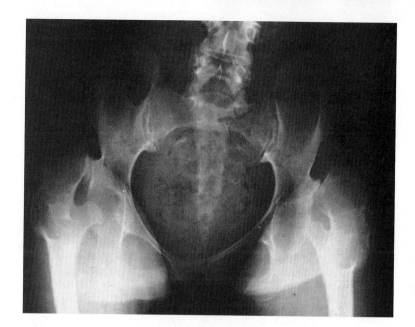

▲ **Figure 7-10.** Case 7-1. A pelvis radiograph in a 25-year-old woman with progressively unbearable hip pain. She always walked abnormally and had some discomfort for as long as she could remember.

7-3. The patient in Case 7-3, whose film is shown in Figure 7-12, most likely suffers from what condition?
A. Acute trauma
B. An inflammatory disorder
C. Acute infection
D. Neuropathic joints

Radiologic Findings

7-1. Both hips in the patient in this case (Figure 7-10) are abnormal. The femoral heads and necks are malformed and dislocated from the acetabula fossae superiorly. The acetabulae are also malformed and

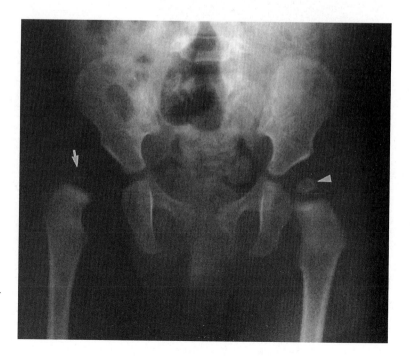

▲ **Figure 7-11.** Case 7-2. A radiograph of the pelvis in a child who was examined by a pediatrician because of developmental delay. He is still crawling at the age of 2 years and has not attempted to walk.

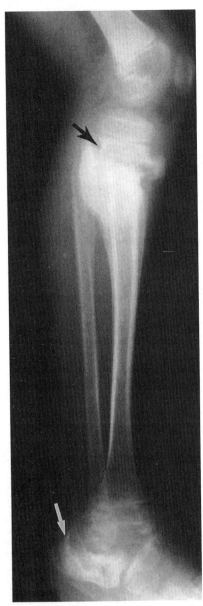

▲ **Figure 7-12.** Case 7-3. A film of the tibia and fibula in this young boy who was examined by a pediatrician because "he walks funny," according to his mother. He denies any pain.

oriented more vertically than normal. The patient had bilateral congenital dislocation of the hips that had been ignored by her parents (A is the correct answer to Question 7-1). This diagnosis should have been made at birth or shortly thereafter so that corrective therapy could have been instituted.

7-2. In this case (Figure 7-11), the capital femoral epiphysis on the right (arrow) is laterally displaced and smaller than the left epiphysis (arrowhead). The acetabular fossa on the right side is also malformed and more vertical than the one on the left. The normal development of the acetabulum is dependent on a normally located femoral head, and this is the explanation for this abnormality. These findings are the classical radiographic features of developmental dysplasia of the hip (DDH). When this finding is encountered, MR imaging is the next most appropriate imaging test (B is the correct answer to Question 7-2).

7-3. In this case (Figure 7-12), the calcaneus is deformed (white arrow). The talus is poorly visualized because of its complete dislocation from its normal position below the tibia, and there are subluxations at the tibiotalar, talocalcaneal, and talonavicular joints. There is overall frank disorganization of this ankle joint, and clinically there was diffuse soft-tissue swelling around the ankle (not appreciated on this lateral film). There is also a metaphyseal fracture of the proximal tibia with exuberant periosteal/callus formation (black arrow). All of these findings in this patient are caused by chronic repetitive trauma in a patient with congenital insensitivity to pain (D is the correct answer to Question 7-3).

Discussion

Congenital joint disorders are uncommonly encountered, but they should be diagnosed as early as possible after birth because delayed diagnosis complicates management. Some of the more common congenital joint disorders include:

1. Congenital dislocation of the hips

2. Arthrogryposis multiplex congenita

3. Congenital insensitivity to pain (asymbolia)

Congenital hip dislocation is actually a bone dysplasia manifesting as a joint disorder. The femoral head is dysplastic and does not provide adequate stimulation for proper development of the acetabulum. Usually, the femoral head is displaced laterally out of an unusually shallow (ie, more vertically oriented) acetabulum (Figure 7-11). Once the diagnosis of DDH is confirmed, treatment should begin at birth or in the perinatal period to minimize complications.

Historically, hip arthrograms were used to define the location of the femoral head in the neonate because the structure is cartilaginous at birth and therefore radiolucent. Ultrasonography is an excellent test to assist in the diagnosis of DDH in utero and in the neonatal period because it requires no ionizing radiation. However, the interpretation of ultrasound is observer dependent, and the diagnosis and characterization of DDH can be difficult at times. MR imaging can show the soft-tissue and osseous structures, as well as the articular cartilage, and is currently the modality of choice in the evaluation of DDH. If patients are not treated or are incompletely treated, they will eventually develop secondary, premature osteoarthritis. MR imaging offers limited diagnostic value over conventional radiographs in late-stage disease.

Proximal focal femoral deficiency (PFFD) is a disease of uncertain etiology that is characterized by congenital absence of a segment or all of the proximal third of the femur. The incidence is higher in children of diabetic mothers, and there is also an association with congenital hip dysplasia. MR imaging is also the imaging modality of choice in evaluating children with these disorders.

Arthrogryposis multiplex congenita is a noninheritable congenital disease of uncertain etiology characterized by multiple joint contractures. It is believed to be due to neuromuscular events occurring in utero. The joints of the lower limb are almost invariably affected. There may be other associated extraskeletal congenital anomalies.

A neuropathic joint is caused by chronic repetitive trauma in the setting of impaired or absent sensation. The characteristic features of neuropathic joint include soft-tissue swelling, fragmentation of the bony structures, and general disorganization of the joint. Joint effusion is often present. The more common causes of neuropathic joints in the lower extremities include diabetes mellitus and tabes dorsalis (neurosyphilis). Asymbolia or congenital insensitivity to pain, as exhibited in Case 7-3 (Figure 7-12), is a group of uncommon congenital disorders in which there is a variable degree of loss of pain sensation and is an unusual cause of neuropathic joints. Patients with asymbolia almost always acquire deformities of the extremities after repeated trauma. This diagnosis should be considered in the young patient with multiple healing fractures with soft-tissue swelling and joint disorganization in whom nonaccidental trauma has been excluded.

EXERCISE 7-2. JOINT TRAUMA

7-4. In Case 7-4 (Figure 7-13), the most likely diagnosis is
   A. lunate dislocation.
   B. perilunate dislocation.
   C. transcaphoid fracture-dislocation.
   D. distal radius fracture.

7-5. The basketball player in Case 7-5 (Figure 7-14) shows which of the following injuries?
   A. Fracture
   B. Dislocation
   C. Osteoarthritis
   D. None of the above

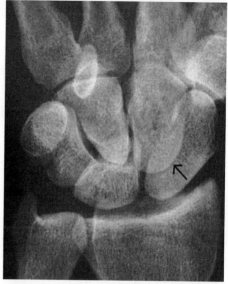

A

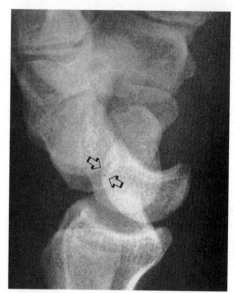

B

▲ **Figure 7-13.** Case 7-4. AP (**A**) and lateral (**B**) radiographs of the wrist in a 25-year-old man who fell on his outstretched hand.

7-6. The basketball player in Case 7-6 (Figure 7-15) has which type of abnormality on the MR image?
   A. Tendon injury
   B. Muscle injury
   C. Ligament injury
   D. Cartilage injury

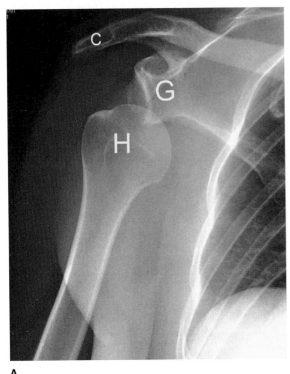
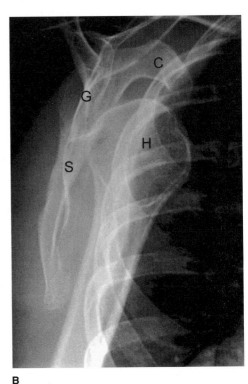

A   **B**

▲ **Figure 7-14.** Case 7-5. AP (**A**) and scapular-Y views of radiograph (**B**) of the shoulder in a 30-year-old basketball player who fell in practice. H, humeral head; G, glenoid; C, coracoid; S, scapula.

7-7. The MR image in Case 7-7 (Figure 7-16) shows which abnormality?
 A. Muscle injury
 B. Ligament injury
 C. Tendon injury
 D. Cartilage injury

Radiologic Findings

7-4. In the frontal projection (Figure 7-13 A), there is disorganization of the carpal arcs. The capitate is no longer articulating with the lunate and partly overlaps the scaphoid (arrow). The scaphoid is elongated on this view but not fractured. On the lateral projection (Figure 7-13 B) the lunate is still in line with the distal radius, but the capitate has been dislocated dorsally (open arrows). Therefore, the patient has a dorsal perilunate dislocation (B is the correct answer to Question 7-4).

7-5. The AP radiograph of the shoulder of a basketball player (Figure 7-14 A) shows inferior displacement of the humeral head out of its normal position within the glenoid. The scapular-Y view of the shoulder (Figure 7-14 B) shows that the humeral head (H) is dislocated anteriorly in relation to the glenoid (G), thus representing an anterior shoulder dislocation. S, scapula; C, coracoid. This is the classic appearance of an anterior dislocation of the shoulder. (B is the correct answer to Question 7-5.)

7-6. The sagittal MR image shows the advantage of MR imaging in this clinical setting. Figure 7-15 shows a tear of the anterior cruciate ligament (ACL) (arrow) (C is the correct answer to Question 7-6).

7-7. Figure 7-16 shows the ends of a torn supraspinatus tendon (arrows) in the squash player (C is the correct answer to Question 7-7).

Discussion

Dislocation or subluxation: The terms subluxation and dislocation are often used interchangeably. However, *subluxation* refers to partial loss of congruity between the articulating ends of bones, whereas *dislocation* denotes complete loss of congruity. Disruption or loss of the integrity of

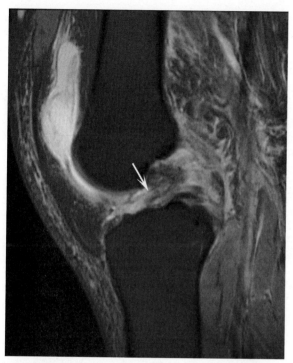

▲ **Figure 7-15.** Case 7-6. A sagittal T2-weighted, fat-saturated MR image of the knee in a 34-year-old athlete who was injured in a basketball game.

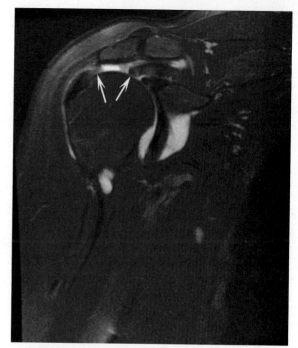

▲ **Figure 7-16.** Case 7-7. A T2-weighted, fat-saturated MR image of the shoulder in a 40-year-old squash player who was having shoulder pain and was referred for an MR scan.

the restraining ligaments around the joint leads to instability and thus permits dislocation to occur. Severe hyperflexion or hyperextension forces often cause traumatic dislocations. Fractures are frequently associated with traumatic dislocations.

Carpal Dislocation

The normal arrangement of the carpal bones of the wrist is seen on the AP view of the wrist (Figure 7-17 A). Note the three smooth, parallel arcs in the proximal and mid-carpal rows (arcs of Gilula). The lateral view of the wrist (Figure 7-17 B) shows that the radius, lunate, and capitate are in an almost straight line. There are two major types of wrist carpal dislocation: perilunate and lunate dislocations. In a perilunate dislocation, the lateral film shows that the lunate maintains its normal articulation with the radius and the capitate is displaced dorsally. In a lunate dislocation, the lunate has a triangular shape on the frontal projection (Figure 7-18 A) and is displaced from its normal articulation and the radius and capitate maintain a linear relationship (Figure 7-18 B). Carpal dislocations are usually produced by a fall on the outstretched hand (foot) and are more common in young adults. The diagnosis is usually

made by radiographic examination, although CT may be used after reduction to evaluate the wrist for joint congruity and for the presence of intraarticular fracture fragments ("loose bodies").

Shoulder Dislocation

The two main directions in which the proximal and humerus dislocates are anterior and posterior. Anterior dislocation, usually caused by falls, is most common and is seen in about 95% of cases. In an anterior dislocation, the humeral head is displaced anteriorly and inferiorly to the scapular glenoid fossa. There are various subtypes of anterior dislocation: subglenoid, subcoracoid, and medial. These subtypes are based on the location of the humeral head relative to the glenoid fossa and coracoid process.

Posterior dislocation is relatively uncommon. It is most commonly associated with severe contraction of the muscles of the shoulder girdle, which may occur in electric shock or convulsions. A diagnosis of posterior dislocation in one shoulder should prompt investigation of the other shoulder, because this injury is often bilateral.

If the postreduction radiographs are normal after a single instance of dislocation, there is usually no need for another

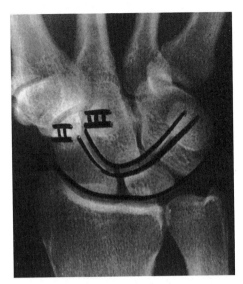

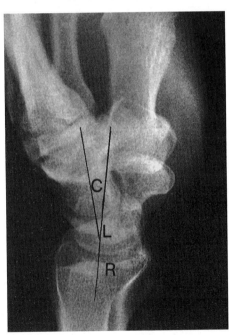

B

▲ **Figure 7-17. (A)** AP view of the normal wrist showing the three parallel arcs of the radiocarpal joint (I) and the midcarpal joint (II and III) (From Poeling G et al: Arthroscopy of the wrist and elbow. New York, Raven Press, 1994; used with permission.) **(B)** Lateral view of the normal wrist showing the almost linear arrangement (straight lines) of the distal radius (R), lunate (L), and capitate (C).

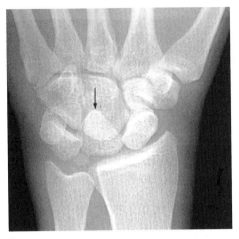

A

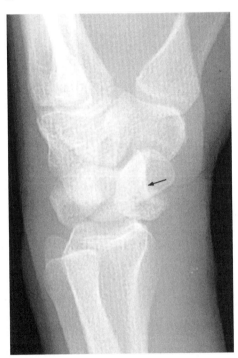

B

▲ **Figure 7-18. (A)** Frontal radiograph of a person who fell on an outstretched hand shows the triangular shape of the lunate (arrow) seen with lunate dislocation. **(B)** Lateral radiograph shows the displacement of the lunate volarly (arrow) with maintenance of the normal linear relationship between the distal radius and capitate.

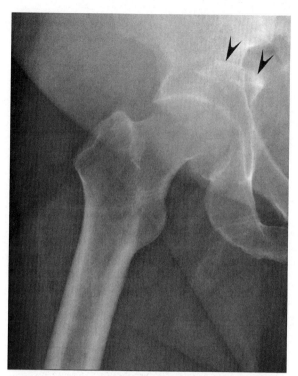

▲ **Figure 7-19.** Radiograph of the right hip in a person who had been involved in an automobile accident. The femoral head displaced superiorly and posterior relative to the acetabulum, representing a posterior hip dislocation. The arrowheads show a fragment of bone (posterior acetabulum wall) that was fractured during the posterior dislocation.

imaging study in the acute setting. However, if there is a recurrence of dislocation or if the patient remains chronically symptomatic, MR imaging or CT arthrography of the shoulder should be obtained to search for the cause of the dislocations and any associated shoulder abnormalities resulting from the dislocation.

CT arthrography and MR imaging are used to investigate the shoulder for cartilage and soft-tissue injuries resulting from shoulder dislocation. After an anterior dislocation, there is frequently associated injury of the anterior glenoid labrum. This is produced by impaction of the posterior and lateral aspect of the humeral head against the anterior and inferior portion of the glenoid. There may also be an accompanying compression fracture of the humeral head, referred to as a Hill-Sachs deformity.

Hip Dislocation

The hip is a relatively stable joint because of the surrounding strong muscles and joint capsule, and significant trauma is required for dislocations to occur. One of the most common mechanisms of injury causing hip dislocation is the "dashboard injury." This is caused by deceleration when the knee is impacted on the dashboard, driving the femoral head posteriorly in relation to the acetabulum. As the femoral head is driven posteriorly, it comes to be superior and lateral to the acetabulum. There is almost always an associated fracture of the posterior aspect of the acetabular rim or the femoral head with posterior dislocation (Figure 7-19). Anterior hip dislocation is uncommon and is produced by a blow to the hip when the femur is internally rotated and abducted. Central dislocation of the hip usually occurs with direct lateral forces, and there is an associated fracture of the quadrilateral plate (medial aspect) of the acetabulum.

Knee Ligament Tears

Tears of the ligaments of the knee are commonly seen in athletic individuals. The function of the anterior cruciate ligament (ACL) is to limit the anterior translation of the tibia in relation to the femur. Any sport that requires pivoting and planting of the feet places an enormous stress on the ACL and may cause injury to it. The normal ACL originates on the inner aspect of the lateral femoral condyle and extends anteriorly and slightly obliquely to insert adjacent to the anterior tibial spine. It has a fascicular arrangement with individual bands that can easily be seen by MR (Figure 7-20). The most

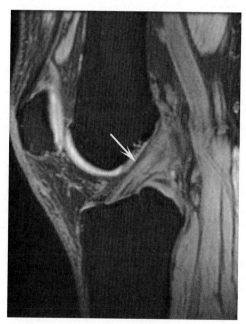

▲ **Figure 7-20.** Sagittal T2-weighted fat-saturated MR image of the knee showing a normal ACL (arrow). Notice the fascicular arrangement.

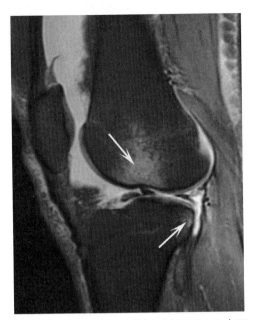

▲ **Figure 7-21.** Sagittal T2-weighted fat-saturated MR image of the knee in a patient with an ACL tear shows the classic contusion pattern of the lateral femoral condyle and the lateral tibial plateau (arrows). These contusions are caused by the transient dislocation of the knee that occurs during this injury. Typically, this pattern is associated with an ACL tear.

common mechanism of injury to the ACL is the "clipping" injury with valgus stress and internal rotation of the knee. On MR, the injured ACL is diagnosed by high signal intensity within the substance of the ligament (the so-called pseudomass). There may also be other associated abnormalities such as bone contusions (usually on the posterolateral aspect of the tibia and the anterolateral aspect of the femur that result from the transient dislocation that occurs at the time of injury, the so-called kissing contusions) and medial collateral ligament injury from the valgus stress (Figure 7-21). There may also be associated meniscal tears, usually vertical tears in the acute setting (Figure 7-22).

The posterior cruciate ligament (PCL) serves to limit the posterior translation of the tibia in relation to the femur. The PCL is commonly injured in kicking sports such as soccer and is also injured in automobile accidents if the tibia impacts on the dashboard and is translated posteriorly in relation to the femur in a flexed knee.

The normal PCL on MR is a homogeneous structure that originates from the inner aspect of the medial femoral condyle and extends far posteriorly to insert onto the posterior aspect of the tibia (Figure 7-23). The PCL should easily be seen on all knee MR studies. Tears of the PCL are diagnosed using MR imaging. Partial tears are identified by increased T2

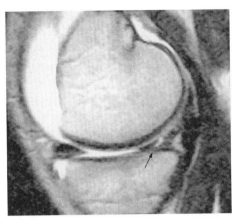

▲ **Figure 7-22.** Sagittal MR image in a patient with an ACL tear showing a vertical tear of the posterior horn of the medial meniscus (arrow). These vertical tears are often seen in the acute setting.

signal and swelling within the ligament. Complete tears of the ligament are diagnosed by discontinuity of the ligament fibers at some point along its course (Figure 7-24). MR imaging is extremely important in the evaluation of the knee of the injured athlete and is used frequently in this setting.

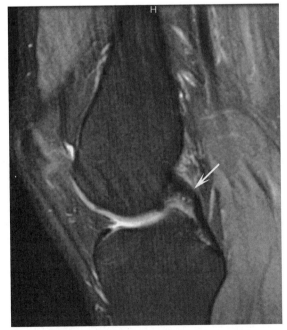

▲ **Figure 7-23.** Sagittal T2-weighted fat-saturated MR image of the knee showing the normal homogeneously low-signal-intensity PCL (arrow).

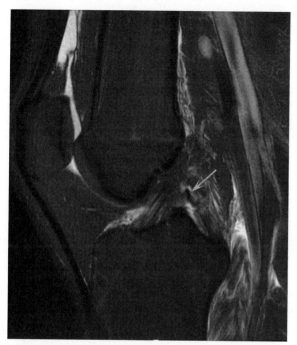

▲ **Figure 7-24.** Tear of posterior cruciate ligament (PCL). Sagittal T2-weighted fat-saturated MR imaging of the knee shows a typical example of a tear of the posterior cruciate ligament (arrow).

Supraspinatus Tendon Tears

The supraspinatus, infraspinatus, teres minor, and subscapularis muscles (SITS muscles) comprise the rotator cuff. Despite being the most unstable joint in the body, the rotator cuff muscles help to stabilize the joint. The most commonly torn tendon in the shoulder is the supraspinatus, and it usually tears approximately 1 centimeter proximal to its insertion onto the anterior aspect of the greater tuberosity of the humeral head. The supraspinatus tendon is easily seen on MR imaging as a low-signal-intensity structure, and tears of the supraspinatus tendon are well demonstrated on MR. The most common causes of supraspinatus tendon tears are aging and impingement. Acute rotator cuff tears are unusual. MR imaging is vital in the preoperative evaluation of the patient suspected of having a rotator cuff tear. The morphology of the tendons, the size of the tear, and other associated abnormalities of the joint, including pathology of the glenoid labrum, can be diagnosed with this technique. Importantly, the degree of muscle atrophy associated with chronic tears can be assessed, thereby suggesting the probability of a successful postoperative recovery and rehabilitation.

Achilles Tendon Rupture

The injury of Achilles tendon rupture occurs most frequently in patients in the fourth and fifth decades of life. Although the injury may occur in any person, individuals who do not exercise regularly ("weekend warriors") are more susceptible to this tear.

The clinical history and physical findings are often enough to make a diagnosis of Achilles tendon rupture. Radiographic stress views should not be performed in the setting of a suspected Achilles tendon rupture because the stress may actually make the tear worse. Any question of whether the tear is partial or complete should be resolved, as the treatment for each of these is different. Moreover, the clinician needs to know the level of injury and how far the tendon fragments are separated. MR imaging is currently the imaging technique of choice to evaluate the Achilles tendon, although ultrasound is an excellent alternative and is used more commonly in Europe for this injury. The whole length of the tendon, including its insertion on the calcaneus, and any associated injuries can be shown in detail. In cases of acute complete rupture of the tendon, the MR images show discontinuity of the normally low-signal-intensity fibers of the Achilles tendon, which are replaced by edema and hemorrhage. MRI helps to quantitate the amount of distraction between the ends of the torn tendon. The Achilles tendon may also avulse a small portion of bone from its calcaneous attachment (Figure 7-25). In partial tears, areas of intermediate to high signal, representing regions of partial disruption, are seen within the normally

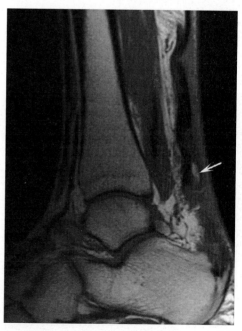

▲ **Figure 7-25.** Sagittal T1-weighted MR image of the hindfoot reveals an avulsion of the Achilles tendon with retraction (arrow points to retracted bony fragment from the calcaneous attachment of the Achilles tendon).

low-signal-intensity tendon, and some of the fibers of the tendon remain intact. Ultrasound may also be used to evaluate the Achilles tendon, and color Doppler examination may be used to follow the process of revascularization and healing of a partially torn tendon.

EXERCISE 7-3. JOINT INSTABILITY

7-8. The most likely diagnosis for Case 7-8 (Figure 7-26) is
    A. dislocation of the shoulder.
    B. myositis ossificans.
    C. tear of the anterior glenoid labrum.
    D. rotator cuff tear.

7-9. Regarding Case 7-9 (Figure 7-27), the arrowheads indicate a
    A. fracture of the patella.
    B. lipohemarthrosis.
    C. tear of the anterior cruciate ligament.
    D. foreign body.
    E. ligament injury.

7-10. The axial MR image for Case 7-10 (Figure 7-28), of a little girl who was injured by tripping on an electrical cord, shows a
    A. meniscal tear.
    B. tendon injury.
    C. medial retinacular injury.
    D. ligament strain.

7-11. The medial pain in the football player in Case 7-11 was most likely caused by (arrow in Figure 7-29)
    A. a medial collateral ligament tear.
    B. a lateral collateral ligament tear.

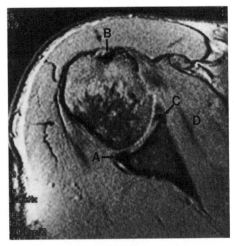

▲ **Figure 7-26.** Case 7-8. A selected axial MR image from his study in a 45-year-old former baseball pitcher who had recurrent dislocations of the shoulder, pain, and inability to reach around to his back pocket. He also feels a click and catching sensation when he moves his arm. Radiographs of his shoulder are normal.

    C. an anterior cruciate ligament tear.
    D. a meniscal tear.

Radiologic Findings

7-8. Figure 7-26 is an axial image. There is a high-signal-intensity line through the triangular anterior glenoid

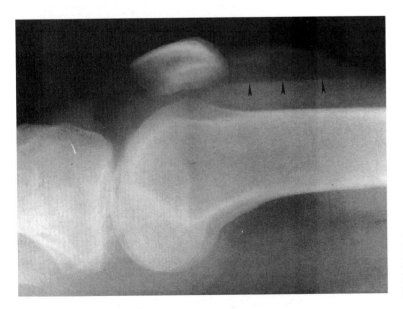

▲ **Figure 7-27.** Case 7-9. A radiograph of the knee in a 20-year-old football player who was examined in the emergency department after being tackled particularly hard.

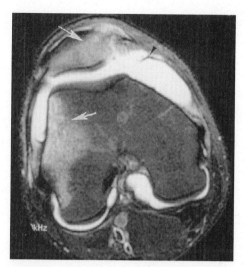

▲ **Figure 7-28.** Case 7-10. A selected axial image from a T2-weighted fat-saturated MR study in a little girl who was running through her house and tripped on an electrical cord. Intense knee pain ensued, and she was referred for an MR examination.

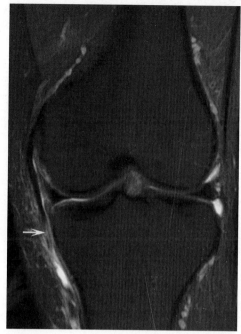

▲ **Figure 7-29.** Case 7-11. A coronal, T2-weighted fat-saturated MR image in a college football player who was injured and was thought to have transiently subluxed his knee when he was hit on the lateral side of the leg. His orthopedic sports medicine physician noted medial laxity and referred him for an MR scan.

labrum representing an anterior glenoid labral tear (C). (C is the correct answer to Question 7-8.) In Figure 7-26, A is the posterior labrum, B is the biceps tendon, and D is the belly of the subscapularis muscle.

7-9.   Figure 7-27 is a lateral radiograph of the knee obtained with a horizontal x-ray beam. There is a joint effusion with a fat-fluid level (arrowheads). This fat-fluid level is called a lipohemarthrosis. It is important to perform horizontal cross-table lateral films in the acute trauma setting in order to demonstrate this. Frequently, there is a fracture to account for the presence of fat within the joint, as the fat has entered the joint space from the bone marrow cavity (B is the correct answer to Question 7-9).

7-10.   Figure 7-28, the axial image on the little girl injured by tripping over the electric cord, shows a large joint effusion and high-signal-intensity areas on the medial aspect of the patella and the lateral aspect of the lateral femoral condyle (arrows). These are corresponding contusions. In this instance, the contusions result from impingement of the medial aspect of the patella onto the lateral femoral condyle as the patella dislocates laterally. For this to happen, there has to be a stretch or tear of the medial retinaculum (arrowhead) (B is the correct answer to Question 7-10). This constellation of findings is diagnostic of patellar dislocation-relocation.

7-11.   Figure 7-29, a coronal image of the football player injured during a game, shows a complete tear of the medial collateral ligament (arrow) (A is the correct answer to Question 7-11). Injuries to the medial side of the knee occur from lateral trauma (valgus stress). The clinician in this instance noticed the medial joint laxity and suspected an MCL tear.

Discussion

Instability Disorders

These are functional joint disorders generally manifested by pain or a sensation of the joint giving way and abnormal motion around the joint. There may be no radiographic evidence of joint abnormality as often only soft-tissue injuries, such as ligamentous or fibrocartilaginous tears, are present. These abnormalities can often only be demonstrated by conventional stress views or MR examinations of the joint in question.

Shoulder Instability

The glenohumeral joint is the most inherently unstable ball-in-socket joint in the body. The major stability of the shoulder joint is provided by the joint capsule, the rotator cuff muscles, and the ligaments and tendons that surround it. The glenoid labrum, a fibrocartilaginous structure, contributes to shoulder joint stability by deepening the socket (glenoid labral complex) for this ball (humeral head).

A variety of soft-tissue injuries are associated with anterior instability syndrome. The most common injuries resulting from anterior glenohumeral dislocation are anteroinferior glenoid labral tears (the Bankart lesion), capsular stripping, Hill-Sachs deformity (compression fracture of the posterolateral aspect of the humeral head), and glenoid labral tears associated with osseous fractures (Figures 7-30, 7-31). Tears of the posterior aspect of the glenoid labrum are seen following posterior dislocation (Figure 7-32). As we discussed in the last section, ruptures or tears of the rotator cuff tendons (supraspinatus, subscapularis, infraspinatus, and teres minor [SITS] muscles) are common causes of shoulder joint dysfunction and instability. The supraspinatus is the most commonly torn tendon in the shoulder. When the subscapularis tendon tears, there is often an associated dislocation of the biceps tendon. This results from a tear of the transverse ligament, a fascial extension across the intertubercular sulcus that holds the biceps in place (Figure 7-33).

The shoulder joint is best evaluated with MR imaging if there is a suspicion of a tendon abnormality. Shoulder arthrography and CT arthrography may also be requested by the orthopedic surgeon as an alternative to MR in those patients who have undergone rotator cuff repairs or who have had surgery to vital structures utilizing ferromagnetic metallic clips, precluding MR imaging. Patients who have aneurysm clips or who have embedded foreign metallic bodies are some examples. This is particularly important for metallic foreign bodies located within or in close proximity to the eyes.

Knee Joint Instability

Stability of the knee, which is a hinge joint, is provided by the muscles and the ligamentous complexes. The most important of these are the anterior and posterior cruciate ligaments and the lateral and medial collateral ligament complexes. The major knee structures that cross the joint anteriorly are part of the extensor mechanism, made up of the quadriceps insertion and the patella ligament. Laterally, the biceps femoris tendon, tensor fascia lata, and popliteus muscles cross the joint. Medially, the pes anserinus tendons, which comprise the sartorius, gracilis, and semitendinosus muscles-(the way to remember this is the phrase, "say grace before tea"). The gastrocnemius and plantaris muscles are posterior to the joint. Rupture of any of the tendons, ligaments, or muscles compromises stability of the knee joint. All of these structures can be exquisitely demonstrated with MR imaging, which is the best imaging test to evaluate instability in this joint.

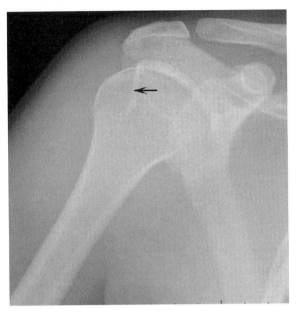

A

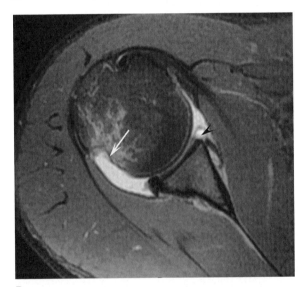

B

▲ **Figure 7-30.** (**A**) Frontal postreduction radiograph of a patient who had an anterior dislocation shows the compression fracture of the posterolateral aspect of the humeral head (arrow). This abnormality is called the Hill-Sachs lesion. (**B**) Axial T2-weighed fat-saturated MR image of the same patient also shows the Hill-Sachs deformity within the posterior/superior humeral head (arrow) and a tear of the anterior glenoid labrum (arrowhead).

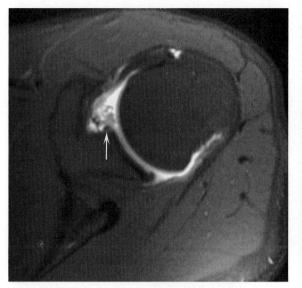

A

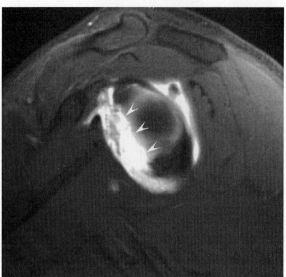

B

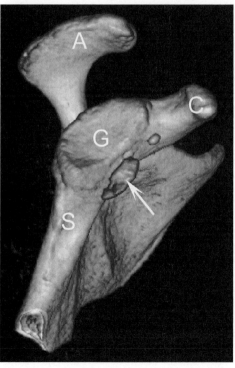

C

▲ **Figure 7-31.** (**A**) Axial, T1 fat-saturated MR image with intraarticular contrast of a patient who had an anterior dislocation showing a fracture of the anterior and inferior aspect of the glenoid (arrow). This is also called the "bony" Bankart lesion. (**B**) Sagittal oblique T1 fat-saturated MR image with intraarticular contrast reveals a large bony defect (arrowheads) within the anterior glenoid representing a bony Bankart lesion secondary to a previous anterior dislocation. (**C**) 3D reformatted CT of a similar case with an anterior bony Bankart lesion. Note the large bony fragment originating from the anterior glenoid (arrow). A, acromion; C, coracoid; G, glenoid; S, scapula.

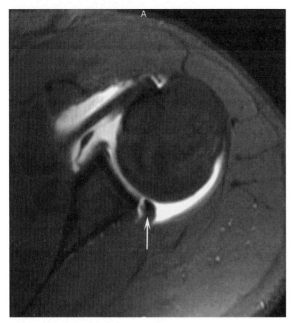

▲ **Figure 7-32.** Axial T1-weighted fat-saturated MR image of the shoulder in a patient with a previous posterior dislocation revealing detachment of the posterior labrum (arrow).

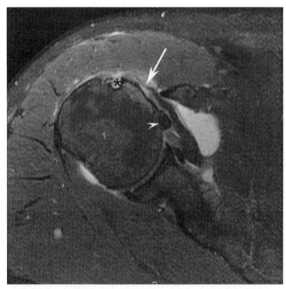

▲ **Figure 7-33.** Axial T2-weighted fat-saturated MR image of a subscapularis tear (arrow) with dislocation of the long head of the biceps tendon (arrowhead) from the intertubercular groove (*).

EXERCISE 7-4. ARTHRITIDES

7-12. The frontal pelvis view for Case 7-12 (Figure 7-34) shows all of the following features except
   A. loss of articular space.
   B. geode formation.
   C. juxtaarticular osteopenia.
   D. bony sclerosis.

7-13. The hands of the 45-year-old woman in Case 7-13 (Figure 7-35) show soft-tissue calcifications that are most consistent with a diagnosis of
   A. osteoarthritis.
   B. scleroderma.
   C. systemic lupus erythematosus (SLE).
   D. psoriasis.

7-14. The radiograph of the right hip in Case 7-14 (Figure 7-36) is most compatible with
   A. osteoarthritis.
   B. gout.
   C. septic arthritis.
   D. scleroderma.

7-15. The imaging findings for Case 7-15, at the first metatarsal phalangeal joint (Figure 7-37), are most likely due to
   A. scleroderma.
   B. ankylosing spondylitis.
   C. gout.
   D. osteoarthritis.

7-16. The linear ossification connecting the cervical vertebral bodies in Case 7-16 (Figure 7-38) are called
   A. osteophytes.
   B. erosions.
   C. soft-tissue swelling.
   D. syndesmophytes.

7-17. The "pencil-in-cup" deformity of the interphalangeal joint of the thumb in Case 7-17 (Figure 7-39) is most compatible with a diagnosis of
   A. psoriasis.
   B. gout.
   C. ankylosing spondylitis.
   D. SLE.

Radiologic Findings

7-12. The frontal radiograph of both hips in this case (Figure 7-34) shows articular space narrowing, sclerosis, and subchondral cyst formation (also called geodes) bilaterally. There is no significant juxtaarticular osteopenia (C is the correct answer to Question 7-12). The findings are most compatible with bilateral osteoarthritis (OA) of the hips.

7-13. In this case (Figure 7-35), the most prominent feature of this lady's hand is soft-tissue calcification and

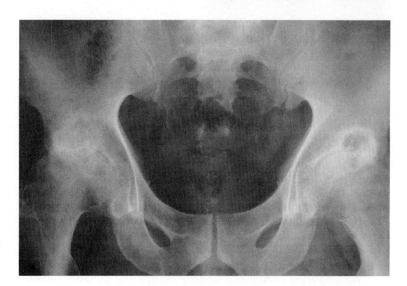

▲ **Figure 7-34.** Case 7-12. A frontal view of the pelvis in a 75-year-old man who presented with bilateral hip pain of several years' duration.

acroosteolysis of the distal tuft. The features are most compatible with a diagnosis of scleroderma (B is the correct answer to Question 7-13).

7-14.   In this case (Figure 7-36), the radiograph of the right hip shows articular space narrowing, bony erosion in the acetabulum and femoral head (arrowheads), and irregular bony sclerosis. The findings are most compatible with septic arthritis (C is the correct answer for Question 7-14).

7-15.   Figure 7-37 shows marked soft-tissue swelling and erosion of the distal aspect of the first metatarsal as well as erosions involving the proximal aspect of the proximal phalanx. These erosions have "overhanging margins." This radiographic appearance and the location of these changes at the first metatarsal phalangeal joint are characteristic of "podagra" associated with the initial attack of gout (C is the correct answer to Question 7-15).

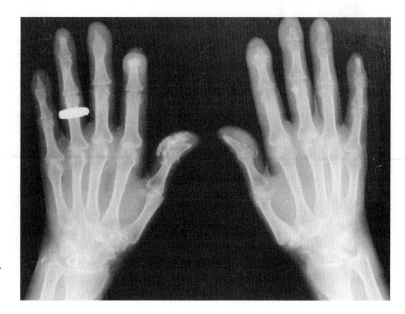

▲ **Figure 7-35.** Case 7-13. A frontal view of both hands in a 45-year-old woman with generalized body "aches and pains" presented to her rheumatologist. Her erythrocyte sedimentation rate (ESR) was elevated at 70 mm.

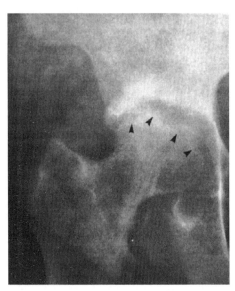

▲ **Figure 7-36.** Case 7-14. Frontal view of the right hip in a 59-year-old woman with renal failure and a long history of hemodialysis who was seen in the emergency department having experienced 2 days of intense right hip pain and fever. She had a fall 8 days ago. She has substantial limitation of motion in the right hip on physical examination.

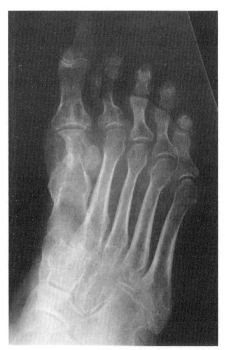

▲ **Figure 7-37.** Case 7-15. An oblique view of right foot in a 60-year-old man who presented to the emergency department with intense foot pain. He was a known alcoholic.

7-16. The lateral view of the cervical spine in Figure 7-38 shows prominent thin vertically oriented connections between the anterior aspects of the vertebral bodies and fusion of the posterior elements of the spine. The thin vertically oriented ossifications are located anatomically in the outer layers of the annulus fibrosis and represent syndesmophytes that are associated with ankylosing spondylitis (D is the correct answer to Question 7-16).

7-17. Figure 7-39 shows a distinct "pencil-in-cup" erosion of the interphalangeal joint of the thumb and severe joint space loss of the distal interphalangeal (DIP) joints with bony ankylosis of the second, third, and fifth DIP joints. Fine periostitis is evident around some of the erosions. Theses findings are most compatible with a diagnosis of psoriasis (A is the correct answer to Question 7-17).

Discussion

Osteoarthrosis (Osteoarthritis)

The frontal view of the pelvis of Case 7-12 (Figure 7-34) shows the classic findings of osteoarthritis. These include joint space narrowing resulting in cartilage loss, subchondral cysts, and osteophyte formation. The findings of osteoarthritis are similar in

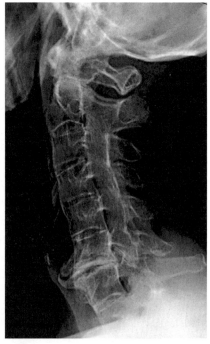

▲ **Figure 7-38.** Case 7-16. A lateral view of cervical spine in a 39-year-old man with a long history of back pain who presented with limitation of movement in his neck. His HLA-B27 antigen was elevated.

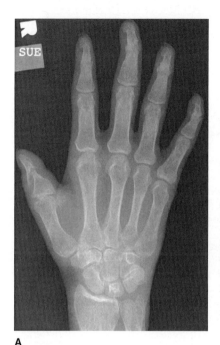

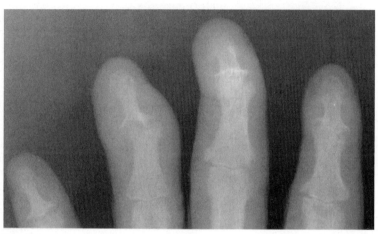

A　　　　　　　　　　　　　**B**

▲ **Figure 7-39.** Case 7-17. A frontal view (**A**) of his hand and a coned-down view of the distal phalanges (**B**) of a different patient with the same diagnosis. A 58-year-old man with a "rash" on his elbows presented to his rheumatologist with hand pain.

all joints. In the knee, the articular space narrowing typically involves the medial compartment initially (Figure 7-40) but may progress to involve the lateral and patellofemoral compartments. In the hands, the articular space narrowing typically involves the distal interphalangeal joints. Another classic "target area" of osteoarthritis in the hand is the first CMC (carpometacarpal joint) and the STT (scaphotrapezo-trapezoidal) joint. There is a variant of osteoarthritis called erosive osteoarthritis. Erosive osteoarthritis usually affects postmenopausal women and can be confused with rheumatoid arthritis. However, erosive arthritis usually affects the distal interphalangeal joints and exhibits predominately subchondral or central erosions as opposed to the marginal erosions seen in rheumatoid arthritis. These central or subchondral erosions have the classic "gull wing" appearance as shown at the proximal interphalangeal joint of the third digit (Figure 7-41).

Connective Tissue Diseases and Seronegative Spondyloarthropathies

Generally, in the clinical setting of polyarticular stiffness and pain, conventional radiographs are used as the initial survey of the affected joints. These images target the most common regions of involvement and usually include films of the hands, wrists, pelvis, knee, feet, and ankles. The findings on these studies, coupled with the ESR value and other laboratory tests, should indicate whether a connective-tissue disorder is

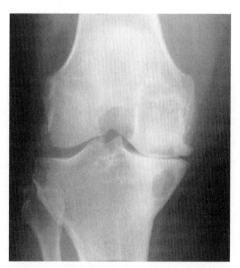

▲ **Figure 7-40.** Frontal view of a 65-year-old man shows the classic features of osteoarthritis of the knee with medial articular space narrowing, subchondral cyst formation, sclerosis, and osteophyte formation. Osteoarthritis of the knee initially involves the medial compartment but may, over time, progress to involve the lateral and patellofemoral compartments.

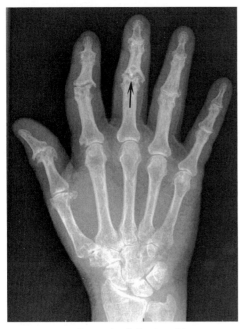

▲ **Figure 7-41.** Radiograph of the hand in a post-menopausal woman exhibits the classic changes of erosive osteoarthritis. Note the "gull-wing" appearance (arrow) of the third proximal interphalangeal (PIP) joint.

the cause of the arthropathy. Often patients will be tested for rheumatoid factor (discussed in the next paragraph). If this test is negative and the patient has symptoms involving the peripheral joints and spine, then a "seronegative spondyloarthropathy" is considered.

Perhaps the most common and characteristic connective tissue disease producing arthritis is rheumatoid arthritis (RA). Females (especially middle-aged women) are more commonly affected by this disease than men. RA is thought to be a malfunction of the immune system, and patients with this disorder usually produce a measurable immune complex called rheumatoid factor (RF). They also characteristically have an elevated ESR. The disease often progresses in a symmetrical fashion. The major initial pathologic process in RA is a synovitis that produces periarticular osteopenia because of the associated hyperemia. Later in the disease, synovial proliferation with pannus formation may then cause erosions in the juxtaarticular regions (the so-called bare areas). These erosions occur at the margins of the joint where the bony cortex and synovium contact each other without interposition of articular cartilage. The articular cartilage provides some protection from erosion in the early stages of the disease. Subsequently, the disease may progress to secondary degenerative changes and eventually to fibrous or bony ankylosis of the joint. In the wrist, the carpal bones will show osteopenia, carpal crowding, or subluxations. In fact, the ulnar styloid is often one of the first sites of erosions and "penciling." Juxtaarticular osteopenia is seen in the bones of the hands and wrists. Symmetric swelling at the proximal interphalangeal joints of the hand is present, and the articular surfaces show erosions, especially at the metacarpophalangeal and proximal interphalangeal joints (Figure 7-42).

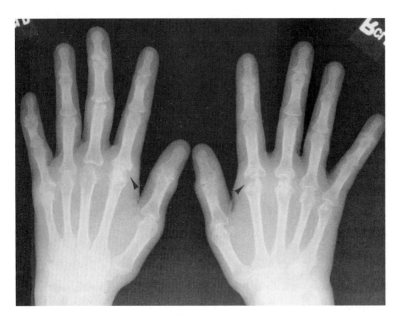

▲ **Figure 7-42.** Frontal view of both hands in a patient with long-standing rheumatoid arthritis showing marked carpal destruction and radiocarpal joint narrowing with substantial erosive change as well as the characteristic "bare area" erosions best exhibited at the second metacarpal phalangeal joint (arrowheads). Also note the soft-tissue swelling at multiple joints.

Systemic lupus erythematosus (SLE) is a connective-tissue disorder that can be seen in conjunction with other connective tissue diseases (the "overlap syndrome"). Patients with SLE may show profound osteopenia, including resorption of the tufts, but it does not characteristically result in erosions. The typical appearance is of joint instability with multiple subluxations at the wrists and metacarpophalangeal joints. In fact, SLE is the most common cause of a nonerosive subluxing arthropathy (Figure 7-43). Subluxations also occur in RA, but the distinguishing factor is that the subluxations in RA are associated with the "bare area" erosions.

Scleroderma (also called progressive systemic sclerosis or PSS) is a disorder characterized by fibrosis and skin thickening. Soft-tissue calcification is a prominent feature of this disorder. The major effects of this disease are not on the joints per se, but are secondary to the diffuse sclerosis with resultant joint stiffness for which the patient may seek treatment initially. About 10% of patients with PSS have synovitis that is indistinguishable from RA at presentation, and many of these patients eventually develop Raynaud's phenomenon. The typical imaging findings are periarticular calcification and resorption of the terminal phalangeal tufts (acroosteolysis). Scleroderma may also be associated with other connective disorders such as rheumatoid arthritis and SLE in the same individual.

Psoriasis, Reiter's disease, ankylosing spondylitis, and inflammatory bowel disease comprise the major seronegative spondyloarthropathies. Psoriasis is a connective tissue disorder that primarily affects the skin. However, about 15% of patients with psoriasis develop bone and joint changes, and these findings may be the initial manifestations of the disease. Radiographic findings of psoriasis include periosteal reaction (periostitis) and/or focal cortical thickening in the digits. The earliest manifestation of the disease is juxtaarticular osteopenia that is less profound than in RA. The disease may then progress to show erosions at the articular surfaces. The distribution of these findings in psoriasis is mainly the distal interphalangeal joints, unlike the findings in patients with RA, which are predominately in the proximal interphalangeal joints, metacarpophalangeal joints, and carpus. The "pencil-in-cup" erosion seen in Figure 7-39 is typical of psoriasis. Patients with psoriasis and other seronegative spondyloarthropathies also develop abnormalities of the spine and sacroiliac joints (hence, the term *spondyloarthropathy*).

Reiter's disease is a postinfective disorder of the immune system that is characterized by the triad of non-gonococcal urethritis, conjunctivitis/iritis, and arthritis. Seen most frequently in male patients, Reiter's disease was originally thought to be caused by *Chlamydia*, but other organisms, including *Escherichia coli* and *Salmonella* organisms, have also been implicated. The imaging findings of Reiter's disease are often indistinguishable from those of psoriatic arthritis except that Reiter's disease most commonly affects the feet and psoriasis most commonly affects the hands. Both diseases show periostitis, erosions, and enthesopathic changes. An *enthesis* is an area of attachment of a ligament or tendon to bone by the perforating fibers of Sharpey. An enthesopathy is, therefore, an abnormality at this site and is seen on the radiograph as bony excrescences in these areas. A typical example of enthesopathy in Reiter's disease is the bony excrescence on the inferior aspect of the calcaneus, which develops at the site of attachment of the plantar fascia and the short flexors in the foot (Figure 7-44).

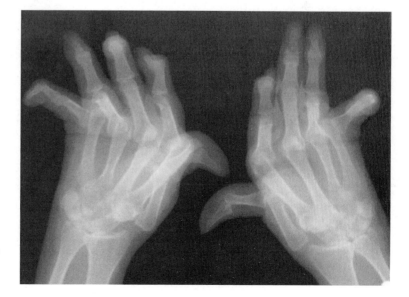

▲ **Figure 7-43.** Frontal view of both hands in a patient with long-standing systemic lupus erythematosus (SLE) shows marked ulna deviation at the metacarpal phalangeal joint as well as subluxation of the thumb. Note the absence of erosions. These findings are classic for this disease.

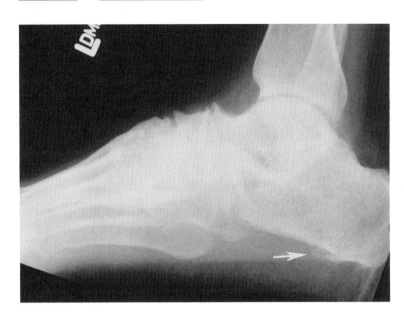

▲ **Figure 7-44.** Lateral foot radiographic in a patient with long-standing Reiter's disease shows marked narrowing of the hindfoot and midfoot, proliferative changes, and sclerosis. Note the prominent calcaneal spur representing enthesopathic change (arrow). Reiter's and psoriasis look identical except that Reiter's more commonly affects the feet.

Ankylosing spondylitis (AS) is a rheumatic disease causing arthritis of the spine and sacroiliac joints and can cause inflammation of the eyes, lungs, and heart valve. The typical clinical scenario is intermittent back pain that occurs throughout life. The pain may progress to severe chronic disease attacking the spine, peripheral joints, and other organs resulting in marked loss of motion and deformity over time. The cause of AS is not known, but most of the spondyloarthritides share a common genetic marker called the HLA-B27 antigen. The disease usually presents in the adolescent and young adults and is most common in Native Americans.

Figure 7-38 shows the typical features of AS in the cervical spine. The thin vertically oriented ossifications connecting the vertebral bodies, syndesmophytes, are anatomically located in the outer layers of the annulus fibrosis. Also typical in this case is the fusion of the posterior elements. In fact, the classic appearance of AS is the "bamboo spine" (Figure 7-45). This appearance is caused by fusion of all the synovial joints of the spine and predisposes the patient to the development of fractures (insufficiency type fractures). This insufficiency fracture (which may lead to a "pseudoarthrosis") is a well-documented complication of ankylosing spondylitis.

The mainstay of treatment for AS is nonsteroidal anti-inflammatory medication to control pain. However, some patients with severe disease may be given methotrexate.

Septic Arthritis

Septic arthritis is usually blood-borne (hematogenous) and is most commonly monoarticular (that is, involving only one joint at any time). A common cause of septic arthritis in the adult is *Staphylococcus aureus*, although other infective agents

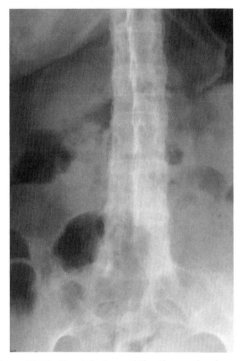

▲ **Figure 7-45.** Frontal view of the thoracolumbar spine showing the classic "bamboo" appearance of the spine in ankylosing spondylitis. This appearance results from fusion of the vertebral bodies and posterior elements.

including *Streptococcus*, *Gonococcus*, and other gram-negative organisms may also be encountered. *Streptococcus* and gram-negative organisms are particularly important in the pediatric age group. Also, tuberculosis has been recently encountered with greater frequency, especially in patients who are immunocompromised.

The radiographic examination of the patient in Case 7-14 (Figure 7-36) provides general anatomic information, helps to determine whether further imaging is necessary, and aids in deciding whether further intervention is appropriate. Her physicians were very worried about septic arthritis in this clinical setting of previous renal transplant (ie, relatively immunocompromised), and a hip aspiration was requested. Twenty milliliters of bloodstained turbid fluid was aspirated and was sent to the microbiology laboratory for Gram's stain, culture, and sensitivity studies. The cultures grew *Staphylococcus aureus*, a common pathogen in septic arthritis.

Figure 7-36 shows the classic radiographic findings of septic arthritis and osteomyelitis. These include articular space narrowing, erosion of bone on both sides of the joint, and sclerosis. An effusion is typically present and can be identified by ultrasound or MR imaging. In addition, MR imaging can be useful if abscesses are suspected in the adjacent soft tissues. Septic joints will exhibit increased uptake on bone scan because of the marked hyperemia and bony proliferation.

Crystal Deposition Diseases

Gout, a disorder more common in middle-aged men, is an inflammatory arthritis caused by abnormal deposition of urates (called tophi) in the soft tissues and cartilage. These deposits cause episodic joint inflammation and are associated with pain and disability. In the earlier stages of the disease, radiographs of the bone and joints may be normal except for soft-tissue swelling and in some instances soft-tissue calcification. The initial classic clinical presentation of gout is podagra, an acute inflammation of a joint, often the first metatarsal phalangeal joint (Figure 7-37). At presentation, the patient will have severe joint pain, and the overlying soft tissues will be swollen and red. With repeated attacks over years, bony erosions with "overhanging edges" (or overhanging margins) may develop adjacent to the joint but not within the joint. When the patient is severely incapacitated by pain and not moving the joint, "disuse" osteopenia can be seen at radiography. The typical areas to screen for gout are the first metatarsophalangeal joint, the heel, the back of the elbow joint (olecranon fossa), and the hands and wrists. Screening for elevated serum levels of uric acid and joint aspiration are the best ways to confirm the clinical suspicion of gout after obtaining conventional radiographs. The joint aspirate will show birefringent uric acid crystals in the synovial fluid on polarized light microscopy.

Calcium pyrophosphate dehydrate crystal deposition (CPPD) disease is another common crystal deposition joint disorders. In CPPD disease, there is calcification in the fibrocartilage and hyaline articular cartilage (so-called chondrocalcinosis). The most common association with chondrocalcinosis is aging, although it may also be seen in pseudogout (CPPD disease), gout, ochronosis, hemochromatosis, and hyperparathyroidism. This finding is most commonly seen in the wrist, symphysis pubis, or knee. So, if one suspects a patient of having CPPD, radiographs of the pelvis, wrist, and knees would be a good start at screening for it. The presence of calcification alone is not diagnostic of CPPD, however. The clinical syndrome of pain from the presence of abnormal cartilage calcification is referred to as the CPPD syndrome, and symptoms may be provoked by various stresses (eg, surgical procedures). Confirmation of the diagnosis may be obtained by identification of calcium pyrophosphate crystals from synovial fluid obtained via percutaneous aspiration of the affected joint.

EXERCISE 7-5. MISCELLANEOUS JOINT DISORDERS

7-18.   The most likely diagnosis for Case 7-18 (Figure 7-46) is
   A. synovial osteochondromatosis.
   B. pigmented villonodular synovitis.
   C. avascular necrosis of the femoral condyle.
   D. osteochondritis dissecans (OCD) of the femoral condyle.

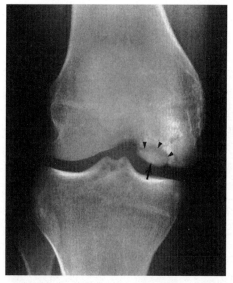

▲ **Figure 7-46.** Case 7-18. A knee x-ray in a 24-year-old male medical student, an avid tennis player, who had intermittent joint swelling and minimal knee pain. Lately, the pain had worsened and was interfering with his tennis game. Nonsteroidal anti-inflammatory agents were not working well.

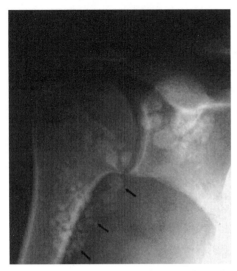

▲ **Figure 7-47.** Case 7-19. A radiograph of the right shoulder in a 20-year-old man who complained of a feeling of fullness and gritty sensations in his right shoulder. He has never had a shoulder dislocation, although on several occasions he has been unable to raise the shoulder and has felt a painful "catch" at times.

7-19. The most likely diagnosis for Case 7-19 (Figure 7-47) is
    A. hemochromatosis.
    B. synovial osteochondromatosis.
    C. pigmented villonodular synovitis.
    D. calcified Heberden's nodes.

7-20. The most likely diagnosis for Case 7-20 (Figure 7-48) is
    A. chronic changes of transient synovitis of the right hip.
    B. chronic changes of slipped capital femoral epiphysis (epiphysiolysis).
    C. chronic changes of Legg-Calvé-Perthes disease of the right hip.
    D. neurofibromatosis.

7-21. Concerning Case 7-21 (Figure 7-49), the observations include all of the following except
    A. osteophyte in both femoral heads.
    B. irregularity and loss of spherocity of the right femoral head.
    C. depression/subchondral fracture of right femoral head.
    D. bilateral acetabular sclerosis.

Radiologic Findings

7-18. The AP view of the right knee (Figure 7-46) shows an ovoid bony fragment on the inner aspect of the medial femoral condyle (arrow) separated from the femur by a lucency (arrowheads). This appearance is diagnostic of osteochondritis dissecans (OCD) of the knee (D is the correct answer to Question 7-18).

7-19. The radiograph of the right shoulder in Figure 7-47 shows multiple rounded calcific bodies overlying the proximal humerus and glenoid process of the scapula. The distribution of these is within the joint and axillary recess (arrows). This appearance is

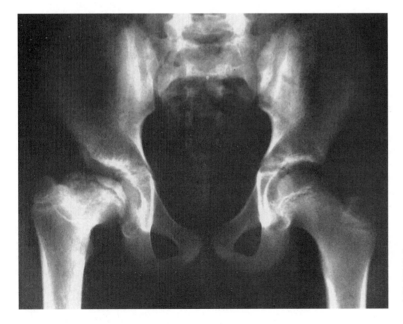

▲ **Figure 7-48.** Case 7-20. A frontal radiograph of the pelvis in a 10-year-old boy who was referred to an orthopedic surgeon for investigation of a limp. There was no reliable history of trauma.

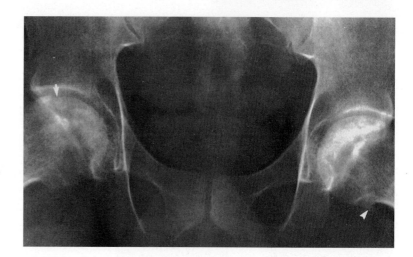

▲ **Figure 7-49.** Case 7-21. A frontal radiograph of both hips in a 35-year-old man with episodic right hip pain that began 4 to 6 months ago who presented with a dull aching pain now in both hips.

classic for synovial osteochondromatosis (SOC) (B is the correct answer to Question 7-19).

7-20. The radiograph of the pelvis in Figure 7-48 shows collapse of the right capital femoral epiphysis, which is broad and short and forms an acute angle with the shaft of the femur. The femoral head is displaced laterally and is not completely covered by the mildly remodeled acetabulum. The left hip is normal. The findings are characteristic of the late changes in Legg-Calvé-Perthes disease (C is the correct answer to Question 7-20).

7-21. The radiograph of both hips in Figure 7-49 demonstrates that the right femoral head is no longer smooth and spherical (loss of spherocity), and this is due to the presence of subchondral collapse in the superiolateral aspect (arrow). The left femoral head is still spherical but shows sclerosis. Also note the marginal osteophytes arising from the inferior and medial aspect of the left femoral head (arrowhead). The acetabuli are normal, and these radiographic features are typical of avascular necrosis (osteonecrosis) of the femoral head (D is the correct answer to Question 7-21).

Discussion

Osteochondritis dissecans is a bone disorder that produces joint symptoms because of the intraarticular location of the abnormality. OCD, as classically demonstrated in Figure 7-46, is seen on the radiograph as a semicircular focus of bone and overlying cartilage separated from the convex articular surface of the native bone by a lucency. The etiology is uncertain, but current opinion favors repetitive microtrauma and vascular insult to the subchondral bone. Almost any joint may be affected, but the knee (distal femur), ankle (dome of the talus), and elbow (capitellum) joints are the most commonly involved

sites. The disease is slightly more common in active young men but is increasingly being encountered in young women because they are more actively involved in athletics today. In the knee, OCD most commonly involves the non-weight-bearing aspect of the medial femoral condyle (ie, the inner aspect and area shown in Figure 7-46) and the lateral femoral condyle. MR imaging is the most appropriate modality to stage the lesion, assess the stability of the fragment, and plan definitive treatment. CT or CT arthrography is an alternate modality to use in patients who cannot undergo MR imaging.

Synovial osteochondromatosis is a joint abnormality characterized by the presence of cartilaginous and osseous loose bodies within the synovial cavity in the joint. The exact cause is not known, but "primary" SOC is thought to be caused by synovial metaplasia. "Secondary" OCD is assumed to be due to fractures of osteophytes or articular cartilage that shed into the joint cavity. If calcified, these intraarticular fragments can be visualized on conventional radiographs (Figure 7-47, arrows). MR imaging is the best modality to use to show both ossified and nonossified intraarticular fragments and to evaluate the other soft-tissue structures around the joint.

Pigmented villonodular synovitis (PVNS) is a condition of unknown etiology characterized by hyperplasia or excessive villous proliferation of the synovium. This condition may occur in a single joint (localized form) or involve multiple joints (diffuse form). Thought to be caused by hemorrhage, PVNS shows hemosiderin-laden macrophages within the synovium best appreciated by gross examination. Radiographs often show a joint effusion with preservation of the articular space and normal bone mineral density. The later stages of the disease result in erosions on both sides of the joint. Joint aspiration yields dark brown fluid ("chocolate" effusion) due to the presence of the hemosiderin-laden macrophages. MR imaging is an excellent preoperative test to evaluate PVNS because the pigmented material (hemosiderin) shows low

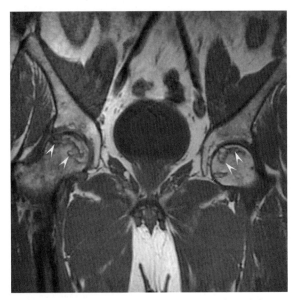

▲ **Figure 7-50.** Coronal T1-weighted MR image of the pelvis in a patient with bilateral hip avascular necrosis. Note the serpiginous low signal abnormality in the subchondral regions of the femoral heads (arrowheads).

signal intensity on both the short TE (T1-weighted) and the long TE (T2-weighted) MR sequences. The gradient echo sequence is particularly sensitive for the detection of hemosiderin. In fact, this finding is a very specific appearance for this disease.

Heberden's node is a disfigurement of the interphalangeal joints as a result of severe osteoarthritis. Initially, it is due to soft-tissue inflammatory changes and is subsequently due to bony changes at the distal interphalangeal joints. It is more commonly seen in female patients.

Osteonecrosis can occur in any bone and is associated with a variety of disorders, including sickle cell hemoglobinopathy, Gaucher's disease, SLE, pancreatitis, alcoholism, steroid treatment, and barotrauma. When the process occurs at an articular surface, it is known as avascular necrosis or osteonecrosis; when it occurs in the metaphysis of the bone, it is commonly referred to as a bone infarct. Eponyms have been used to designate osteonecrosis in certain sites. For example, Perthes' disease (Legg-Calvé-Perthes disease) is the eponym used to refer to idiopathic osteonecrosis of the femoral head occurring in a child as shown in Case 7-20 (Figure 7-48).

Other common eponyms include Freiberg's infarction, (avascular necrosis of the head of the second or third metatarsal), Kohler's disease (tarsal navicular), Panner's disease (capitellum of the humerus), and Kienbock's disease (carpal lunate). The exact mechanism of the development of osteonecrosis is unknown, although bone-marrow edema after thrombosis and occlusion of the osseous capillaries and end arterioles are believed to be primarily responsible.

Conventional radiographs are much less sensitive compared to MR regarding the detection of early osteonecrosis. Increased areas of serpiginous sclerosis and osteolysis can be noted on conventional radiographs; however, these abnormalities found relatively late compared to MR imaging, and therefore treatment outcome of the disease may be delayed or adversely affected (Figure 7-49). Importantly, if the disease is not diagnosed and treated early, the affected bone may go through a phase of subchondral collapse and become deformed. Subsequently, complications of secondary osteoarthrosis will develop in the affected joint. Traditionally, nuclear medicine bone scanning has been used in this setting, but today MR imaging is the most sensitive available modality for the early diagnosis of this disease (Figure 7-50).

Hemochromatosis is a rare disorder of iron metabolism, in which iron is deposited in the skin, parenchymal organs, and articular cartilage. This predisposes the joint to degenerative disease. Arthritis due to hemochromatosis is characterized by loss of joint space and formation of peculiar hooked osteophytes, especially at metacarpal heads.

SUGGESTED READING

1. Pope T, Bloem HL, Beltran J, Morrison W, Wilson DB. *Imaging of the Musculoskeletal System.* New York: Elsevier; 2008.
2. Manaster BJ, May DA, Disler DG. *Musculoskeletal Imaging: The Requisites.* 3rd ed. New York: Elsevier; 2007.
3. Yu JS. *Musculoskeletal Imaging: Case Review Series.* 2nd ed. New York: Elsevier; 2008.
4. Resnick D. *Diagnosis of Bone and Joint Disorders.* 4th ed. Philadelphia: Saunders; 2002.
5. Rogers LF. *Radiology of Skeletal Trauma.* 3rd ed. Philadelphia: Churchill Livingstone; 2002.
6. Berquist TH. *MRI of the Musculoskeletal System.* 4th ed. Philadelphia: Lippincott Williams & Wilkins; 2001.
7. Kaplan P. *Musculoskeletal MRI.* Philadelphia: Saunders; 2001.
8. Greenspan A. *Orthopaedic Imaging.* 4th ed. Philadelphia: Lippincott Williams & Wilkins; 2004.
9. Chew, SF, Roberts CC. *Musculoskeletal Imaging: A Teaching File.* 2nd ed. Philadelphia: Lippincott Williams & Wilkins; 2005.
10. El-Khoury GY, Bennett DL. *Essentials of Musculoskeletal Imaging.* New York: Churchill Livingstone; 2003.

Plain Film of the Abdomen

8

Michael Y. M. Chen, MD

In recent years, new techniques such as ultrasonography, computerized tomography (CT), and magnetic resonance (MR) imaging have been used widely and have altered the use of plain films of the abdomen in the evaluation of abdominal diseases. Plain films of the abdomen are still used primarily to assess intestinal perforation (intraperitoneal air) or bowel obstruction or assessment for catheter placement. The plain radiograph is commonly used as a preliminary radiograph before other studies such as CT and barium enema. The yield of plain radiographs is higher in patients with moderate or severe abdominal symptoms and signs than in those with minor symptoms.

TECHNIQUE AND NORMAL IMAGING

▶ Technique

The most common plain radiograph of the abdomen is an anteroposterior (AP) view with the patient in supine position. The AP view of the abdomen is also called by the acronym KUB film because it includes the kidneys, ureters, and bladder. When acute abdominal disease is suspected clinically, an erect film of the abdomen and a posteroanterior (PA) view of the chest are also required. Digital imaging is becoming more common, and abdominal images may be viewed on a computer monitor rather than on films.

▶ Normal Imaging
Soft Tissue

The abdomen is composed primarily of soft tissue. The density of soft tissue is similar to the density of water, and the difference in density between solid and liquid is not distinguishable on a plain radiograph. The liver is a homogeneous structure located in the right upper quadrant; the hepatic angle delineates the lower margin of the posterior portion of the liver (Figure 8-1). In the left upper quadrant, a similar angular structure, the splenic angle, can be identified by the fat shadow around the spleen (see Figure 8-1).

Organ enlargement can be recognized by the effect of displacement on nearby bowel loops or by obliteration of the adjacent normal fat or gas pattern. Hepatomegaly may compress the proximal transverse colon below the right kidney. Splenomegaly may push the splenic flexure of the colon downward. A large fused renal shadow across the psoas muscle and lumbar spine suggests a horseshoe kidney.

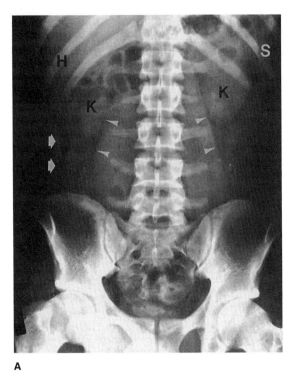

A

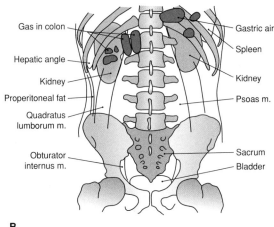

B

▲ **Figure 8-1.** (**A**) Normal plain film of the abdomen. The lower margins of the posterior portion of the liver, the hepatic angle (H), and the lower part of the spleen (S) are delineated by a fat shadow. Both kidneys (K) and the psoas muscle shadows (arrowheads) are outlined by a fat shadow. The properitoneal fat stripe is also shown bilaterally (arrows). (**B**) Diagram of normal abdominal plain film.

Fat Shadow

Fat density, which is between that of soft tissue and that of gas, outlines the contour of solid organs or muscles. In obese patients, fat may not be distinguishable from ascitic fluid on plain abdominal film. The flank stripe, also called the properitoneal fat stripe, is a line of fat next to the muscle of the lateral abdominal wall (see Figure 8-1). The flank stripes are symmetrically concave or slightly convex in obese people and are located along the side of the abdominal wall. The normal properitoneal fat stripe is in close proximity to the gas pattern seen in the ascending or descending colon. Widening of the distance between the properitoneal fat stripe and the ascending or descending colon suggests fluid, such as abscess, ascitic fluid, or blood within the paracolic gutter.

Fat is present in the retroperitoneal space adjacent to the psoas muscle (see Figure 8-1). The psoas muscle shadow may be absent unilaterally or bilaterally as a normal variant or as a result of inflammation, hemorrhage, or neoplasms of the retroperitoneum. Unilateral convexity of the psoas muscle contour suggests an intramuscular mass or abscess. The quadratus lumborum muscles may be delineated by fat located

lateral to the psoas shadow (see Figure 8-1). In the pelvis, the fatty envelope of the obturator internus muscle is seen on the inner aspect of the pelvic inlet (see Figure 8-1). The dome of the urinary bladder may be delineated by fat.

Gas Pattern

Gas has the lowest density (radiolucency) in the abdomen. It is seen in the stomach and colon, but it is rarely seen in the normal small bowel because the air rapidly traverses the organ. Presence of more than a minimal amount of gas in the small bowel should be considered abnormal and is indicative of a functional ileus or mechanical obstruction. Identification of the differences between the gas shadows of the jejunum, ileum, or colon helps to assess the location of bowel obstruction (Figure 8-2). A gas pattern in distended intestinal loops is usually limited above the point of mechanical obstruction, but functional ileus has a more diffuse distribution in both the small intestine and the colon. If the gas shadow in the intestine is displaced to an unusual location, a soft-tissue mass, either inflammatory or neoplastic, may be suspected. The presence of air-fluid levels in a distended small intestine on

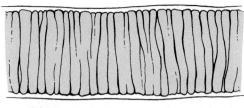

Jejunum

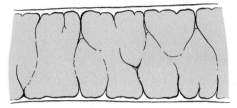

Ileum

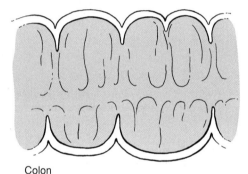

Colon

▲ **Figure 8-2.** Schematic illustration of portions of bowel. The jejunum shows numerous mucosal folds, and the ileum has fewer folds. Both serosa of the jejunum and the ileum are smooth. The colon has serosa indented by haustra, and mucosal folds do not cross the lumen.

upright films suggests either functional ileus or mechanical obstruction. Fluid levels within the stomach or colon are ordinarily of no pathologic importance, because fluid may be introduced by oral agents or by cleansing enemas. The presence of solid material with a mottled appearance and small bubbles of gas surrounded by the colonic contour suggests feces in the colon.

A large amount of gas seen in the peritoneal cavity indicates postoperative status or bowel perforation. Air bubbles in the peritoneal cavity indicate a perforated viscus, abscess, or necrotic tumor. In the right upper quadrant, air that is seen in the biliary tree or around the gallbladder suggests cholecystoenteric fistula or emphysematous cholecystitis. A finely arborizing gas pattern over the right upper quadrant that extends peripherally to the edge of the liver is characteristic of hepatic portal vein gas. In the bowel wall, multiple air bubbles may indicate pneumatosis cystoides intestinalis. Extraluminal gas also may appear within the retroperitoneal structures, including the lesser omental bursa, a subhepatic site, the paraduodenal fossa, and the pericecal or periappendiceal areas. A gas pattern seen below the bony pelvis indicates an inguinal or femoral hernia.

Bony Structure or Calcification

Bony structures or calcifications have the highest density (radiopacity) that is seen on the plain film. Bony structures comprise the ribs superiorly, the lumbar spine, and the pelvis. Calcifications in the abdomen include calcified arteries, calculi in the urinary or biliary tract, prostatic calculi, pancreatic calcifications (which are usually indicative of chronic pancreatitis, with or without carcinoma), appendicolith, or ectopic gallstone in the small bowel associated with mechanical obstruction from gallstone ileus. Some foreign bodies, including ingested foreign bodies, bullets, or surgical clips, may be seen in the abdomen. Other rare structures, such as parasitic, metastatic, or heterotopic bone formations, also may be seen in the abdomen.

Suspicion of urinary calculi is a indication for abdominal radiography. About one-half of calculi in the urinary tract that are shown on unenhanced helical CT can be detected on plain abdominal films. On the other hand, about 15% of gallstones are radiopaque and are seen on abdominal plain radiograph. Ultrasonography is the better choice in evaluating gallstones.

TECHNIQUE SELECTION

The routine abdominal films consist of supine and upright views. If the patient cannot stand for an erect abdominal film and a PA view of the chest, the cross-table lateral projection with the right side elevated may be used to assess pneumoperitoneum and air-fluid levels. As little as 1 to 2 mL of free air in the peritoneal space may be identified if the films are appropriately obtained. The PA view of the chest is usually obtained as part of an acute abdominal series because an abnormality in the chest may have symptoms referred to the abdomen. Oblique views of the abdomen may be obtained, if needed.

Plain abdominal radiography is less sensitive in evaluating solid organs or metastases. In recent years, increased use of cross-sectional techniques, such as ultrasonography and CT, has shown them to be more sensitive in assessing disorders of the abdominal solid organs and metastatic diseases. Acute cholecystitis is better assessed by ultrasonography or nuclear medicine studies.

EXERCISE 8-1. UPPER ABDOMINAL CALCIFICATIONS

8-1. What is the most likely diagnosis in Case 8-1 (Figure 8-3)?
A. Adrenal calcification
B. Calcified gallstones
C. Kidney stones
D. Milk-of-calcium bile in the gallbladder

8-2. What is the most likely diagnosis in Case 8-2 (Figure 8-4)?
A. Adrenal calcification
B. Calcified gallstones
C. Kidney stones
D. Medullary nephrocalcinosis

8-3. What is the most likely diagnosis in Case 8-3 (Figure 8-5)?
A. Adrenal calcification.
B. Calcified hepatic metastases.
C. Pancreatic calcification.
D. Primary calcified mucoproducing adenocarcinoma in the colon.

8-4. What is the most likely diagnosis in Case 8-4 (Figure 8-6)?
A. Adrenal calcification
B. Calcified hepatic metastases
C. Pancreatic calcification
D. Primary calcified mucoproducing adenocarcinoma in the colon

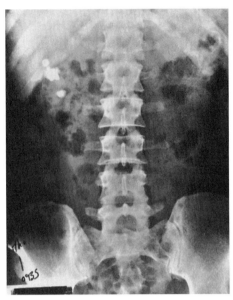

▲ **Figure 8-4.** Case 8-2. A 36-year-old woman presents with flank pain.

Radiologic Findings

8-1. This case demonstrates multiple faceted calcifications in the right upper quadrant that are characteristic for gallstones (B is the correct answer to Question 8-1).

8-2. This case shows three separate deposits of calcified density confined to the right renal shadow. The largest one measures 2 cm in greatest diameter (C is the correct answer to Question 8-2).

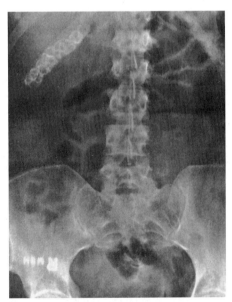

▲ **Figure 8-3.** Case 8-1. A 44-year-old woman presents with right upper quadrant pain.

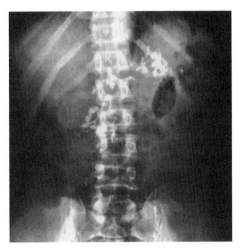

▲ **Figure 8-5.** Case 8-3. A 48-year-old alcoholic man presents with epigastric pain.

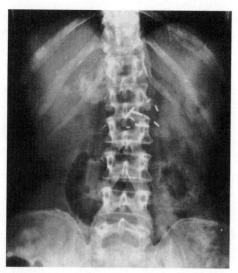

▲ **Figure 8-6.** Case 8-4. A 59-year-old woman is seen who underwent colectomy surgery for colon cancer 10 years ago.

8-3. This case shows multiple stippled calcifications in the upper abdomen adjacent to the lumbar spine. In a patient with a history of alcoholism, pancreatic calcification from chronic pancreatitis would be the most likely diagnosis (C is the correct answer to Question 8-3).

8-4. This case shows stippled and discrete calcifications overlying the right twelfth rib, just above the renal outline. When calcification in the lung base, skin, retroperitoneum, pancreas, kidney, and adrenal glands is excluded, hepatic calcification should be considered in a patient with a history of colon cancer (B is the correct answer to Question 8-4).

Discussion

About 15% to 20% of gallstones are calcified sufficiently to be seen on plain abdominal film. Most gallstones comprise mixed components, including cholesterol, bile salts, and biliary pigments. Pure cholesterol and pure pigment stones are uncommon. Calcified gallstones vary in size and shape. Most gallstones have thin, marginal calcification with central lucency and are laminated, faceted, or irregular in shape. Some gallstones contain gas in their fissures, whether calcified or noncalcified. Milk-of-calcium or "limy" bile occurs in patients with long-standing cystic duct obstruction. The bile contains a high concentration of calcium carbonate and is densely radiopaque on plain radiograph (Figure 8-7). Calcification of the gallbladder wall (porcelain gallbladder) develops in patients with chronic cholecystitis, cholelithiasis, and cystic duct obstruction. Porcelain gallbladder is characterized

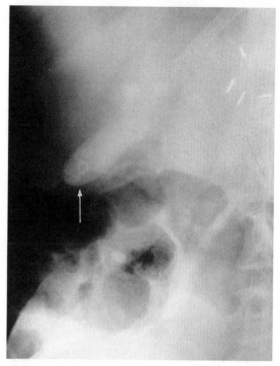

▲ **Figure 8-7.** Milk-of-calcium bile. Plain radiograph shows homogenous density of the gallbladder. A small gallstone is also seen within the gallbladder (arrow) (From Chen MY et al: Abnormal calcification on plain radiographs of the abdomen, *The Radiologist* 1999;7:65-83, used with permission).

by curvilinear calcification in the muscular layer of the gallbladder mimicking a calcified cyst (Figure 8-8). In general, ultrasonography is the primary modality now used to evaluate the gallbladder (Figure 8-9).

Nephrolithiasis is the most common cause of calcification within the kidneys. Most renal calculi (85%) contain calcium complexed with oxalate and phosphate salts. Any process that creates urinary tract stasis may cause the development of urinary calculi. Renal calculi are usually small and lie within the pelvicalyceal system or in a calyceal diverticulum. They may remain and increase in size, or they may pass distally. When calcifications are seen projecting over the renal shadows on routine films of the abdomen, an oblique view may be obtained to localize the densities in relation to the kidneys. A staghorn calculus contains calcium mixed with magnesium, ammonium, and phosphate and forms in the environment of recurrent urinary tract infection with alkaline urine. CT is more sensitive than plain radiography in evaluating urinary calculi.

The adrenal gland is located at the superomedial part of the adjacent kidney. The right gland is lower than the left.

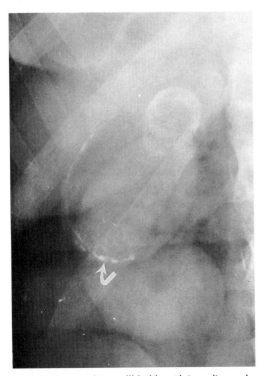

▲ **Figure 8-8.** Porcelain gallbladder. Plain radiograph shows curvilinear discontinuous calcification in the gallbladder wall (arrow). (From Chen MY et al: Abnormal calcification on plain radiographs of the abdomen, *The Radiologist* 1999;7:65-83, used with permission).

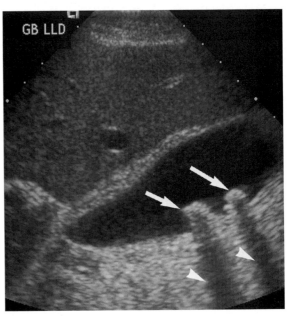

▲ **Figure 8-9.** Gallstones. Sonography shows two echogenic foci (arrows) located dependently in the gallbladder with posterior acoustic shadowing (arrowheads).

Normally the adrenal gland measures less than 2.5 × 3 cm. Stippled, mottled, discrete, or homogeneous calcifications may appear as a portion of the adrenal gland or may occupy the entire organ, forming a triangular clump in the adrenal glands (Figure 8-10). Most adrenal calcifications are incidental findings in normal-sized glands. They are caused by neonatal adrenal hemorrhage, prolonged hypoxia, severe

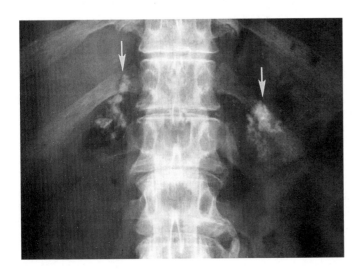

▲ **Figure 8-10.** Solid adrenal calcifications. Bilateral discrete, stippled adrenal calcifications (arrows) in the normal-sized glands in an asymptomatic patient with a history of complicated childbirth (From Chen MY et al: Abnormal calcification on plain radiographs of the abdomen, *The Radiologist* 1999;7:65-83, used with permission).

neonatal infection, or birth trauma. Less than one-fourth of patients with Addison's disease have adrenal calcifications.

In the United States, 85% to 90% of patients with pancreatic lithiasis are alcoholics. Conversely, less than half of patients with chronic pancreatitis ever develop pancreatic calcifications visible on plain radiograph. Although gallstones passing through the biliary tract can cause acute pancreatitis, chronic pancreatitis or pancreatic calcification is rarely caused by cholelithiasis.

Hepatic calcifications are caused primarily by neoplasms, infections, or parasitic infestations. Primary hepatic tumors, both benign and malignant, may have calcifications. Colonic carcinoma and papillary serous cystadenocarcinoma of the ovary are the most frequent primary tumors causing calcified metastases in the liver. Other primary neoplasms in the thyroid gland, lung, pancreas, adrenal gland, stomach, kidney, and breast may cause calcified hepatic metastases. Inflammatory calcified granulomas related to tuberculosis or histoplasmosis are common in miliary calcifications. Calcified cystic lesions, such as *Echinococcus* disease in the liver, are commonly seen in areas of the world where the causative organism is endemic.

EXERCISES 8-2. PELVIC CALCIFICATIONS

8-5.   What is the most likely diagnosis in Case 8-5 (Figure 8-11)?
    A. Appendicolith
    B. Ectopic gallstone
    C. Pelvic phlebolith
    D. Right ureteral calculus

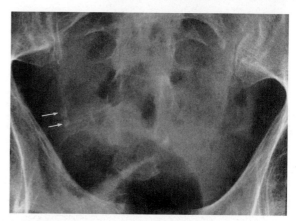

▲ **Figure 8-12.** Case 8-6. A 64-year-old man presents with hematuria.

8-6.   What is the most likely diagnosis in Case 8-6 (Figure 8-12)?
    A. Calcified ovarian tumor
    B. Multiple phleboliths
    C. Multiple ureteral calculi
    D. Uterine fibroid calcification

8-7.   What is the most likely diagnosis in Case 8-7 (Figure 8-13)?
    A. Bladder calculus
    B. Chondrosarcoma of the sacrum
    C. Cystadenoma of the ovary
    D. Uterine fibroid calcifications

8-8.   What is the most likely diagnosis in Case 8-8 (Figure 8-14)?
    A. Bladder calculi
    B. Calcified vas deferens
    C. Ovarian dermoid cyst
    D. Uterine fibroid calcification

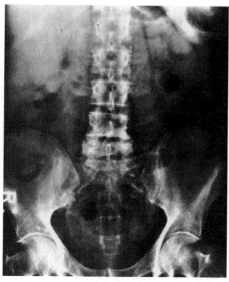

▲ **Figure 8-11.** Case 8-5. A 15-year-old boy presents with right lower quadrant pain and fever.

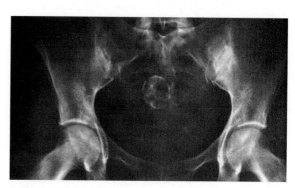

▲ **Figure 8-13.** Case 8-7. A 48-year-old woman presents with lower abdominal fullness.

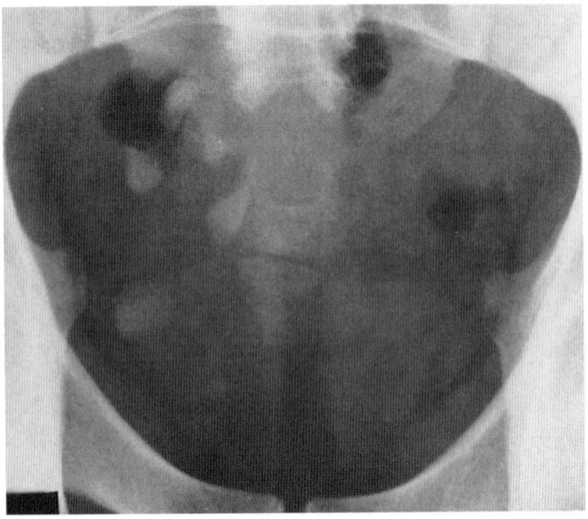

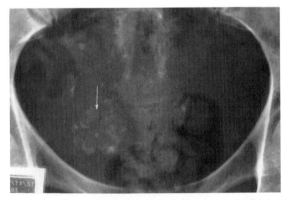

▲ **Figure 8-14.** Case 8-8. A 14-year-old girl presents with lower abdominal pain and a palpable mass in the pelvis.

Radiologic Findings

8-5. This case is that of a boy with acute appendicitis (A is the correct answer to Question 8-5). An oval calcification measuring 0.8 cm in diameter projects over the iliac bone and laterally to the right sacroiliac joint with a distended appendiceal lumen filled with gas. At surgery, gangrenous appendicitis with perforation and an obstructing appendicolith were found.

8-6. This case demonstrates 5 × 5 mm and 4 × 4 mm calcified densities (arrows) along the expected course of the right distal ureter. These densities were formerly identified in the right kidney and have migrated inferiorly to the current position, indicating right ureteral calculi. With the history of hematuria, the most likely choice would be right ureteral calculi (C is the correct answer to Question 8-6).

8-7. This case shows large, 2-cm-diameter mottled and curvilinear calcifications in the midpelvis. These calcifications overlie the sacrum and are consistent with calcification in uterine fibroids (D is the correct answer to Question 8-7).

8-8. This case shows several "teeth-like" calcifications in the right side of the pelvis. With a palpable pelvic mass, the most likely diagnosis is ovarian dermoid cyst. (C is the correct answer to Question 8-8.)

Discussion

Calcified appendiceal stones are present in only about 10% of patients with appendicitis; however, in a symptomatic child, an appendicolith indicates at least a 90% chance of acute appendicitis. Prophylactic appendectomy has been recommended in the child with an incidentally discovered appendicolith because of a high incidence of gangrene and perforation. CT or ultrasound are better choices in evaluating appendicitis.

Ureteral calculi are always a consideration in patients with hematuria. About 50% of urinary calculi are radiographically opaque and shown on the plain abdominal radiograph. Close scrutiny of the abdominal film is crucial because ureteral calculi may be elusive when they project over the lumbar transverse processes or the sacroiliac region. To confirm a ureteral calculus, CT is often needed to localize the density to the ureter. CT is more sensitive in evaluating ureteral calculi. Phleboliths are thrombi within the pelvic veins, and this location accounts for their circular shape. Calcification within these thrombi starts peripherally with a typical radiolucent center that is seen radiographically. Phleboliths have little clinical significance except that they can be confused with other pelvic densities, particularly distal ureteral calculi. In general, ureteral stones lie above and medially to the ischial spines, and they lack a radiolucent center.

Most uterine leiomyoma calcifications appear as multiple mottled or speckled calcifications or as dense, smooth, curvilinear calcifications around the mass. The real soft-tissue mass is often larger than the area of calcification. Other calcifications in the pelvis include calcified ovarian tumors (Figure 8-15), foreign material, lymph nodes, or prostate.

Ovarian dermoid cyst accounts for about 10% of ovarian neoplasms. Ovarian dermoid cyst range from 6 to 15 cm in diameter and contain teeth, abortive bone, and curvilinear capsular calcification, which may be seen on plain radiograph. Dermoid cyst may contain sebaceous material

▲ **Figure 8-15.** Calcifications in ovarian tumor. Multiple sporadic calcifications (arrow) in the central pelvis from an ovarian cystadenocarcinoma (From Chen MY et al: Abnormal calcification on plain radiographs of the abdomen, *The Radiologist* 1999;7:65-83, used with permission).

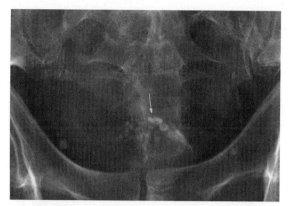

▲ **Figure 8-16.** Prostate calculi. Diffuse and symmetric coarse calcifications (arrow) in an enlarged prostate (From Chen MY et al: Abnormal calcification on plain radiographs of the abdomen, *The Radiologist* 1999;7:65-83, used with permission).

simulating low-density fat compared to surrounding soft tissue.

Bladder stone is often seen in association with bladder outlet obstruction. Bladder calculi are composed of mixed calcium oxalate and phosphate salts that are radiopaque. Other calcifications in the bladder include foreign body, transitional cell carcinoma, urachal carcinoma, *Schistosoma* infestation, tuberculosis, or alkaline encrusting cystitis. Calcifications in the same area include prostatic calculi (Figure 8-16) and calcified vas deferens (Figure 8-17). The prostate gland may be calcified. If enlarged, it may protrude into the bladder.

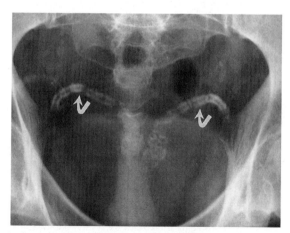

▲ **Figure 8-17.** Calcifications of vas deferens. Calcifications (arrows) in the tortuous ampullary segment of the vas deferens (From Chen MY et al: Abnormal calcification on plain radiographs of the abdomen, *The Radiologist* 1999; 7:65-83, used with permission).

EXERCISE 8-3. INCREASED ABDOMINAL DENSITY OR MASSES

8-9. What is the most likely diagnosis of this soft-tissue mass (arrows) in Case 8-9 (Figure 8-18)?
A. Ascites
B. Cirrhosis
C. Hepatomegaly
D. Nephromegaly

8-10. What is the most likely diagnosis of this soft-tissue mass (arrows) in Case 8-10 (Figure 8-19)?
A. Adrenal carcinoma
B. Gastric outlet obstruction
C. Renal cell carcinoma
D. Splenomegaly

8-11. What is the most likely diagnosis of this soft-tissue mass (arrows) in Case 8-11 (Figure 8-20)?
A. A pseudotumor sign of small bowel obstruction
B. Gastric outlet obstruction
C. Hepatomegaly
D. Horseshoe kidney

8-12. What is the most likely diagnosis in Case 8-12 (Figure 8-21)?
A. Ovarian cyst
B. Pelvic abscess
C. Pelvic hematoma
D. Pelvic kidney

Radiologic Findings

8-9. In this case, the right side of the abdomen shows increased density and is relatively free of gas.

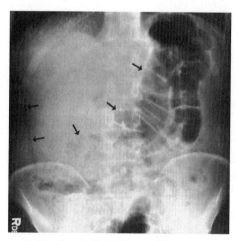

▲ **Figure 8-18.** Case 8-9. A 57-year-old man presents with history of hepatitis.

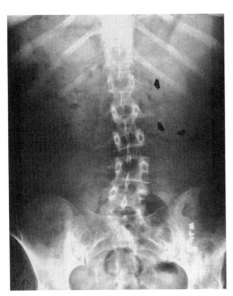

▲ **Figure 8-19.** Case 8-10. A 35-year-old woman presents with fever and anemia.

Displacement of the gas pattern in the duodenum and jejunum to the left side is indicative of hepatomegaly (C is the correct answer to Question 8-9). Hepatic metastases from lung cancer were later confirmed.

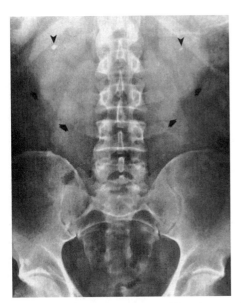

▲ **Figure 8-20.** Case 8-11. A 40-year-old man presents with back pain.

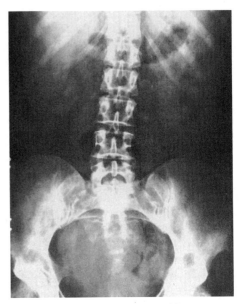

▲ **Figure 8-21.** Case 8-12. A 45-year-old woman presents with lower abdominal fullness.

8-10. In this case, a soft-tissue mass in the left upper quadrant displaces the gas in the splenic flexure of the colon downward. Left adrenal or renal cell carcinoma rarely presents as a large mass to the left of the midline. The most likely diagnosis is splenomegaly (D is the correct answer to Question 8-10).

8-11. In this case, a mass in the midabdomen delineates the lower poles of both kidneys, which are fused at the midline, consistent with horseshoe kidney (D is the correct answer to Question 8-11). Small renal calculi (arrowheads) are present bilaterally.

8-12. This case shows a soft-tissue mass in the pelvis. In a middle-aged woman, an ovarian or uterine mass would be the most likely considerations. Ultrasonography of the pelvis showed a large, fluid-filled mass, confirmed surgically as an ovarian cyst (A is the correct answer to Question 8-12).

Discussion

Although abdominal plain radiographs are useful in detecting hepatomegaly or splenomegaly, they are of little use in diagnosing hepatic disease, particularly if hepatomegaly is not present. Other imaging modalities, such as ultrasonography, CT (Figures 8-22, 8-23), MR imaging, and radionuclide liver scans, are more sensitive and accurate for evaluating hepatic primary diseases or metastases. In addition, barium studies of the gastrointestinal tract and CT may be helpful in excluding gastric outlet obstruction, carcinoma, or renal cell carcinoma.

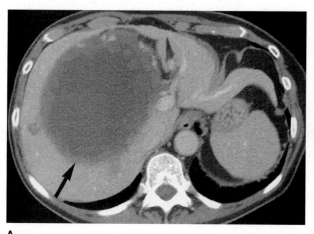
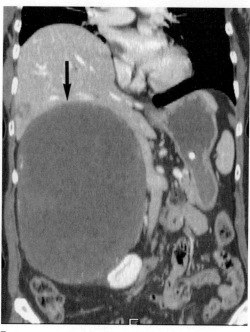

A   **B**

▲ **Figure 8-22.** Hepatomegaly. Axial (**A**) and coronal (**B**) CT scans shows a large oval well-circumscribed hypoattenuating mass (arrow) in the liver secondary to a cavernous hemangioma.

Fusion of the kidneys may occur in the embryologic stage during the second month of gestation. Most (95%) of these fusions occur at the lower poles of the kidneys. CT shows the kidney to be vertical or even in the reverse oblique direction and its position to be lower than normal. Horseshoe kidney may be associated with other congenital anomalies, as well as a high incidence of urinary tract obstruction, infection, or stone formation. A horseshoe kidney may also deviate the upper ureters laterally.

When the plain film suggests the presence of a pelvic mass, a specific diagnosis is often not possible. Pelvic ultrasonography, CT (Figure 8-24), or MR imaging better demonstrates the pelvic organs and their interrelationship and will differentiate between solid and fluid content in the mass.

EXERCISE 8-4. INTESTINAL DISTENTION

8-13. What is the most likely diagnosis in Case 8-13 (Figure 8-25)?
  A. Functional ileus of the bowel
  B. Mechanical obstruction of the colon
  C. Mechanical obstruction of the small bowel
  D. Pneumoperitoneum

8-14. What is the most likely diagnosis in Case 8-14 (Figure 8-26)?
  A. Functional ileus of the bowel
  B. Gastric outlet obstruction
  C. Mechanical obstruction of the small intestine
  D. Pneumoperitoneum

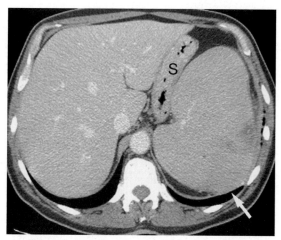

▲ **Figure 8-23.** Splenomegaly. CT shows a massively enlarged spleen (arrow) that displaces the stomach (S) medially in a patient with chronic myelogenous leukemia.

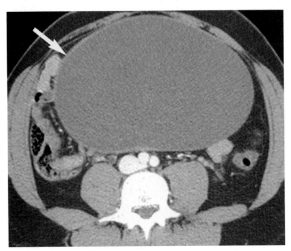

▲ **Figure 8-24.** Pelvic mass. CT shows a large intraperitoneal mass (arrow) that arose from a clear cell carcinoma of the right ovary.

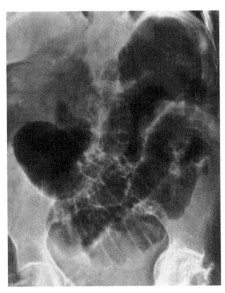

▲ **Figure 8-26.** Case 8-14. A 65-year-old woman presents with abdominal distention and a history of abdominal surgery.

8-15. What is the most likely cause of the distended bowel loop (arrowheads) in Case 8-15 (Figure 8-27)?
   A. Cecal volvulus
   B. Functional ileus of the bowel
   C. Pneumoperitoneum
   D. Sigmoid volvulus

8-16. What is the most likely diagnosis in Case 8-16 (Figure 8-28)?
   A. Ascites
   B. Functional ileus of the bowel
   C. Mechanical obstruction at the colon
   D. Mechanical obstruction at the small bowel

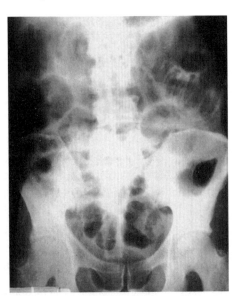

▲ **Figure 8-25.** Case 8-13. A 66-year-old man presents with fever, chills, and abdominal pain.

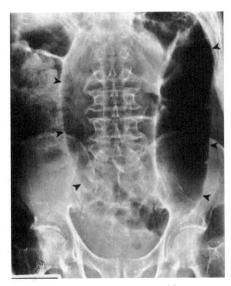

▲ **Figure 8-27.** Case 8-15. A 70-year-old man presents with abdominal distention.

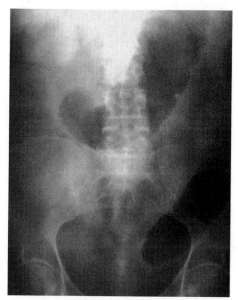

▲ **Figure 8-28.** Case 8-16. A 66-year-old woman presents with abdominal distention and constipation for 3 days.

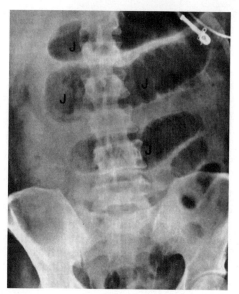

▲ **Figure 8-29.** Two days later, a follow-up abdominal plain film in the same patient as in Figure 8-25 shows a gas pattern in several separated loops of the jejunum (J) at midabdomen indicative of bowel wall thickening, which is confirmed as enteric ischemia.

Radiologic Findings

8-13. In this case, a diffuse abnormal gas pattern with distention of the small bowel, colon, and rectum suggests functional ileus. Two days later the patient underwent laparotomy, and small-bowel ischemia was found (Figure 8-29) (A is the correct answer to Question 8-13). Separation of bowel loops may indicate bowel wall thickening but is a nonspecific sign.

8-14. This case shows gaseous distention of the stomach, duodenum, and jejunum on the supine film, but no gas is seen in the colon, suggesting mechanical small-bowel obstruction. Gastric outlet or duodenal obstruction is unlikely because many jejunal loops are dilated. At surgery, an obstructing jejunal adhesion was found (C is the correct answer to Question 8-14).

8-15. This patient has a huge distended and folded colonic loop in the midabdomen and pelvis (the "coffee bean" sign). The most likely consideration is a sigmoid volvulus (D is the correct answer to Question 8-15).

8-16. This case shows distended transverse colon and descending colon and no gas in the sigmoid colon and rectum. The small bowel is not distended. Mechanical obstruction of the colon distal to the level of descending colon is likely (C is the correct answer to Question 8-16). Barium enema (Figure 8-30) shows

an irregular narrowing at the rectosigmoid region, indicative of sigmoid carcinoma.

Discussion

Generalized or diffuse distribution of gas, both in the small bowel and in the colon, is more indicative of a functional

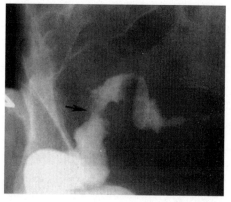

▲ **Figure 8-30.** Barium enema in the same patient as in Figure 8-28 shows a narrowing (arrow) with an irregular contour at the rectosigmoid region, suggesting sigmoid carcinoma as the cause of colonic obstruction.

ileus. The most common causes of functional ileus are post-operative status, neuromuscular diseases, ischemia, and intrinsic or extrinsic inflammations. Air-fluid levels may be seen in patients with functional ileus when plain films are obtained with the patient in upright or decubitus position.

Limited distribution of abnormal gas in the intestine favors a mechanical obstruction. Air-fluid levels may also be seen in patients with mechanical obstruction when an upright abdominal radiograph is obtained. The most common causes of mechanical obstruction in the small bowel are adhesions, internal or external hernias, neoplasms, or intussusceptions. Ileocolic intussusception is common in children.

When the small bowel is filled with a large amount of fluid, a row of small gas bubbles may be trapped between the valvulae conniventes. The row of gas bubbles is called the "string of beads" or "string of pearls" sign and is seen on the decubitus or upright view of the abdomen (Figure 8-31). A fluid-filled, closed-loop small bowel obstruction may appear as an oval mass in the abdomen and is known as the "pseudo-tumor sign" (Figure 8-32). These signs suggest a mechanical obstruction and possible strangulation.

Sigmoid volvulus may twist along the mesenteric axis and the long axis of the bowel. The twisted and overdistended sigmoid colon may appear as an inverted U shape or a coffee bean shape, without haustra or septa, at the upper

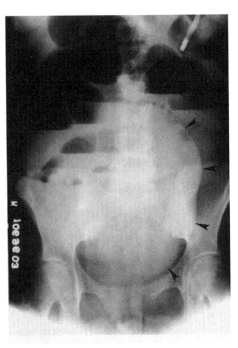

▲ **Figure 8-32.** Small-bowel obstruction shows a huge mass (arrowheads, pseudotumor sign) in the midabdomen with several adjacent fluid levels. (From Chen MYM, Zagoria RJ, Ott DJ, Gelfand DW. *Radiology of the Small Bowel,* New York, Igaku-Shoin, 1992, used with permission)

pelvis and abdomen crossing the transverse colon. The colon above the sigmoid may be distended; however, the small bowel is rarely distended in a patient with sigmoid volvulus. Barium enema may show a beaking sign adjacent to the twisted point. Vascular insufficiency may occur if volvulus cannot be corrected.

A small-bowel volvulus may be caused by internal hernia or adhesion similar to that of sigmoid volvulus. Small-bowel volvulus may be located outside the pelvis with no proximal colonic dilatation. Cecal volvulus is the cause of 1% to 2% of intestinal obstructions. Most often a cecal volvulus is twisted and relocated in the midabdomen or left upper quadrant (Figure 8-33).

Mechanical obstruction of the colon is commonly caused by colonic neoplasm, volvulus, or inflammatory mass caused by diverticulitis of the left colon. All colonic segments proximal to the mechanical obstruction are distended with gas or a combination of gas and feces. When intestinal secretions and fecal matter fill the distended bowel loop, solid and liquid contents produce a mottled appearance. Whether the small bowel becomes distended from a colonic obstruction depends on its duration and severity, and also on the

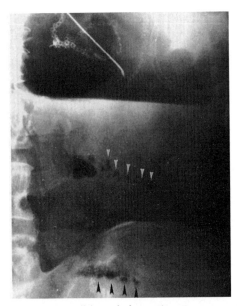

▲ **Figure 8-31.** Small-bowel obstruction. Two rows of air bubbles (arrowheads) with fluid levels in the left midabdomen are indicative of mechanical obstruction in the small intestine.

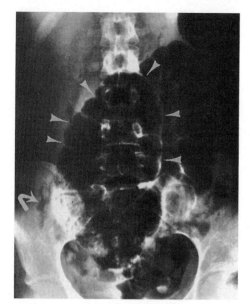

▲ **Figure 8-33.** A distended cecum and right colon (arrowheads) are seen at midabdomen. The terminal ileum (curved arrow) is located laterally to the cecal volvulus. Barium enema may delineate the twisted point in the ascending colon.

competency of the ileocecal valve. Abdominal radiographs are often of limited value in differentiating the cause of bowel distention, and CT is more useful for locating a mechanical obstruction (Figure 8-34).

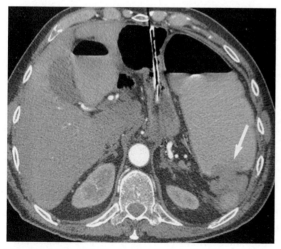

▲ **Figure 8-34.** Colonic mechanical obstruction. CT shows a large intraluminal mass (arrow) in a dilated transverse colon due to adenocarcinoma of the splenic flexure.

EXERCISE 8-5. INCREASED OR DECREASED DENSITY IN THE ABDOMEN

8-17. What is the most likely diagnosis in Case 8-**17** (Figure 8-35)?
   A. Bullous emphysema
   B. Colon interposition
   C. Pneumoperitoneum
   D. Tension pneumothorax

8-18. What is the most likely diagnosis in Case 8-18 (Figure 8-36)?
   A. Functional ileus of the bowel
   B. Mechanical obstruction of the colon
   C. Mechanical obstruction of the small bowel
   D. Pneumoperitoneum

8-19. What is the most likely diagnosis in Case 8-19 (Figure 8-37)?
   A. Ascites
   B. Functional ileus
   C. Gallstone ileus
   D. Mechanical obstruction in the small bowel

8-20. What is the most likely diagnosis in Case 8-20 (Figure 8-38)?
   A. Ascites
   B. Hemoperitoneum
   C. Pelvic teratoma
   D. Uterine fibroma

Radiologic Findings

8-17. This case shows crescent-shaped lucencies beneath both hemidiaphragms outline the liver on the right

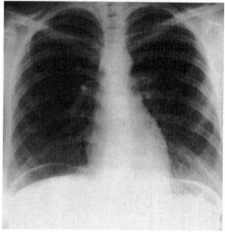

▲ **Figure 8-35.** Case 8-7. A 35-year-old man is seen who underwent laparotomy 2 days earlier.

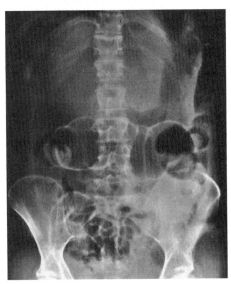

▲ **Figure 8-36.** Case 8-18. A 49-year-old woman presents with acute abdominal pain.

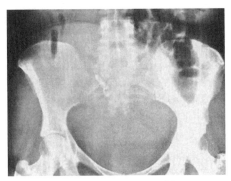

▲ **Figure 8-38.** Case 8-20. A 45-year-old woman is seen who had a motor vehicle accident.

double-wall sign is seen on the supine film of the abdomen because there is air within the intestinal lumen and in the peritoneal cavity, caused by rupture of a viscus (D is the correct answer to Question 8-18).

8-19. In this case, the hepatic angle (arrowheads) and the descending colon (D) are displaced medially, the small bowel (S) is located centrally in the abdomen, and there is increased density in the pelvis, suggesting ascites (Figure 8-40) (A is the correct answer to Question 8-19).

and the spleen on the left in the PA chest film, suggesting pneumoperitoneum (C is the correct answer to Question 8-17).

8-18. This case shows both the inner and outer walls of the transverse colon (arrows) (Figure 8-39). This

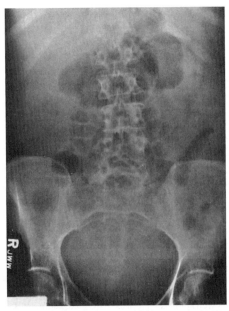

▲ **Figure 8-37.** Case 8-19. A 40-year-old woman presents with abdominal distention.

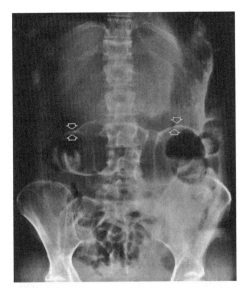

▲ **Figure 8-39.** In a patient with pneumoperitoneum (same patient as in Figure 8-36), the double-wall sign shows inner and outer walls of the transverse colon (arrows) delineated by air in the colon and in the peritoneal cavity.

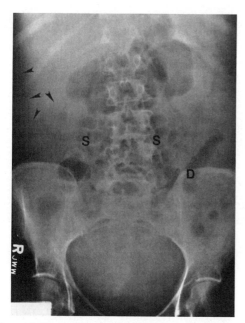

▲ **Figure 8-40.** Ascites shows hepatic angle (arrowheads, Hellmer's sign) and descending colon (D) displacing medially, small bowel loops (S) located centrally, and increased density in the pelvis.

8-20.   In this case, the soft-tissue density with no gas pattern in the pelvis is consistent with hemoperitoneum in this motor vehicle accident victim. CT better evaluates hemoperitoneum (Figure 8-41) (B is the correct answer to Question 8-20).

Discussion

In adults, the most common causes of pneumoperitoneum are postoperative status, ruptured abdominal viscus, and peritoneal dialysis. Residual air in the abdomen after surgery may persist for 1 to 2 weeks. Serial abdominal films, however, should show a gradual reduction in the amount of free peritoneal air. A persistent or increasing amount of air on postoperative serial films suggests a perforated viscus or ruptured surgical anastomosis. Spontaneous pneumoperitoneum is commonly caused by the perforation of a duodenal ulcer. Less common causes include pneumomediastinum, pulmonary emphysema, pneumatosis intestinalis, and entrance of air per vagina.

Pneumoperitoneum is most readily detected on the upright film of the chest, even if only a small amount of air is present. The left lateral decubitus view is useful and may show small amount of free air accumulating between the right lateral margin of the liver and the peritoneal surface. Normally, the interface between the air and inner intestinal wall is visible, but the serosal surface is not appreciated because its density is similar to that of the adjacent peritoneal contents. When gas is present in the peritoneal cavity, however, both inner and outer walls will be delineated; this is called the "double-wall sign" or "Rigler's sign". A visible serosal margin of bowel can also be simulated by normal adjacent omental fat or adjacent contiguous loops of small or large bowel (Figure 8-42). If in doubt, the upright or left lateral decubitus film may confirm pneumoperitoneum. CT is more sensitive than plain radiograph in assessing pneumoperitoneum (Figure 8-43). Colon interposition occurs on the right between the liver and hemidiaphragm, and haustrations are usually recognized that aid differentiation from pneumoperitoneum.

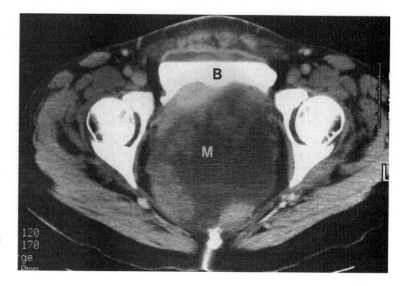

▲ **Figure 8-41.** CT shows a large soft-tissue mass (M) shadow with different attenuation in the pelvis, pushing the bladder (B) anteriorly. Hemoperitoneum was the diagnosis in this patient with a history of trauma.

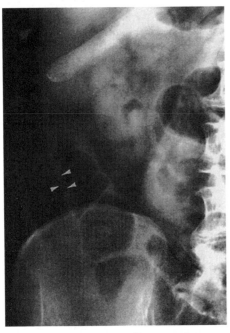

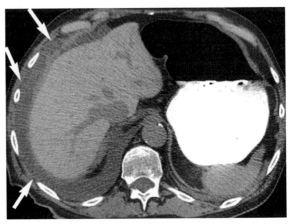

▲ **Figure 8-44.** Ascites. CT shows the presence of perihepatic ascites (arrows) in a patient with heart failure.

▲ **Figure 8-42.** False double-wall sign. Both inner and outer walls of the ascending colon (arrowheads) are outlined by air inside the colon and fat shadow outside.

Although plain film of the abdomen is not sensitive in assessing small amounts of intraperitoneal fluid, the plain film can demonstrate moderate and large amounts of fluid collection. In ascites, the hepatic angle may be obscured or

displaced medially (Hellmer's sign). The ascending or descending colon may be displaced medially by fluid in the paracolic gutter. A large amount of fluid may accumulate in the pelvis, causing increased density and symmetrical bulges. Other signs, such as separation of the small bowel loops and overall higher density in the abdomen, are also seen, but not often. CT (Figure 8-44) and ultrasonography (Figure 8-45) more accurately assess intraperitoneal fluid and coexistent masses.

Blood and pus have a similar density to that of ascitic fluid in the peritoneal cavity; therefore, hemoperitoneum may

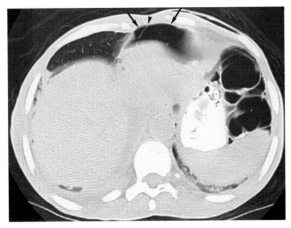

▲ **Figure 8-43.** Pneumoperitoneum. CT confirms free air (arrows) in the peritoneal cavity showing falciform ligament (arrowhead).

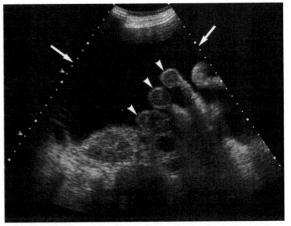

▲ **Figure 8-45.** Ascites. Ultrasonography shows anechoic fluid (arrows) and floating bowel loops (arrowheads).

produce signs similar to those found in ascites. High density in the pelvis is a sign of hemoperitoneum in patients with a history of trauma. CT better evaluates hemoperitoneum.

EXERCISE 8-6. EXTRALUMINAL GAS PATTERN

8-21. What is the most likely diagnosis in Case 8-21 (Figure 8-46)?
   A. Colonic diverticulitis
   B. Mechanical obstruction of the colon
   C. Pneumatosis cystoides intestinalis
   D. Pneumoperitoneum

8-22. What is the most likely diagnosis in Case 8-22 (Figure 8-47)?
   A. Abscess
   B. Functional ileus
   C. Gallstone ileus with gas in the biliary tree
   D. Hepatic portal vein gas

8-23. What is the most likely diagnosis in Case 8-23 (Figure 8-48)?
   A. Gallstone ileus with gas in the biliary tree
   B. Hepatic portal venous gas
   C. Pneumoperitoneum
   D. Right subdiaphragmatic abscess

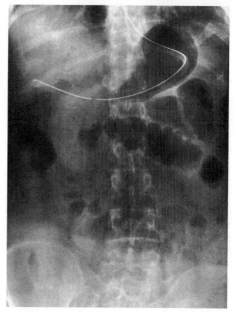

▲ **Figure 8-47.** Case 8-22. A 66-year-old woman is admitted with vague abdominal pain and vomiting.

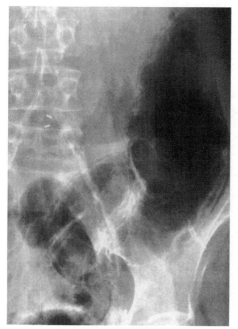

▲ **Figure 8-46.** Case 8-21. A 42-year-old man presents with mild abdominal pain.

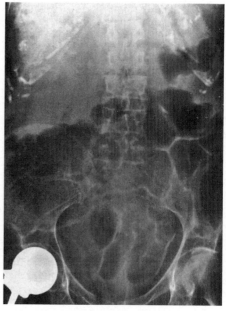

▲ **Figure 8-48.** Case 8-23. A 77-year-old woman presents with fever and a 1-week history of abdominal pain.

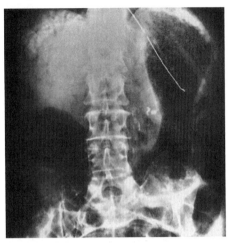

▲ **Figure 8-49.** Case 8-24. A 64-year-old man presents with fever, abdominal pain, and distention.

8-24. What is the most likely diagnosis in Case 8-24 (Figure 8-49)?
   A. Gallstone ileus with gas in the biliary tree
   B. Hepatic portal venous gas
   C. Pneumoperitoneum
   D. Subdiaphragmatic abscess

Radiologic Findings

8-21. This case shows linear air streaks along the descending and sigmoid colon in a patient with mild abdominal pain. These streaks indicate pneumatosis cystoides intestinalis (C is the correct answer to Question 8-21).

8-22. This case shows a distended proximal jejunum and a few air bubbles in the right upper quadrant, indicating gallstone ileus with mechanical obstruction and air in the biliary tree (Figure 8-50 A). An upper gastrointestinal study demonstrates a distended proximal small bowel, a fistula (Figure 8-50B) between the biliary tree and the duodenum, and three gallstones in the small bowel (Figure 8-50 C). CT shows air in the biliary tree (Figure 8-50 D) (C is the correct answer to Question 8-22).

8-23. In this case, multiple air bubbles in the right upper quadrant in a patient with fever are consistent with a subdiaphragmatic abscess (Figure 8-51). Bilateral linear rib calcifications and right hip replacement are also seen (D is the correct answer to Question 8-23).

8-24. This case shows a fine arborizing linear gas pattern in the right upper quadrant extends to the periphery of the liver, indicating portal venous gas (B is correct answer to Question 8-24).

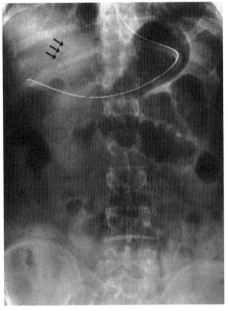

A

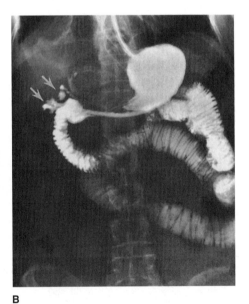

B

▲ **Figure 8-50.** (**A**) Gallstone ileus, in the same patient as in Figure 8-47, is seen as distended small-bowel loops and air bubbles at the right upper quadrant (arrows). (**B**) Upper gastrointestinal series shows reflux of barium suspension into the biliary tree through a cholecystoduodenal fistula (arrows).

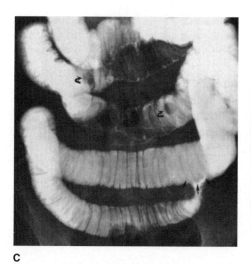

C

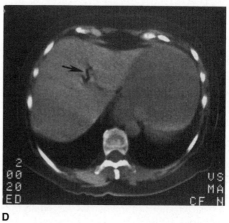

D

▲ **Figure 8-50.** *(Continued)* (**C**) Small-bowel examination shows three gallstones in the small bowel (arrows), with the distal stone (straight arrows) causing obstruction. (**D**) CT study demonstrates air (arrow) in the biliary tree in the same patient. (A-D from Chen MYM, Dyer RD, Zagoria RJ, et al: CT of gallstone ileus. *Appl Radiol* 1991;20:37-38, used with permission).

Discussion

Pneumatosis cystoides intestinalis appears as linear streaks of gas or intramural cystic collections of gas in the small bowel or colon. The cysts range in size from 0.5 to 3 cm and may extend into the adjacent mesentery. Pneumatosis intestinalis is an incidental finding in most patients, usually with a self-limited benign course; simple bowel obstruction, volvulus, and air from the mediastinum or retroperitoneum are commonly associated. Pneumatosis intestinalis may be caused by ischemic and necrotizing enterocolitis in patients with leukemia or non-Hodgkin lymphoma and in those who have had bone marrow transplantation.

Gallstone ileus, the mechanical obstruction of the small bowel by an impacted gallstone, is commonly seen in elderly women. Clinical presentation in gallstone ileus is nonspecific,

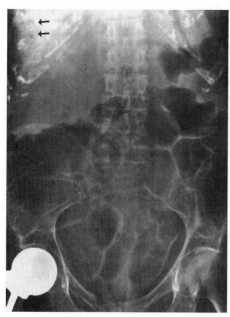

▲ **Figure 8-51.** Multiple air bubbles (arrows) (same patient as in Figure 8-48) in the right upper quadrant indicate a subdiaphragmatic abscess.

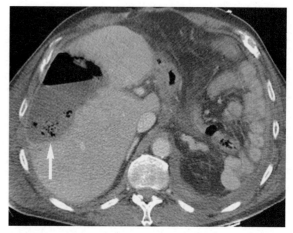

▲ **Figure 8-52.** Pyogenic liver abscess in a 55-year-old man with 3 days of fever, chill, and productive cough after right lobectomy. CT shows mottled gas collection (arrow) in the right lobe indicating liver abscess.

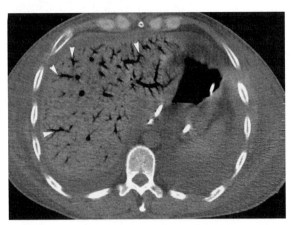

▲ **Figure 8-53.** Portal venous gas. CT shows tiny numerous branching gas collections (arrowheads) extending toward the periphery of the liver.

and the mortality rate is high (15%). A gallstone enters the intestinal lumen via a cholecystoenteric fistula. Major radiographic signs include small-bowel obstruction, air in the biliary tree, and an ectopic gallstone seen on plain abdominal film, upper gastrointestinal series, or CT study.

Abscess in the subphrenic and subhepatic spaces is a serious problem, with a mortality rate of 30%. Subphrenic abscess may arise spontaneously or as a complication of abdominal surgery, pancreatitis, diverticulitis, or appendicitis. A cluster of gas may be seen on plain film in 70% of abscesses. Left-sided abscess is difficult to discern because gas in the splenic flexure, stomach, or jejunum may mimic gas within

the abscess. Other radiographic findings include elevation of the adjacent hemidiaphragm, pleural effusion, and basilar atelectasis. CT is more accurate in assessing hepatic and extra-hepatic abscess (Figure 8-52).

In the right upper quadrant, when multiple tubular lucencies are seen reaching the lateral hepatic margins, portal venous gas is a likely consideration (Figure 8-53). Biliary tree gas is located in the central hepatic zone near the porta hepatis. Benign portal venous gas has been noted in sigmoid diverticulosis, nonobstructed splenic flexure carcinoma, ulcerative colitis, and bronchopneumonia. Mesenteric vascular insufficiency and necrotizing intestinal infection are common causes of hepatic portal venous gas. In children, necrotizing enterocolitis produces intramural gas within mesenteric veins to the liver; the mortality rate in patients with the sign of hepatic portal venous gas is higher than in those without portal venous gas.

Acknowledgments *Special thanks to my colleague Dr. Michael Oliphant, MD, for providing me with the CT images used in this chapter.*

SUGGESTED READING

1. Baker SR, Cho KC. *The Abdominal Plain Film with Correlative Imaging.* 2nd ed. New York: McGraw-Hill, 1998.
2. Chen MYM, Bechtold RE, Bohrer SP, Zagoria RJ, Dyer RB. Abnormal calcification on plain radiographs of the abdomen. *Crit. Rev. Diagn. Imaging.* 1999;40:63-202.
3. Meyers MA. *Dynamic Radiology of the Abdomen: Normal and Pathologic Anatomy.* 5th ed. New York: Springer-Verlag; 2000.
4. Gore RM, Levine MS. *Textbook of Gastrointestinal Radiology.* 3rd ed. Philadelphia: WB Saunders; 2007.

Radiology of the Urinary Tract

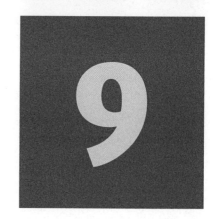

Jud R. Gash, MD

Jacob Noe, MD

Techniques and Normal Anatomy
Abdominal Radiography
Computed Tomography
Ultrasonography
Magnetic Resonance Imaging
Nuclear Medicine
Retrograde Pyelography/Cystography/Urethrography
Angiography

Technique Selection
Exercises

Five years is a long time in radiology, and the pace of change in imaging has even quickened since the prior edition of this text. The increasing availability and technical capability of cross-sectional modalities such computed tomography (CT), magnetic resonance imaging (MRI), and ultrasound (US) now dominate imaging of the urinary system with multidetector (spiral) CT having the greatest impact. In our department, CT is called the "temple of truth" for good reason. These cross-sectional modalities have essentially eliminated the intravenous pyelogram (IVP), which after 70 years of being the backbone of urinary tract imaging, has had its epitaph written, and has little if any role in modern-day urinary imaging. The result of these progressive advances in imaging continues to be improved, earlier, and more accurate diagnosis of genitourinary tract disease.

This chapter introduces the basic concepts in imaging of the urinary tract. First, the imaging modalities currently in clinical practice and principles of their interpretation are discussed, especially regarding normal anatomy and its variants. The importance of choosing the most appropriate study for a given clinical scenario cannot be overemphasized, and the next section of the chapter reviews technique selection. A series of clinical exercises and case examples follow, demon-

strating important imaging concepts and diseases of the urinary tract. Finally, suggested readings is provided at the end of the chapter.

TECHNIQUES AND NORMAL ANATOMY

This section introduces the common radiologic techniques used in evaluation of the urinary tract, with emphasis on an overview of each technique as it applies to the urinary tract. A discussion of normal anatomy and some important fundamental concepts of interpretation are included. A basic knowledge of the gross anatomy is assumed, with emphasis placed on the radiographic anatomic correlations.

▶ Abdominal Radiography

Conventional radiographs, or "plain films," are an inexpensive, quick overview of the abdomen and can occasionally provide useful diagnostic information for selected urinary tract indications. A radiograph of the abdomen when used to evaluate the urinary tract is often referred to as a KUB (kidney, ureter, and bladder). "Gas, mass, bones, stones" can be used as a reminder of main areas to examine on the abdominal radiograph. On the normal abdominal radiograph, the renal outline may be visible adjacent to the upper lumbar spine and should be bilaterally symmetric and measure between 3 and 4 lumbar vertebrae in length. The ureters are not discernable, although knowledge of their normal course, between the tips of lumbar transverse process tips and pedicles, along the mid sacral ala, and finally gently coursing laterally below the sacrum to enter the bladder, allows for potential stone identification. The distended bladder may also be visible, if outlined by fat, on the KUB. The most common genitourinary findings seen on abdominal radiography will be in the form of urinary tract calcifications (Figure 9-1). Unfortunately, the KUB suffers from poor sensitivity and specificity regarding urinary tract calcifications. In the past, it was reported that 80% of calculi were radiopaque and could be identified on conventional radiographs. However, recent studies suggest that no more than 40% to 60% of urinary tract stones are detected and accurately diagnosed on plain radiographs. The sensitivity for detection of stones is limited when the calculi are small, of lower density composition, or when there is overlapping stool, bony structures, or air obscuring the stones. Additionally, the specificity of conventional radiography is somewhat limited because a multitude of other calcifications occur in the abdomen, including arterial vascular calcifications, pancreatic calcifications, gallstones, leiomyomas, and many more (more than 200 causes of calcification in the abdomen have been described). Phleboliths, which are calcified venous thromboses, are especially problematic because they frequently overlap the urinary tract and are difficult to differentiate from distal ureteral stones. Lucent centers are a hallmark of phleboliths, whereas renal calculi are often most dense centrally. Rarely, the conventional radiograph may suggest a soft-tissue mass or abnormal air (gas) within the urinary tract. Emphysematous pyelonephritis, a urologic emergency with high mortality, is the result of a renal infection by gas-producing organisms and may be diagnosed on plain films by mottled or linear collections of air within the renal parenchyma. Bony lesions, such as sclerotic bony changes, can suggest metastatic prostate cancer, and lytic bony lesions can be seen with disseminated renal cell carcinoma. Additionally, the bony changes of renal osteodystrophy (diffuse bony sclerosis) may be identified on plain radiographs. Vertebral anomalies are associated with congenital malformations of the urinary tract. Thus, although the KUB is limited by low sensitivity and specificity, close examination of the "gas, mass, bones, stones" may yield important, sometimes critical, diagnostic information.

▶ Computed Tomography

Multidetector (spiral) CT is now the dominant radiologic imaging modality for evaluation of the urinary tract and adrenal glands. Several factors make CT quite effective. The high contrast and spatial resolution afforded by CT allow detection and evaluation of subtle differences in very small structures. Mathematical calculations of the attenuation of the CT x-ray beam allow quantitative evaluation of the relative density of structures (ie, their Hounsfield units) and by using these "CT numbers," much unique diagnostic information on the urinary tract is gained. Examinations can be performed quickly and reproducibly with thin CT slices of the entire urinary tract now obtainable in just a few seconds. With these advances, CT can now be used to evaluate much of the urinary tract, including vascular, parenchymal, and urothelial components as well as adjacent structures including the adrenal glands.

Careful techniques and protocols are critical to CT accuracy. CT scans of the urinary tract may be performed with and/or without intravenous iodinated contrast material depending on the indications. CT performed without contrast is typically used for the detection of renal or ureteral calculi, for which it is exquisitely sensitive. Additionally, noncontrast views of the kidneys serve as a baseline to evaluate for lesion enhancement after contrast administration, a critical factor in mass evaluation. Intravenously administered iodinated contrast is excreted by the kidney primarily by glomerular filtration, opacifying the urinary tract progressively from the

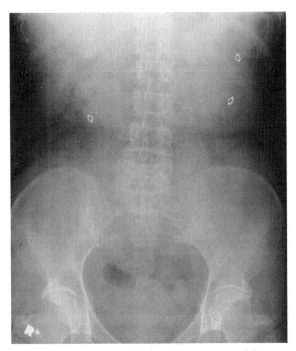

▲ **Figure 9-1.** Normal KUB. Note that portions of the normal renal contours (arrows) are visible and should be evaluated. There are no abnormal calcifications, soft-tissue densities, or bony lesions evident.

kidney through the ureter and to the bladder. Contrast "opacification" during CT is most accurate, exquisitely demonstrating and evaluating the urinary tract. One of the major advances in the past 5 to 10 years has been advent of CT urography (CTU), a superior replacement of the IVP. CTU is most often indicated for evaluation of hematuria and typically consists of three scanning phases—noncontrast, nephrographic (90 seconds), and delayed (8 to 10 minutes) excretory phase. The noncontrast phase allows for stone detection and serves as a baseline to assess possible mass enhancement. The nephrographic phase is predominately used to evaluate the kidneys for mass lesions. Finally, the excretory phase allows assessment of the collecting system, particularly for the detection of urothelial carcinoma (Figure 9-2). Frequently, the axial CT images are augmented with multiplanar and three-dimensional reconstructions (Figure 9-3).

The kidneys, which enclose the renal sinus and are surrounded by retroperitoneal fat, are well delineated on CT. The renal parenchyma is composed of outer cortex, containing much of the nephron, as well as the pyramid-shaped collecting duct containing inner medulla. On noncontrast examinations, the kidneys are homogeneous and have a density similar to most soft tissue (Figure 9-4 A). With rapid scanning after contrast administration, several sequential

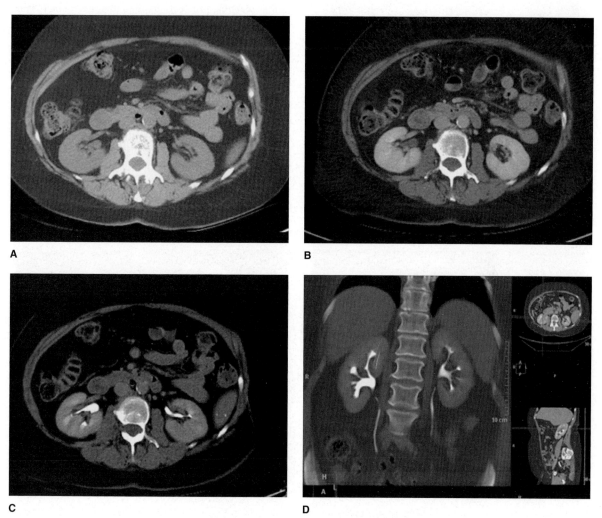

A   B

C   D

▲ **Figure 9-2.** Normal CT urogram. Note the homogeneous renal density on the noncontrast images (**A**), with bright enhancement of the renal parenchyma during the nephrographic phase (**B**), followed by intense opacification of the collecting system during the excretory phase (**C**). Multiplanar reformats are often very helpful (**D**).

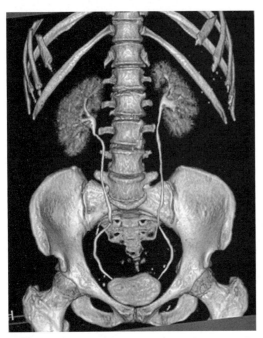

▲ **Figure 9-3.** 3-D reconstruction. Three-dimensional postprocessed volume-rendered image of the urinary tract beautifully demonstrate the kidneys, ureters, and bladder.

phases of opacification within the kidney can be delineated by CT including the corticomedullary, nephrographic, and excretory phases. The corticomedullary phase can be seen if scanning is performed during the first 20 to 70 seconds after contrast administration and represents the early preferential blood flow to the renal cortex (Figure 9-4 B). Subsequently, contrast begins to pass into the distal collecting tubules within the renal medulla, resulting in a more homogeneous opacification of the renal parenchyma termed the CT nephrographic phase (Figure 9-4 C). This generally occurs around 90 to 120 seconds after contrast medium injection. Finally, the excretory phase is seen when contrast opacifies the collecting system. Each different phase of opacification may better demonstrate different disease processes, and thus various scanning protocols are used to evaluate the kidneys depending on the clinical indication.

On CT, the kidneys should be evaluated for size, location, orientation, and contour (Figure 9-5). The kidneys are typically located at the level of the upper lumbar spine with the right kidney slightly lower than the left. They generally lie with their axes along the psoas muscles with the upper pole slightly more medial than the lower pole. Alterations in position and orientation of the kidneys may be related to congenital anomalies such as pelvic kidneys or may be secondary to mass effect from an adjacent lesion. The size of the kidneys is somewhat variable depending on the age, sex, and size of the patient, but generally range from 11 to 14 cm. Although the right is often slightly smaller than the left, the kidneys should be relatively symmetric in size, with a discrepancy

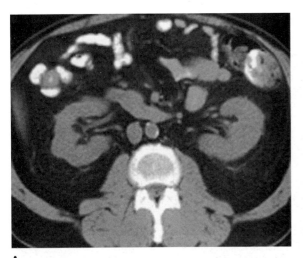

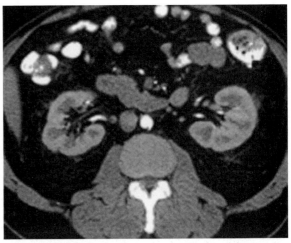

A   B

▲ **Figure 9-4.** Normal CT renal phases. Note the homogeneous density of the noncontrast portion (**A**), the distinction of cortex and medulla of the corticomedullary phase (**B**), and the once again homogeneous enhancement during the nephrographic phase (**C**).

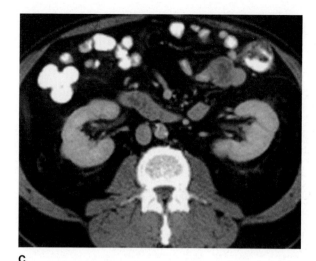

C

▲ **Figure 9-4.** *(Continued)*

greater than 2 cm suggesting pathology. There are a number of causes of abnormal renal size, ranging from incidental anomalies such as congenital renal hypoplasia to clinically significant conditions such as renal artery stenosis (small kidney) or infiltrating renal neoplasm (large kidney). The kidneys should have a reniform shape and a smooth contour. Clefts suggest scarring, which most often results from chronic vesicoureteral reflux/chronic bacterial pyelonephritis or from

renal infarcts. Additionally, the kidneys should be evaluated for calcifications, hydronephrosis, and inflammation. A critical role for CT is mass/cyst detection and characterization. CT is very specific in identifying a lesion as a simple cyst when the lesion is homogenous and of water density, typically <10 HU. Lesions of higher density may represent hyperdense (complex) cysts or solid masses, and further evaluation with contrast CT to detect enhancement may be needed to differentiate these causes. Fat within a solid mass generally allows a confident diagnosis of angiomyolipoma. A solid, non-fat-containing mass in the adult should be considered a renal cell carcinoma until proven otherwise. CT is also useful in staging renal neoplasms. Non-neoplastic renal disease, such as trauma and complicated infections, is accurately demonstrated on CT, providing specific information regarding the extent and severity of the process. The remainder of the retroperitoneum, containing fat, the normal occupants of the retroperitoneum (kidneys, adrenal glands, pancreas, duodenum, and parts of the colon), and vascular structures, is well seen by CT, and diseases such as inflammation, infection, and neoplasms are readily demonstrated. Additionally, the thin section and rapid imaging of modern CT also allows noninvasive evaluation of the vascular system, including the major renal arterial and venous structures (Figure 9-6).

As previously mentioned, the unenhanced CT of the urinary system, commonly referred to as the urinary tract CT or "stone study," is the procedure of choice for the detection of urolithiasis and associated obstruction, with unmatched specificity and sensitivity. There are many other advantages

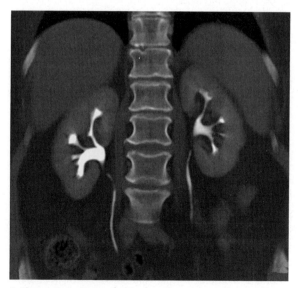

▲ **Figure 9-5.** Normal size, location, orientation, and contour of the kidneys.

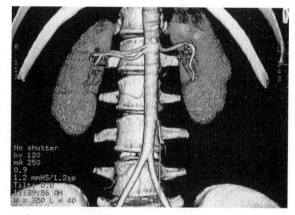

▲ **Figure 9-6.** Normal CT angiogram of the renal arteries, 3-D reconstruction. Note that this image clearly demonstrates that there are two right renal arteries. This is a normal variant. In this case, the renal arteries are patent without evidence of significant stenosis.

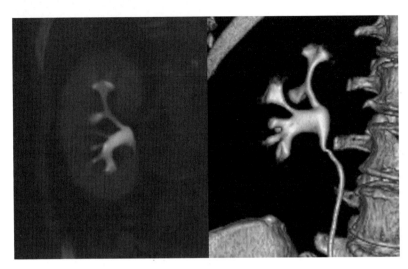

▲ **Figure 9-7.** Normal intrarenal collecting system. Coronal reformat and volume-rendered CT images demonstrate the normal intrarenal collecting system anatomy.

to using CT to evaluate suspected ureteral stones, including speed of the examination, identification of alternative explanations for the pain (appendicitis, diverticulitis, aneurysm, etc), and elimination of intravenous contrast complications. Scans no thicker than 5 mm are performed from the top of the kidneys to the symphysis pubis. The ureter can be visualized and followed from the renal pelvis to the bladder in most cases and appears as a tubular 2- to 3-mm fluid structure surrounded by retroperitoneal fat. Stones can be diagnosed by their high density and location within the ureter. Secondary signs of obstruction have been described, including dilation of the proximal ureter. As on the KUB, phleboliths can prove troubling because of their frequent close approximation with the distal ureter; however, their central lucency, lack of surrounding inflamed ureteral wall, and lack of secondary signs of obstruction usually allow their distinction.

Although visible without contrast material, the intrarenal collecting system, ureters, and bladder are conspicuous and nicely demonstrated when contrast material has been administered and delayed images obtained. Collecting system anatomy is now visible in fine detail with the use of modern high-resolution (<1 mm) spiral CT and multiplanar (coronal, sagittal) and three-dimensional reformat methods. The intrarenal collecting system consists of calyces, infundibula, and the renal pelvis. Normally, each kidney consists of 7 to 14 evenly distributed calyces (Figure 9-7). The individual renal calyx, from the Latin for "chalice," is a delicate-appearing cup-shaped structure. Not uncommonly, partial fusion of the calyces occurs, especially in the renal poles, creating the compound calyx. Other calyceal variants occur, including variants of number (polycalycosis, unicalyx kidney) and size (megacalycosis, microcalyx) and must be differentiated from true pathology. The normal delicate, cuplike appearance can be distorted or irregular in conditions such as papillary necrosis, tuberculosis, or urothelial (transitional cell) carcinoma. Diverticula may arise from the calyces creating a haven for stone formation, recurrent infection, or even transitional-cell malignancy. The renal pelvis is also quite variable in appearance. A common variation is the so-called extrarenal pelvis, where the pelvis lies outside the renal sinus. In this setting, the pelvis tends to be more prominent and rounded, mimicking hydronephrosis. This can be differentiated from true obstruction by normal-appearing calyces. The ureters appear as contrast-containing, rounded structures in the retroperitoneum (Figure 9-8). Because of peristalsis, portions of the ureters may be collapsed. On CT, the bladder appears as a rounded water or contrast density structure in the pelvis.

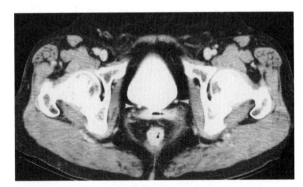

▲ **Figure 9-8.** Normal CT showing the distal ureters and urinary bladder opacified with intravenous (IV) contrast. After a 5-minute delay, the distal ureters (arrowheads) and bladder are easily identified. Delayed images may be necessary to evaluate the ureter or bladder in certain circumstances.

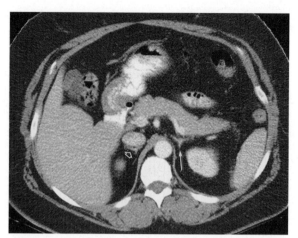

▲ **Figure 9-9.** Normal CT of the adrenals. The left adrenal has the characteristic inverted Y shape (arrow) while the right, located immediately behind the inferior vena cava, is somewhat more linear in appearance (open arrow) in this case.

Detection of malignancy arising from the urinary tract epithelium is a major concern, particularly with the advent of CT urography. Urothelial neoplasia generally appears as papillary solid lesions arising from the urothelial mucosa. Occasionally, urothelial neoplasm may appear as a more flat area of mucosal thickening. The urethra is not normally seen on CT.

The adrenal glands are well seen on CT, appearing as linear, arrowhead, or inverted Y-shaped structures usually consisting of body and medial and lateral limbs (Figure 9-9). The adrenal glands are normally less than 1 cm in thickness and 3 to 4 cm

in length. They lie cephalad to the kidneys, with the right just posterior to the inferior vena cava (IVC) and the left antero-medial to the upper pole of the left kidney. Note that the embryological and functionally distinct outer cortex and inner medulla are not visibly separable. Although occasionally affected by trauma or infection, the adrenal mass evokes the most attention, and for this CT evaluation is well suited.

▶ Ultrasonography

Ultrasound is a useful technique for evaluation of the urinary tract, with its principal advantages including wide availability, no need for intravenous contrast material, and lack of ionizing radiation. The kidneys are generally well seen by a posterior or lateral approach in all but the largest of patients (Figure 9-10). The renal medulla is hypoechoic (darker) relative to renal cortex and can be identified in some adults as cone-shaped central structures. In some patients, this corticomedullary distinction is not visible and should not be considered pathologic. The renal cortex is isoechoic or slightly hypoechoic compared with the echogenicity of the adjacent liver. Renal echogenicity exceeding that of the liver is abnormal and requires explanation. Most commonly, hyperechoic kidneys are the result of medical renal disease, such as end-stage hypertensive glomerulosclerosis. In addition to echogenicity and as with CT evaluation, the kidneys should be assessed for size, location, and symmetry. Scarring and masses can be evaluated. US assessment is often specific in identifying simple or mildly complicated cysts and differentiating these lesions from a solid mass. Solid masses, however, remain nonspecific and generally require further evaluation. There are normal variants that can mimic mass lesions, including dromedary humps, as well as central prominences of normal

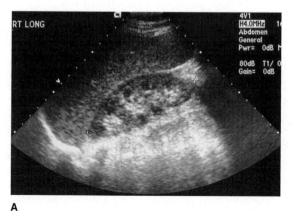

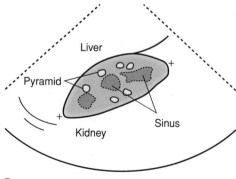

A   **B**

▲ **Figure 9-10.** Normal renal ultrasound, long axis view (**A**) and drawing (**B**). Note the smooth contour of the kidney. The rounded to cone-shaped medullary pyramids are hypoechoic to the cortex and should not be mistaken for a mass or dilated collecting system. The renal cortex should be similar to or slightly hypoechoic compared with liver. In addition, notice the hyperechoic fat of the renal sinus—the central echo complex.

renal tissue interposed between lobes referred to as persistent columns of Bertin. Additionally, the parenchyma near the renal hila may appear prominent as well, occasionally mimicking a mass. Each of these variants may be distinguished by its normal echogenicity, lack of mass effect, and characteristic location. Occasionally, additional imaging with CT or MR may be required in equivocal masses. The renal sinus is the area engulfed by the kidney medially, harboring the renal pelvis, arteries, veins, nerves, and lymphatics that enter and exit the kidney, all contained within a variable amount of fat. Fat is typically brightly echogenic on ultrasound, and fat within the renal sinus dominates the ultrasonographic appearance, creating what is known as the "central echo complex." The size of the central echo complex is variable, often more prominent in the elderly and minimal in the child. Absence of the central echo complex may suggest a mass such as a urothelial carcinoma replacing the normal fat. Alternatively, the complex may be very prominent in the benign condition of renal sinus lipomatosis. Calcifications often have a typical appearance on ultrasound, being brightly echogenic and resulting in shadowing posteriorly as the sound waves are attenuated. Renal stones or calcifications may be detected within the renal parenchyma or in the intrarenal collecting system. The echogenicity of the normal renal sinus, however, may be problematic by obscuring or mimicking small stones. Ultrasound is also excellent for detecting hydronephrosis, with the distended collecting system easily recognized within the central echo complex. The ureters are not normally seen on ultrasound because of obscuring overlying tissue and their small size. Evidence of their patency may be verified by Doppler detection of urine rapidly entering the bladder from the distal ureters that is, distal ureteral jets (Figure 9-11). The bladder is seen as a rounded or oval anechoic (fluid)

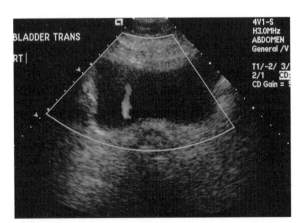

▲ **Figure 9-11.** Normal ultrasound image of a ureteral jet. Color Doppler image shows the stream of urine entering the urinary bladder through the ureteral orifice, consistent with an unobstructed normal ureter.

structure in the pelvis. The bladder may demonstrate mass lesions, such as transitional-cell carcinoma, or stones. The urethra is not typically seen by ultrasound, although urethral diverticula may occasionally be demonstrated.

▶ Magnetic Resonance Imaging

Just as with CT, technical advances in MR imaging have led to increasing use in urinary tract imaging. Fast scanning techniques allowing breath-hold imaging, combined with the spectacular tissue contrast of MR imaging and the ability to directly image in any plane, make this an attractive modality for evaluating the urinary tract. Lack of ionizing radiation adds to its appeal, although cost, availability, claustrophobia, and the contraindication of certain materials including pacemakers remain major drawbacks. Finally, MR imaging of the kidney is performed with gadolinium as the contrast agent, not iodinated contrast material. The risk of contrast-induced nephropathy is minimal because of the very low concentrations of gadolinium chelate used in a typical MR study. A new phenomenon, however, has been described known as nephrogenic systemic fibrosis (NSF), which is a systemic disorder associated with significant morbidity and mortality, almost always seen in end-stage renal disease patients with a glomerular filtration rate (GFR) of less than 30 mL/min. Previously, MR was used as a primary modality in patients with renal insufficiency to avoid iodinated contrast nephropathy, but the advent of NSF as a clinical entity has contraindicated contrast-enhanced MR in these patients.

On MR imaging, the kidneys appear of variable signal intensity depending on the imaging factors, and as in CT, contrast-enhanced phases of imaging (arterial, corticomedullary, nephrographic, and excretory) are all visible (Figure 9-12). Specific imaging sequences are designed to manipulate imaging factors to allow for optimum evaluation of the particular clinical concern. The ability to image in any plain is advantageous for MR imaging. The kidneys should be evaluated in a similar fashion to that of other modalities. Finally, the adrenal glands are well seen by MRI, similar to CT; the normal shape is the same as described for CT, and the signal intensity depends on particular imaging parameters. The ureters and bladder can also be evaluated and are well depicted.

MR urography is an emerging modality that promises to offer, or perhaps exceed, many of the benefits of CT urography without the use of ionizing radiation or the need for contrast administration (in some protocols). No consensus protocol for MR urography exists at this time. Many protocols, referred to as "static-fluid MRU," use T2-weighted techniques only, analogous to MR cholangiopancreatography (MRCP). Techniques using IV gadolinium, "excretory MRU," use multiphase T1 imaging in a manner similar to CT urography to evaluate the renal parenchyma and collecting system. Interpretation of the renal collecting system, ureters, and bladder with MR urography is similar to that of

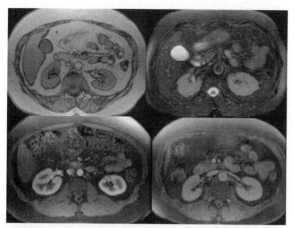

▲ **Figure 9-12.** Normal MRI of the kidneys. The appearance of the kidneys is variable on MRI depending on imaging factors. The top left image is a T1-weighted sequence, and the top right is T2 weighted, whereas the bottom images were obtained after gadolinium injection and demonstrate corticomedullary and nephrographic phases.

CT urography. A major limitation of MR urography is the limited sensitivity for calculi relative to CT. MR urography is equally sensitive for congenital or acquired structural anomalies. Relative sensitivity and specificity of MR versus CT urography for urothelial neoplasm is not well established. Although MR urography is proving effective for many of the indications of CT urography, the excellent availability, reproducibility, and performance of CTU as well as the cost, time, and insensitivity to stone disease has limited the utility of MRU.

Note should also be made of the developing use of MR in the staging of prostate cancer. MR of the prostate with the use of an endorectal coil is now in clinical use as a staging tool for diagnosed prostate cancer, assessing size of lesions, adenopathy, and involvement of other pelvic structures. Other benign prostatic processes mimic the signal characteristics of carcinoma, limiting the specificity of MR for screening and initial diagnosis. Correlation of MRI findings with prostate-specific antigen levels and with MR spectroscopy yields higher specificities; however, in clinical practice sonographically guided transrectal biopsy remains the standard of care for initial diagnosis.

▶ Nuclear Medicine

The basic technique of a nuclear medicine study is discussed in Chapter 1, whereas here we briefly examine the more specific role in evaluation of the urinary tract. In general, the value of nuclear imaging in the urinary tract is severalfold: functional information related to the quantifiable collected

data, lower radiation dose than traditional radiographic techniques, and very low incidence of complications. Renal evaluation is typically performed by intravenous bolus injection of renal specific agents such as technetium-labeled mercaptoacetyltriglycine (Tc-MAG$_3$). Images are acquired every few seconds demonstrating renal blood flow with additional images obtained over several minutes showing renal uptake and excretion. The recorded data can be used to produce images, but it also is quantifiable and is employed to generate time-activity curves (Figure 9-13). Information about renal perfusion, morphology, relative function of each kidney, and excretion can be extremely useful in evaluation of conditions such as renovascular hypertension, obstruction, and renal transplant examination. Although anatomically oriented data can be obtained with other radioisotopes that aggregate more in the renal parenchyma, in general, nuclear medicine renal studies suffer from fairly low spatial resolution and are therefore often used in conjunction with other imaging studies. Radionuclide cystography is another useful test used to diagnose and monitor vesicoureteral reflux. Here, technetium pertechnetate is mixed with saline and infused into the bladder with subsequent images obtained over the urinary tract. This study is quite sensitive for the detection of significant reflux, but at a considerably lower radiation dose than conventional cystography, making it particularly useful in children, especially in those needing follow-up and repeated imaging. Another important study is the radioactive

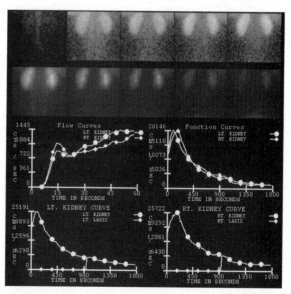

▲ **Figure 9-13.** Normal ^{99m}Tc-MAG$_3$ renogram. Images are shown in the upper portion of the figure demonstrating the radioisotope progressing through the urinary tract. In the bottom portion of the figure, quantitative data are expressed in renogram curves.

iodine labeled metaiodobenzylguanidine (MIBG) examination. MIBG collects in adrenal medullary tissue and is useful in diagnosis and evaluation of pheochromocytoma. Positron emission tomography (PET) is evolving as a powerful imaging tool, especially when combined with CT (PET/CT), combining the functional data of PET with the anatomic CT information. Unfortunately, fluorine-labeled deoxyglucose (FDG), which is the primary agent used in PET/CT, is normally excreted by the kidneys, obscuring urinary tract pathology and limiting utilization. PET/CT has, however, shown promise in evaluation of possible metastatic disease.

▶ Retrograde Pyelography/ Cystography/Urethrography

Direct injection of water-soluble iodinated contrast material is a useful method of examining various regions of the urinary tract. The advantage of this method of evaluation is the direct control over the contrast injection rather than reliance on secondary excretion from the kidney.

Retrograde pyelography, often carried out in conjunction with cystoscopy, is performed by placing a small catheter into the distal ureter. Contrast material is then injected through this catheter into one or both ureters. Fluoroscopy and conventional radiographs should then be obtained. This study usually results in excellent evaluation of the ureter and intrarenal collecting system. The ureter is typically seen in its entirety, which rarely occurs with other imaging studies. Interpretation is similar to that of CT urography, with the caveat that the contrast within the collecting system is under greater pressure than physiologic conditions and mild ballooning of the calyces as well as occasional extravasation can occur normally.

Imaging of the bladder is performed with a cystogram, where a catheter is placed into the bladder and contrast material is then injected. The contrast material is optimally injected under fluoroscopic observation but occasionally is performed with only static conventional radiographs, such as in the trauma setting. One advantage to cystography is that vesicoureteral reflux can be evaluated during the conventional cystogram. The urethra may be evaluated with contrast material via two methods. In one, the urethra is evaluated during voiding, often following a cystogram (voiding cystourethrogram or VCUG). Alternatively, a retrograde study may be performed (retrograde urethrogram). The urethra in the male consists of four portions, including the prostatic, membranous, bulbous, and penile portions. During voiding, the urethra is fairly uniformly distended and tubular in appearance. On a retrograde study, the more posterior urethra (prostatic and membranous) is often contracted and seen as a thin wisp of contrast. The female urethra appears as a short, slightly funnel-shaped tubular structure during voiding (Figure 9-14). The urethra in males is generally evaluated for injuries and strictures but may also be examined for filling defects, masses, and fistulas.

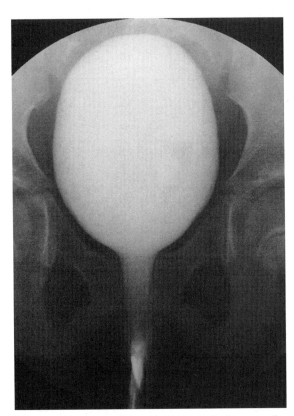

▲ **Figure 9-14.** Normal female VCUG. Note the smooth contour of the urinary bladder and the short, conical-appearing urethra.

▶ Angiography

The role of angiography as a diagnostic tool continues to diminish with the increasing accuracy of noninvasive techniques to evaluate the vascular system. The renal arteriogram is performed after puncture of a more peripheral vessel such as the common femoral artery, with advancement of a catheter into the renal artery origin. Contrast material is injected via the catheter and rapid, typically digital, conventional radiographic images are obtained. The renal arterial vessels are well demonstrated, along with nephrographic images of the kidney and views of the venous drainage (Figure 9-15). Delayed images may be obtained to demonstrate the renal collecting system. The angiogram plays little role in diagnostic evaluation of the renal parenchyma, having been supplanted by cross-sectional imaging techniques. However, the still superior spatial resolution of angiography permits detailed evaluation of the renal arterial supply and has a small but important diagnostic role in evaluating the small vessels of the kidney for such diseases as vasculitis and fibromuscular dysplasia. The

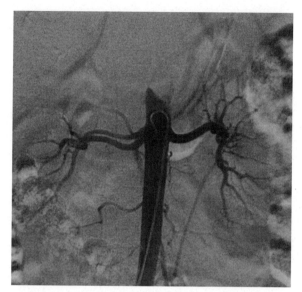

▲ **Figure 9-15.** Normal renal arteriogram. The renal arterial system is visualized in detail with spatial resolution superior to that of other techniques. Delayed images can be obtained to show the venous phase and/or the collecting system filling with contrast material.

main role for angiography today, as discussed later, is aiding and guiding interventional, therapeutic techniques.

TECHNIQUE SELECTION

No one ideal technique is yet available for the comprehensive evaluation of the urinary tract. Each technique has strengths and weaknesses that affect its thoroughness and accuracy in evaluating urinary tract diseases, and also patient complaints. Importantly, imaging techniques are not necessarily exclusive and in some circumstances are complementary—taken alone, they may not provide enough information, but together they allow a correct clinical diagnosis. A knowledge of which tests is most appropriate for a given clinical question is paramount for physicians involved with the treatment of urinary tract disease. Issues of cost, complications, and time are consequences of an injudicious study choice. However, most importantly, the diagnosis of a patient's condition may not be made unless the appropriate test has been used to evaluate the condition. This section discusses technique selection.

The plain radiograph (KUB) has fairly limited use for evaluating the genitourinary (GU) tract. Although abnormal "stones, bones, gas, and masses" may be demonstrated by the KUB, the utility of the study is limited by its lack of sensitivity and specificity. The KUB can be used effectively to follow radiographically visible stone disease such as assessing stone

burden or ureteral stone passage; it is also used to assess stent position, especially with ureteral stents.

The conventional radiographic techniques that utilize direct contrast injection (retrograde pyelogram, cystogram, and urethrogram) have specific roles. Two particular studies of choice include the voiding cystogram for evaluating ureteral reflux and the retrograde male urethrogram in suspected urethral injuries and stricture evaluation.

Nuclear medicine sustains its role in functional evaluation of the urinary tract, especially the kidney. Renal scintigraphy is an important tool in the assessment of renal function and can be useful in evaluating renovascular hypertension. The ability to quantitatively assess relative renal function is frequently an important issue for the surgeon, determining whether nephrectomy or attempted renal sparing surgery is most appropriate. The nuclear medicine cystogram, because of its high sensitivity and lower radiation dose, remains a key tool in evaluating and following ureteral reflux, particularly in the young. The MIBG study plays a unique role regarding the pheochromocytoma. The diagnosis of pheochromocytoma is generally made with a classic clinical history combined with confirmatory biochemical evidence, along with confirmatory imaging, typically CT or MRI demonstrating an adrenal mass. MIBG is most often used in detecting metastatic or recurrent disease, or locating extraadrenal lesions. Although PET/CT is limited in primary evaluation of the urinary tract, it has shown strong utility in evaluating metastatic disease; however, its exact role is yet to be determined.

The safety and availability of ultrasound solidify the utility of this modality. Ultrasound is useful in evaluating the kidney for masses, scarring, and hydronephrosis. Several common indications include evaluation of the patient with acute renal failure to exclude postobstructive (hydronephrosis) etiologies, to evaluate for sequelae (scarring) of vesicoureteral reflux in children, and to diagnose simple renal cysts. Ultrasound is generally the study of choice in evaluating the renal transplant as well. However, the relatively small and sometimes technically limited (in large patients) field of view, lack of visualization of the ureters, and lack of functional assessment limit the use of ultrasound in some circumstances. For instance, in the setting of obstruction, ultrasound may demonstrate hydronephrosis, but often the etiology of the obstruction, such as ureteral stone or mass, is not identified. Additionally, solid renal masses are nonspecific on ultrasound and require further imaging, usually with CT. Ultrasound has only moderate sensitivity for detecting renal stone disease. Although the retroperitoneal position of the kidneys usually provides an excellent window for ultrasound, patients with a large habitus continue to become more common, and in these patients sensitivity for small masses or calculi may be markedly diminished.

The diagnostic role of conventional angiography has been nearly eliminated with the use of noninvasive CT and MR angiography. However, two main factors allow for a persistent important role for the angiogram. As described in the technique section, conventional angiography still has superior resolution compared to CT and MRI for small-vessel evaluation. Thus, diagnostic angiography may play a role in diagnosis of small-vessel renal disease such as polyarteritis nodosa. More importantly, catheter angiography allows for the ability to simultaneously treat abnormalities diagnosed at the time of angiography. For example, although many modalities are used to evaluate for renovascular hypertension, angiography alone allows for treatment at the time of diagnosis as in the patient with fibromuscular dysplasia whose hypertension may be cured with transluminal angioplasty at the time of arteriography. The angiogram is similarly used in acute renal hemorrhage, acute arterial obstruction, and occasional renal mass management. The important and wide-ranging role of the interventional radiologist in the management of urinary tract disease is beyond the scope of this chapter.

MR imaging continues to grow in utility for evaluating the urinary tract and is the study of choice in certain instances. Like CT, MR imaging has excellent spatial and contrast resolution and can evaluate the renal vasculature and renal and adrenal anatomy, characterize lesions, and evaluate the bladder and prostate. Fluid/contrast enhancing techniques allow evaluation of the ureters and the remainder of the collecting system. MR imaging is thus an excellent choice to screen for renovascular hypertension and to problem solve difficult renal masses, and it is gaining favor in evaluation of certain ureteral and bladder conditions. However, high cost, limited availability, and contraindications such as pacemakers and claustrophobia limit the use of routine genitourinary MR imaging. In addition, the advent of NSF as a clinical entity has limited the use of contrast-enhanced MRI in patients with advanced chronic renal disease, a population that previously was specifically indicated for MR to avoid iodinated contrast.

Finally, CT is now the examination of choice for urinary tract imaging. The CT scan is the preferred study for many GU conditions and indications including trauma, flank pain, complicated infections, renal and adrenal masses, neoplastic conditions, retroperitoneal disease, and more. CT may be the sole study needed or may serve as an adjunct to other studies. CT urography has become the first-line procedure for evaluation of the urothelium, including hematuria evaluation, replacing the last indications for the IVP. As discussed previously, CT benefits from wide availability, speed, high contrast and spatial resolution, and patient ease. CT is limited when iodinated contrast is contraindicated or radiation exposure is of special concern, such as in pregnancy.

In summary, there is as yet no one comprehensive best imaging examination for the urinary tract; each has its advantages and disadvantages, and their value depends on indications of the study. The physician must combine evidence-based knowledge of the accuracy and utility of various studies with the art of medicine, combining science with finesse to ultimately result in the best possible evaluation and care of the individual patient. Finally, although the requesting physician should be well informed about the utility, accuracy, strengths, and weaknesses of available tests, the best care, especially in the fast-changing field of imaging, is provided by close consultation between the referring physician and radiologist.

EXERCISE 9-1. ADRENAL MASSES

9-1. In Case 9-1 (Figure 9-16), the most likely diagnosis is
   A. adrenal metastasis.
   B. renal angiomyolipoma.
   C. adrenal myelolipoma.
   D. retroperitoneal liposarcoma.

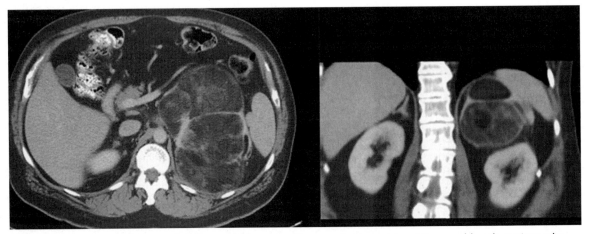

▲ **Figure 9-16.** Case 9-1. CT scan of the upper abdomen with coronal reformat in a 52-year-old male patient who presented with vague left upper abdominal pain.

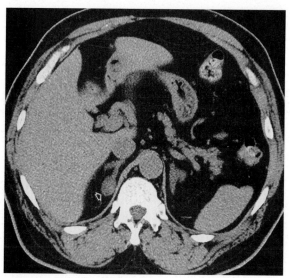

▲ **Figure 9-17.** Case 9-2. CT scan without contrast at the level of the adrenal glands in a 47-year-old patient with newly diagnosed lung cancer who presented to the emergency department for right flank pain.

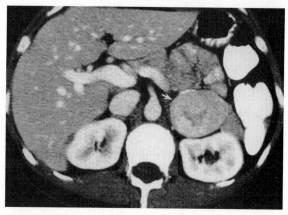

▲ **Figure 9-18.** Case 9-3. CT scan with contrast of the abdomen in a 39-year-old male patient who presented with refractory hypertension and episodes of headaches and palpitations.

9-2. Regarding Case 9-2 (Figure 9-17), in a patient with a primary neoplasm elsewhere, the most common adrenal mass is
   A. metastasis.
   B. adenoma.
   C. adrenal carcinoma.
   D. acute adrenal hemorrhage.

9-3. In Case 9-3 (Figure 9-18), the most likely diagnosis is
   A. pheochromocytoma.
   B. metastasis.
   C. adrenal cyst.
   D. adrenal lymphoma.

Radiologic Findings

In Case 9-1 (Figure 9-16), a 10-cm mass in the left upper abdomen contains areas of macroscopic fat. The mass lies just medial to the spleen and on coronal images is separated from the kidney by a plane of retroperitoneal fat (B is incorrect). Although subtle, the thin rim of tissue surrounding the lesion demarcates the mass and differentiates it from normal adjacent retroperitoneal fat. The fatty nature of the lesions is confirmed by the low-density tissue within the mass, similar to that of adjacent normal retroperitoneal and subcutaneous fat. Fat is rare within adrenal metastasis (A is incorrect). Although the retroperitoneal sarcoma is a differential consideration for a heterogenous retroperitoneal fatty mass, the location of the lesion and commonality of myelolipoma make adrenal

myelolipoma the most likely diagnosis (C is the correct answer to Question 9-1).

Regarding Case 9-2 (Figure 9-17), the diagnosis or exclusion of metastatic adrenal disease is one of the most important issues facing the radiologist in daily practice. The diagnosis of metastatic disease allows appropriate therapy for the patient including the possible prevention of unnecessary surgery. Perhaps more importantly, misdiagnosing a benign lesion as metastatic disease may mistakenly prevent potentially curative therapies such as surgery. In Case 9-2, there is a small 2-cm homogeneous mass arising from the medial limb of the adrenal gland. Recall that the density of a lesion can be quantitated on CT with Hounsfield unit measurements (although not shown, the Hounsfield unit measurements of the mass was 8 HU). Acute adrenal hematomas are high-density masses on non-contrast CT scan measuring between 50 and 90 Hounsfield units (D is incorrect). Adrenal carcinomas are typically large heterogeneous lesions and are quite rare (C is incorrect). The distinction between adrenal metastasis and adenoma is a critical one. Although there can be overlap in their appearances, certain imaging characteristics of adrenal adenomas allow a confident diagnosis in the vast majority of cases, as we see later. Even with a known primary malignancy, however, statistically the most likely etiology of a small adrenal mass is benign adrenal adenoma (B is the correct answer to Question 9-2). There are methods to more confidently differentiate adenoma from metastasis which are covered later.

Case 9-3 (Figure 9-18) demonstrates a 4-cm solid appearing just anterior to the left kidney. Note the fat plane that clearly shows that the mass does not arise from the kidney. No specific characteristics such as fat are seen. The lesion is denser than surrounding muscle, making a cyst unlikely (C is incorrect). Adrenal lymphoma is typically bilateral, usually shows diffuse enlargement of the adrenal glands, and is typically accompanied by retroperitoneal adenopathy (D is incorrect). Although metastatic disease can have variable appearances and cannot be radiographically excluded, the lesion is also typical for a pheochromocytoma and, given the clinical history, this is the most likely diagnosis (A is the correct answer to Question 9-3).

Discussion

The adrenal mass is a common problem for the radiologist and is being incidentally diagnosed with greater frequency with the increased utilization of cross-sectional imaging techniques, especially CT and MRI. In fact, the term "adrenal incidentaloma" has been coined for the small adrenal mass identified on imaging studies obtained for other reasons. Although there are many causes of adrenal masses, the most common include benign adenomas, metastatic disease, adrenal carcinoma, and myelolipomas.

The most common adrenal mass is the adrenal adenoma. Although they can be hyperfunctioning and result in clinical syndromes, the majority of adrenal adenomas are nonhyperfunctioning and are diagnosed incidentally. Distinguishing these "incidentalomas" from more significant pathology is critical. Fortunately, most adenomas have specific characteristics that allow a confident diagnosis. Many adenomas are similar to normal adrenal cortical tissue in that they contain a high proportion of cellular lipid material. This results in a low-density appearance and Hounsfield measurements on unenhanced CT that are highly specific for adenoma. Certain adenomas have a paucity of lipid, however, and may be otherwise differentiated from other masses by their enhancement characteristics. Specifically, contrast enhancement is rapidly lost in adenomas on delayed images, a phenomenon known as "washout." MRI can be used to demonstrate lipid-rich adenomas by using special imaging sequences that reveal intracellular lipid. MRI is no better than CT for demonstrating the characteristic washout of the adenoma. Given the widespread availability and reliability of CT, CT remains the primary modality for evaluating a nonspecific adrenal lesion.

The adrenal gland is a common site of metastatic disease, with breast and lung being the most common sources. The imaging characteristics of metastatic disease are quite variable. Lesions may be unilateral or bilateral, homogeneous or heterogeneous in appearance (Figure 9-19). The larger the metastatic lesion, generally, the more necrosis and hemorrhage and the more heterogeneous the lesion appears. Smaller lesions tend to be more uniform. Fortunately, unlike adenomas, metastatic disease does not contain high intracellular lipid and thus does not show the lipid-type imaging changes that characterize adenomas. However, metastatic disease can be indistinguishable from other adrenal pathology and histologic confirmation with biopsy may be necessary.

Pheochromocytomas are an unusual catecholamine-producing tumor arising from the sympathetic innervation

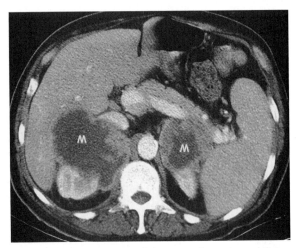

▲ **Figure 9-19.** CT scan with contrast shows large bilateral adrenal masses (M) with extensive central necrosis typical of advanced adrenal metastatic disease.

of the adrenal gland most commonly originating in the adrenal medulla, although in 10% of cases they may arise in an extraadrenal location. Most tumors arise sporadically, although a small percentage occur in certain syndromes. Most pheochromocytomas produce a constellation of symptoms referable to their catecholamine production, including hypertension and episodic headaches and palpitations. Most pheochromocytomas appear as a nonspecific adrenal mass on CT. Many of these lesions are fairly homogeneous solid masses. However, necrosis, calcification, and cystic formation all occur. On MRI, the diagnosis may be suggested by the fairly specific finding of a very bright adrenal mass on T2-weighted images. Finally, MIBG, which collects in adrenal medullary-type tissue, can provide important information about these tumors. Although they may be used to confirm the diagnosis of a suspected adrenal pheochromocytoma, a more important role for MIBG imaging is in the evaluation of metastatic disease or recurrent tumor, or for the localization of extraadrenal lesions. The MIBG scan typically shows a brightly intense area of activity at the site of the lesion (Figure 9-20).

EXERCISE 9-2. RENAL MASS

9-4. Based on the MR images for Case 9-4 (Figure 9-21), what is the most likely diagnosis?
A. A dromedary hump
B. A malignant primary renal neoplasm
C. A simple renal cyst
D. A metastatic lesion from a distant primary malignancy

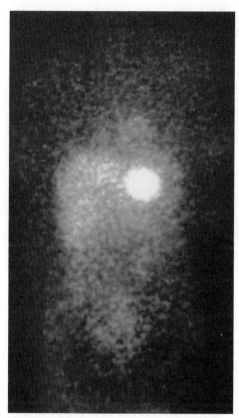

▲ **Figure 9-20.** MIBG scan showing an intense area of increased activity within this proven left adrenal pheochromocytoma.

9-5. Which is *not* true of the lesion shown in Case 9-5 (Figure 9-22)?
  A. This lesion contains fat.
  B. CT is the key to definitive diagnosis.
  C. The ultrasound finding is nonspecific.
  D. The lesion shown is the most common malignant renal neoplasm.

9-6. Which of the following is *not* true of the lesion seen in Case 9-6 (Figure 9-23)?
  A. This is the most common primary renal malignancy.
  B. This lesion is classically associated with the clinical triad of flank pain, hematuria, and a palpable mass.
  C. This type of lesion often contains fat.
  D. This lesion does not enhance with IV contrast.

9-7. How can one differentiate the lesion in Case 9-7 (Figure 9-24) from that seen in Case 9-6?
  A. By CT densitometry
  B. By ultrasonographic characteristics
  C. These lesions cannot be distinguished by imaging.
  D. By MR signal characteristics

Radiologic Findings

Regarding Case 9-4 (Figure 9-21), the MRI images show a rounded, exophytic T2-intense lesion with heterogeneous internal signal on T1 sequences. This appearance is highly suspicious for renal cell carcinoma (B is the correct answer to Question 9-4). Patients with VHL (Von Hippel-Lindau) have a 70% risk of developing renal cell carcinoma by 60 years of age. This lesion clearly differs in signal characteristics from

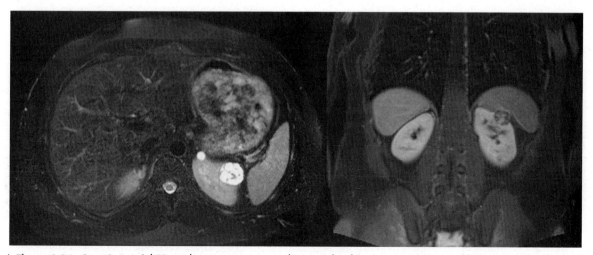

▲ **Figure 9-21.** Case 9-4. Axial T2- and postcontrast coronal T1-weighted images in a 40-year-old woman with history of Von Hippel-Lindau who undergoes MRI after a renal contour abnormality is seen on a urinary tract CT at an outside facility.

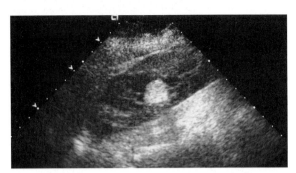

A

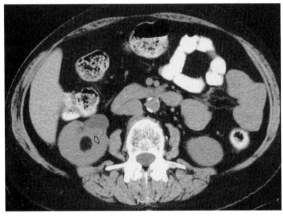
B

▲ Figure 9-22. **(A)** Case 9-5. A 45-year-old woman presents for a right upper quadrant ultrasound to evaluate for gallbladder disease. An image of her right kidney obtained during this study is displayed. **(B)** Case 9-5. A subsequent CT following the ultrasound.

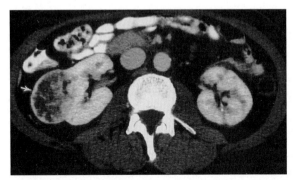

▲ Figure 9-23. Case 9-6. A CT scan with intravenous and oral contrast of the abdomen in a 55-year-old man who presented with a history of right flank pain and hematuria.

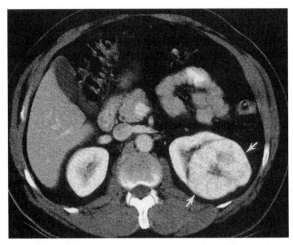

▲ Figure 9-24. Case 9-7. A CT scan of the abdomen in a 60-year-old man who presented with left flank pain and hematuria.

normal renal parenchyma (A is incorrect). Renal cysts would be homogenously T2 intense, with only thin septation at present, and would not demonstrate diffusely heterogeneous T1 signal (C is incorrect). A metastasis could imitate renal cell carcinoma (RCC) in signal, but would be less likely (D is incorrect).

In Case 9-5, the ultrasound image (Figure 9-22 A) reveals a hyperechoic lesion with echogenicity similar to that of adjacent perirenal fat. However, this appearance on ultrasound is nonspecific and requires further evaluation, and a CT scan should generally be obtained. The CT results (Figure 9-22 B) show that this lesion (arrow) does indeed contain fat. The presence of definitive fat within a renal mass is virtually pathognomonic for the diagnosis of angiomyolipoma (AML), which is a benign lesion containing fat, blood vessels, and smooth muscle (D is the correct answer to Question 9-5).

For Case 9-6, the lesion seen (Figure 9-23) is an inhomogenous soft-tissue mass (arrow) arising from the right kidney, which proved to be a renal cell carcinoma. It displays many of the common CT characteristics of RCC, including a somewhat rounded shape with irregular margins, enhancement with IV contrast material, and inhomogeneity (which can be due to hemorrhage, proteinaceous debris, and even calcifications). Renal cell carcinomas almost never contain fat (C is the correct answer to Question 9-6).

Regarding Case 9-7, the lesion has imaging and clinical characteristics indistinguishable from those of RCC. However, the lesion (arrows) (Figure 9-24) is an oncocytoma, a benign tumor arising from the distal tubule or collecting ducts. Classically, oncocytoma is often associated with a characteristic central stellate scar. However, scarring can be seen in a RCC as well, and these lesions cannot be reliably distinguished by imaging alone (C is the correct answer to Question 9-7).

Discussion

These cases demonstrate examples of the most common renal masses, both benign and malignant. In general, all of these renal masses expand and displace normal renal parenchyma and normal collecting-system structures. They are distinguished from infiltrating processes (such as infiltrating neoplasms, infections, and infarctions), which tend to preserve normal renal morphology. Expansile or exophytic renal masses may be seen by cross-sectional imaging and occasionally by conventional radiography if the mass is large. Imaging is used primarily to differentiate between those lesions that are clearly benign, those that are probably benign but require surveillance, and those that may be malignant and require tissue diagnosis.

The simple cyst is the most common renal mass, present in up to 50% of the population over the age of 50. They are almost always asymptomatic and discovered incidentally. Although they occasionally may become infected, hemorrhage, or cause pain, their main importance lies in differentiating the lesions from renal tumors. Cysts can be single or multiple, unilateral or bilateral, and vary greatly in size. Pathologically they are thought to be acquired lesions arising from blocked collecting ducts or tubules. They have thin fibrous capsules lined with epithelial cells and contain clear serous fluid. Only the largest of renal cysts may be evident on plain x-rays. On cross-sectional imaging modalities, cysts are sharply demarcated from adjacent parenchyma, homogenous in appearance, rounded with imperceptible walls, and do not enhance with the administration of contrast material. By ultrasound, a clearly anechoic lesion demonstrating enhanced through-transmission of sound as well as the foregoing criteria can be diagnosed as a simple cyst. On unenhanced CT, cysts measure near water density (<10 HU). No mural nodularity or thick septation should be seen by CT. Internal hemorrhage often makes cysts appear complex, and in these cases, contrast must be administered to evaluate for enhancement that would indicate a mass. An exception is in homogenous lesions measuring greater than 70 HU in attenuation. Recent studies have indicated that these hyperdense lesions almost always represent a hyperdense cyst. Lesions not fulfilling these criteria for cyst, such as those with thick enhancing walls, those containing internal debris, or those with calcifications, may represent cystic neoplasms and must be evaluated further by serial imaging and/or histological diagnosis.

Solid renal masses are of even greater concern. One such lesion, the angiomyolipoma, is most easily distinguished from other renal masses by the presence of internal fat. These lesions are hamartomatous tumors of mesenchymal origin that are usually well differentiated and benign. In addition to fat, they contain sheets of smooth muscle and thick-walled blood vessels. Incidence is highest in middle-aged females. Although these are usually asymptomatic, they are predisposed to spontaneous hemorrhage, especially when large. They can occur as sporadic solitary lesions or in association with tuberous sclerosis, in which case multiple AMLs are often present. Twenty percent of patients with an AML will have tuberous sclerosis, and up to 80% of patients with tuberous sclerosis will have an AML. Macroscopic fat in a renal mass by CT is essentially diagnostic of AML. Although these lesions are benign, they are often removed when greater than 4 to 5 cm because of the increased risk of hemorrhage, and for this reason smaller AMLs require follow-up to monitor the lesion for growth.

Another benign renal neoplasm that deserves comment is the oncocytoma, which originates from the epithelium of the distal tubules or collecting ducts. A central stellate scar is a characteristic, although nonspecific, pathologic feature of these lesions. They are typically asymptomatic and discovered incidentally, though they occasionally may be associated with a flank mass, pain, or hematuria. On cross-sectional imaging studies, oncocytomas appear as a well-defined renal mass. The diagnosis of oncocytoma may be suggested by a central stellate scar. However, even when classic, the imaging characteristics described earlier cannot be used to reliably differentiate them from malignant renal cell carcinoma, and excision is generally indicated. Note that biopsy is usually not recommended because the cytologic appearance of oncocytoma and renal cell carcinoma may be indistinguishable.

Renal cell carcinoma (RCC) is the most common primary renal malignancy, originating from the epithelium of the proximal tubule, having a male predominance and a peak incidence in adults in their 50s. Any renal mass lesion that cannot be definitively identified as one of the benign entities mentioned earlier must be assumed to be RCC until proven otherwise, most often by tissue diagnosis. Classically, RCC is associated with the clinical triad mentioned earlier of flank pain, a flank mass, and hematuria, although all three are present in less than 10% of cases. More commonly, these lesions are being discovered incidentally before symptoms have developed. They may demonstrate calcifications in up to 30% of cases. On ultrasound, a nonspecific renal mass is seen. RCC may be hyperechoic and mimic AML or have central necrosis mimicking the central scar of oncocytomas. By CT, they tend to be rounded soft-tissue masses, enhancing after the administration of IV contrast. When small, they are often homogeneous, though when larger they are more heterogeneous, frequently with necrosis and often with calcifications. One important role for imaging beyond detecting renal cell carcinoma is evaluating the extent of tumor spread. RCC can extend locally and invade adjacent soft tissues, especially when large and extensive. In addition, renal cell carcinoma has a propensity to spread into the renal veins and beyond, and the extent of this must be delineated prior to surgery. Enlarged lymph nodes and spread to liver, lung, bones, and other areas, suggesting metastatic disease, should be sought. Surgical excision is the treatment of choice for resectable lesions, making accurate staging to determine surgical candidacy all the more important.

EXERCISE 9-3. STONE DISEASE

9-8. What is the most likely diagnosis for the patient in Case 9-8 (Figure 9-25)?
  A. Acute appendicitis
  B. Right ureteral calculus
  C. Ruptured aortic aneurysm
  D. Pelvic phlebolith

9-9. What is the most likely diagnosis for the patient in Case 9-9 (Figure 9-26)?
  A. Medullary nephrocalcinosis
  B. Cortical nephrocalcinosis
  C. Renal tuberculosis
  D. Emphysematous pyelonephritis

Radiographic Findings

Case 9-8 (Figure 9-25) is a CT scan of the abdomen obtained without intravenous contrast. Stranding in the fat planes can be seen on the right in the retroperitoneum. Stranding within the fat planes on a CT is a nonspecific finding resulting from many conditions. In general, the stranding can be related to inflammation such as recent surgery, infection, or abnormal fluid collections such as blood or urine. Thus, the stranding seen in this case could result from any of the three listed possible answers. However, within the right ureter is a high-density rounded structure (arrow) consistent with a ureteral calculus (B is the correct answer to Question 9-8). Two main parame-

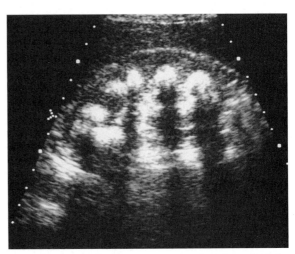

▲ Figure 9-26. Case 9-9. An ultrasound of the right kidney in a 41-year-old female with a history of vague flank pain and recurrent urinary tract infections.

ters that should be noted are the size and location of a stone, as these two factors are directly related to the likelihood of stone passage. Additionally, once the diagnosis of a ureteral stone is made, the radiologist must continue to evaluate the remainder of the scan, because additional abnormalities may also exist.

In Case 9-9, a renal ultrasound (Figure 9-26) demonstrates rounded highly echogenic areas throughout the central parenchyma of the kidney. Several important additional observations include strong uniform shadowing posteriorly from the echogenic areas consistent with sound attenuation and suggesting calcification. Although attenuation of the ultrasound beam occurs with air, such as might occur with emphysematous pyelonephritis, the shadowing in those cases is often "dirty" in appearance, being somewhat inhomogeneous (D is incorrect). Also, the calcifications are located in the medullary area of the kidney, unlike the cortical location of cortical nephrocalcinosis (A is correct answer to Question 9-9).

Discussion

Suspected stone disease is a common indication for urinary tract imaging. Calcifications occurring in the kidney can be dystrophic, related to abnormal tissue such as within tumors, cysts, or infection. This type of calcification is to be distinguished from nephrocalcinosis and nephrolithiasis. Nephrocalcinosis refers to the development of calcification within the renal parenchyma, generally unrelated to an underlying renal pathology. Furthermore, nephrocalcinosis should be distinguished from nephrolithiasis, in which there are stones within the collecting system. Note that nephrocalcinosis and nephrolithiasis may coexist.

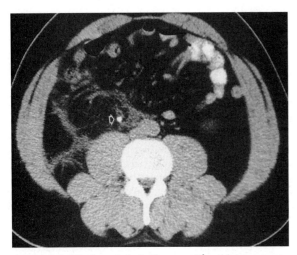

▲ Figure 9-25. Case 9-8. A CT scan without intravenous contrast in a 36-year-old female who presented with acute right flank pain.

Nephrocalcinosis is additionally subdivided into two categories depending on location. That which occurs in the renal cortex is termed cortical nephrocalcinosis, and that within the medulla is called medullary nephrocalcinosis. Cortical nephrocalcinosis is less common and occurs most frequently in the setting of chronic glomerulonephritis or acute cortical necrosis. Acute cortical necrosis most often occurs in the setting of hypotensive shock or toxic ingestion. Cortical nephrocalcinosis may be detected on plain radiographs or cross-sectional imaging modalities such as CT or US. The diagnosis is usually made by demonstrating thin linear bands of calcification at the extreme periphery of the kidney that may extend into the columns of Bertin but should not involve the renal medulla. Medullary nephrocalcinosis is more frequently observed than cortical disease and is most often due to hypercalcemic states such as hyperparathyroidism, renal tubular acidosis, or medullary sponge kidney. On plain films and CT studies, medullary nephrocalcinosis appears as speckled or dense calcifications within the renal medulla, sparing the cortex. In medullary sponge kidney, an anatomic condition of abnormally dilated collecting tubules, the condition may be unilateral or even focal, although medullary nephrocalcinosis from other causes is typically bilateral and diffuse. On ultrasound, shadowing echogenic foci are noted within the renal medulla.

Nephrolithiasis (better known as "kidney stones") is much more common than nephrocalcinosis. In fact, urinary tract calculi occur in as many as 12% of the population of the United States. Although there are clearly definable causes in some cases (hereditary conditions, metabolic diseases such as gout, certain urinary tract infections, and predisposing anatomic conditions), the vast majority of patients have idiopathic stone disease. Many small stones that are located within the intrarenal collecting system are asymptomatic; however, stones that pass into the ureter (ureterolithiasis) may obstruct the urinary tract and result in excruciating pain. Additionally, stones may cause hematuria or be a nidus for recurrent infection. Conventional radiographs have long been used to evaluate stone disease; in fact, the first description of urinary calculi was in April 1896, only a few months after the discovery of the x-ray by Roentgen. Stones appear as calcific densities on x-rays overlying the urinary tract (Figure 9-27). Urinary tract calculi are variably opaque and visible depending on their size, composition, and location. The accuracy of conventional radiographs for detecting stones has long been overestimated. Perhaps only 50% of stones are identified prospectively, and one can never be certain that an individual calcification on an isolated plain radiograph is within the urinary tract or simply overlies it. Confusing calcifications are many, including phleboliths, arterial calcifications, calcified lymph nodes, and other calcified masses. Stones on ultrasound appear as brightly echogenic structures and often with posterior shadowing. However, not all stones shadow, and as there are many small noncalcific echogenic

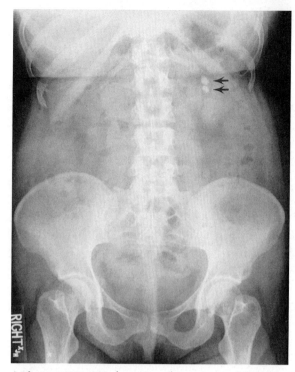

▲ **Figure 9-27.** KUB shows two dense 1-cm calcifications (arrows) projecting over the mid left kidney consistent with nephrolithiasis.

foci (vessels, fat) normally within the kidney, the accuracy for detecting renal calculi is only moderate with ultrasound. Additionally, ultrasound suffers from its ability to visualize only the most proximal and distal ureters and must rely on nonspecific indirect signs such as hydronephrosis and absent ureteral jets to suggest ureteral stones and obstruction. CT is now the imaging examination of choice for evaluation of renal stone disease. Virtually all urinary tract stones are dense on CT and show up as bright foci. Even stones as small as 1 mm are visible with modern scanners. Additionally, the entire urinary tract can be visualized on CT without overlapping or obscuring structures. In patients who present acutely with flank pain and are suspected of having ureteral stones, CT has become the study of choice. The diagnosis is confirmed by directly identifying a stone within the ureter. Secondary findings of obstructing may also be identified on CT, helping to confirm the diagnosis. Renal enlargement, perinephric stranding, and dilation of the ureter and intrarenal collecting system are frequently present in ureteral obstruction. One major additional advantage to CT is the ability to identify alternative explanations for the cause of a patient's acute flank pain. In fact, as many as one-third of all patients originally felt to have ureteral stones are shown by

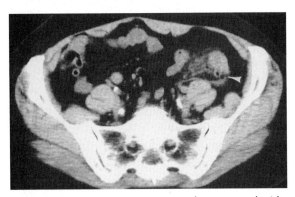

▲ **Figure 9-28.** CT scan in a patient who presented with acute left abdominal pain. The study shows inflammatory stranding surrounding the descending colon on the left with a few colonic diverticula evident (arrowhead). The findings are typical for diverticulitis. No stones were seen along the course of the ureters.

CT to have an alternative diagnosis (Figure 9-28). At this point, MRI performs little role in the evaluation of stone disease.

In pregnant patients with suspected obstructing calculi, CT is not contraindicated. By using a low-dose CT technique with lowered tube current and increased pitch, fetal dose can be lowered to as little as 3 mGy. This is well below the threshold for fetal anomalies of 50 mGy, and below the threshold for increased risk of childhood malignancy of 10 mGy. A similar technique can also be used in other situations where low dose is desired, such as in patients who have multiple scans

for recurrent calculi. It should be remembered that the lowest exposure achievable should always be pursued, and these studies should only be used in situations where they will affect clinical decision making.

Bladder stones may occur secondary to transport from the ureter or arise de novo. Most cases of bladder stones are secondary to urinary stasis such as occurs with bladder outlet obstruction from neurogenic bladders or prostatic enlargement. The diagnosis of bladder stones is similar to those in the upper urinary tract. Finally, urethral stones occur, and in males the vast majority are present as a result of passage from the bladder or above. In women, urethral stones are most frequently the result of urethral diverticula, which result in urinary stasis and stone formation.

EXERCISE 9-4. HEMATURIA

9-10. Based on the two images from Case 9-10 (Figure 9-29), what is the most likely diagnosis?
A. Squamous cell carcinoma
B. Renal stone
C. Urothelial cell carcinoma
D. Blood clot

9-11. What would be the recommended next step in the evaluation and management of the lesion in Case 9-11 (Figure 9-30)?
A. Cystoscopy
B. Retrograde cystogram
C. PET/CT
D. MRI

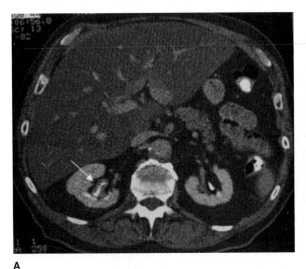

A

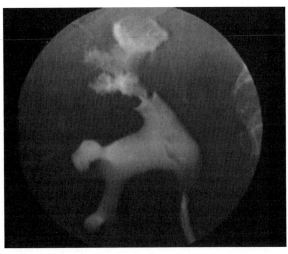

B

▲ **Figure 9-29.** Case 9-10. **(A)** Initial evaluation with CT urography in a 50-year-old male who presented with hematuria but no prior history of urinary stone disease. **(B)** Subsequent retrograde pyelogram performed.

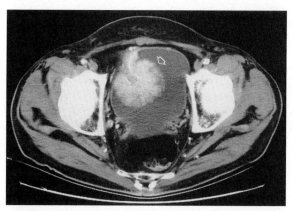

▲ **Figure 9-30.** Case 9-11. A 55-year-old male has a CT abdomen and pelvis performed for vague lower abdominal pain with the following finding. Further examination yielded microscopic hematuria and history of frequent urination.

Radiographic Findings

In Case 9-10, the first image from the excretory phase of a CT urogram (Figure 9-29 A) shows thickening of the mucosal surface (arrow) of the right renal pelvis, compared to the contralateral kidney where the wall is imperceptibly thin. On the retrograde pyelogram (Figure 9-29B), the upper pole calyces are irregular in contour, having a "moth-eaten" appearance.

Blood clots are typically intraluminal filling defects (D is incorrect). Although squamous cell carcinoma is a differential consideration, this is much less common than urothelial cell carcinoma. Additionally, clots often are associated with calcifications and recurrent infections (A is incorrect). This lesion is highly suggestive of urothelial cell carcinoma, the most common malignancy of the urinary collecting tract and bladder (C is the correct answer to Question 9-10). Therefore, further urologic evaluation with cystoscopy and ureteroscopy is recommended.

Regarding the patient in Case 9-11, the image taken from a CT scan (Figure 9-30) of the pelvis shows an enhancing, pedunculated mass (arrow) arising from the anterior wall of the urinary bladder. A retrograde cystogram would effectively demonstrate the presence of a bladder mass, but would do little to narrow the differential (B is incorrect). PET/CT can prove useful for the detection of metastatic disease, but is of limited use for evaluating a primary uroepithelial neoplasm because of the presence of FDG in the excreted urine, which can mask lesion uptake (C is incorrect). MRI is coming into use to establish depth of invasion into the bladder wall, but this would be at the discretion of the surgical oncologist following the establishment of a diagnosis. The gold standard for evaluation of a known bladder mass is cystoscopy (A is the correct answer to Question 9-11), which allows direct visualization and biopsy for a definitive diagnosis.

Discussion

Urothelial cell carcinoma (formally known as transitional cell carcinoma or TCC) is the most common neoplasm of the urinary tract, and up to 90% of all neoplasms of the bladder itself. Although TCCs can occur anywhere that there is transitional epithelium, from the renal collecting system to the urethra, they are most commonly found in the urinary bladder. This is felt to be due to several factors, including the large surface area of the bladder. Also, because the bladder acts as a temporary storage site prior to excretion, carcinogens remain in contact with the epithelium of the bladder for a longer period of time than they do with that of the remainder of the urinary tract. TCC is associated with numerous chemical carcinogens as well as cigarette smoking. Bladder urothelial cell carcinoma usually initially presents with hematuria, which is most commonly microscopic. A TCC can obstruct the vesicoureteral junction and cause obstructive symptoms as well. TCC of the bladder spreads by local invasion and by lymphatic and hematogenous spread. Most TCCs are superficial at presentation, with only about 1 in 4 displaying muscle invasion and 1 in 20 having distant metastases at the time of diagnosis.

Plain films are most often unremarkable in urothelial carcinoma of the bladder, with less than 1% displaying some stippled calcifications. TCCs can be seen as filling defects in a contrast-filled bladder, particularly when greater than 1 cm in size. Filling defects within the bladder on cystography are somewhat nonspecific, with considerations including tumor, radiolucent stones, fungus balls, and blood clots. However, transitional cell cancers have a characteristic stippled and frondlike appearance. Ultrasound can show exophytic soft-tissue lesion within the bladder. CT urography is the imaging modality of choice for evaluation of possible bladder masses, because the size of the mass itself, as well as the extent of invasion through the bladder wall into adjacent pelvic structures, can be evaluated. The use of urographic phase imaging and reformats allows the detection of even small, sessile lesions in the bladder, ureters, or renal pelvis. CT also allows evaluation of abdominal and pelvic lymph nodes and posttreatment examination for tumor recurrence. MRI can assess depth of bladder tumor invasion, but is not currently routinely used in tumor staging. Although the foregoing imaging findings strongly suggest the diagnosis of TCC, cystoscopy is important to confirm the histologic diagnosis. Cystoscopy is also indicated when CT urography does not demonstrate a source for hematuria. Other less common tumors of the bladder include malignancies such as squamous cell carcinoma and adenocarcinoma, uncommon benign lesions, and some masslike manifestations of inflammatory processes.

SUGGESTED READING

1. Dyer RB, Chen MY, Zagoria RJ. Abnormal calcifications in the urinary tract. *RadioGraphics*. 1998;16:123-142.
2. Dalrymple NC. Pearls and pitfalls in the diagnosis of ureterolithiasis by unenhanced helical CT. *RadioGraphics*. 2000;20:439-447.
3. Silverman SG, Israel GM, Herts BR, Richie JP. Management of the incidental renal mass. *Radiology*. 2008;249:16-31.
4. Raghunandan V, Sandler CM, Chaan SN. Imaging and staging of transitional cell carcinoma. *AJR Am J Roentgenol*. 2009;192:1481-1487.
5. Tsai IC, Chen MC, Lee WL, et al. Comprehensive evaluation of patients with suspected renal hypertension using MDCT: from protocol to interpretation. *AJR Am J Roentgenol*. 2009;192:W245-W254.
6. Silverman SG, Leyendecker JR, Arnis ES. What is the current role of CT urography and MR urography in the evaluation of the urinary tract? *Radiology*. 2009;250:309-323.
7. Johnson PT, Horton KM, Fishman EK. Adrenal imaging with multidetector CT: pathologic conditions, pearls, and pitfalls. *RadioGraphics*. 2009;29:1333-1351.
8. Israel GM, Bosniak MA. Pitfalls in renal mass evaluation and how to avoid them. *RadioGraphics*. 2008;28:1325-1338.
9. Gash R, Taylor C. Key concepts in imaging. *Clin. Imaging*. 1989;5:30-31.

Gastrointestinal Tract

10

David J. Ott, MD

Imaging of the hollow organs of the gastrointestinal tract began over a century ago with the use of heavy metal salts. Barium sulfate suspensions emerged as the contrast agent of choice for examination of the gastrointestinal tract. By the 1970s, other imaging modalities, including endoscopy and computed tomographic (CT) examination, appeared and have developed into alternate ways of imaging the hollow gastrointestinal organs.

The emergence and advancements in these newer technologies have dramatically affected the use of luminal contrast examinations of the gastrointestinal tract. In this chapter, I first describe the examination techniques that are currently available to evaluate the gastrointestinal tract. Normal imaging of the hollow organs as seen on a variety of examining modalities is discussed and illustrated. Technique selection is reviewed, with its effects on patient preparation and clinical indications. Finally, a series of exercises based on the more common clinical presentations of gastrointestinal tract disorders shows a wide variety of pathologic conditions.

EXAMINATION TECHNIQUES

▶ Luminal Contrast Studies

Luminal contrast examinations of the gastrointestinal tract can be performed with a variety of contrast materials. Barium sulfate suspensions are the preferred material for most examinations. A variety of barium products are available commercially, and many are formulated for specific examinations depending on their density and viscosity. Water-soluble contrast agents, which contain organically bound iodine, are used less often, primarily to demonstrate perforation of a hollow viscus or to evaluate the status of a surgical anastomosis in the gastrointestinal tract. The details and various options available for luminal contrast examination depend on the organ(s) being evaluated and are further elaborated in the normal imaging section.

▶ Computed Tomographic Imaging

CT imaging of the chest and abdomen can portray the various hollow organs of the gastrointestinal tract. Mucosal disease, such as ulcers, and small neoplasms will not be shown with this imaging modality. Larger gastrointestinal neoplasms, thickening of the walls of the hollow organs, and extrinsic processes can be easily detected. Also, with the use of luminal distention and intravenous contrast material, a variety of gastrointestinal disorders are more readily evaluated.

A major role of CT scanning, especially in the esophagus and colon, is staging malignancy of these organs. In the colon, for example, CT examination is used for initial staging, especially for distant metastases, and for evaluation of recurrence following surgery. Recurrent masses appearing after surgery may also be biopsied percutaneously. CT colonography (CTC) is yet another expanding application for colon cancer screening and detection of polyps and malignancies of the large bowel.

▶ Magnetic Resonance Imaging

Magnetic resonance (MR) imaging is the newest modality developed for cross-sectional imaging of the body and nearly all organ systems can be evaluated with this technique. MR imaging of the hollow organs of the gastrointestinal tract is increasingly being used to evaluate a wide assortment of gastrointestinal tract disorders. As with CT imaging, mild mucosal diseases and small focal lesions are not well detected with this technique; however, malignancies can be similarly evaluated and staged.

Also, with the use of luminal distention and intravenous agents of various types, assessment of obstructive and inflammatory bowel disease has shown dramatic results. Small-bowel obstruction and Crohn disease in particular have become common indications for use of MR imaging. With the newer technologies, both CT and MR imaging offer multiple options for viewing the gastrointestinal tract, including multiplanar viewing and 2-D and 3-D reconstructions. Dynamic MR imaging has also emerged with application in several areas, such as assessment of pelvic floor dysfunction in women.

▶ Abdominal Ultrasound

Abdominal ultrasound has had an increasing impact on evaluation of the hollow organs of the gastrointestinal tract, although in the United States, this modality is used mainly to examine the solid organs of the abdomen and the biliary tract, including the gallbladder. The location of the hollow organs and the presence of gas interference remain technical problems; however, inflammatory disorders can be evaluated, such as acute appendicitis, especially in pediatric patients. Endoluminal ultrasound using blind probes or those attached to an endoscope has been used in the upper gastrointestinal tract and the colorectum to detect and stage malignancy; other indications include fine-needle aspiration (FNA) of pancreatic masses through the gastroduodenal wall.

▶ Endoscopy

Upper gastrointestinal endoscopy visualizes the mucosal surfaces of the esophagus, stomach, and duodenum. The pharynx and often the distal portion of the duodenum are not evaluated with this technique. Also, endoscopy does not assess functional abnormalities of these organs, such as pharyngeal dysfunction and esophageal motility disorders. The major advantages of endoscopy compared to barium examination of the upper gastrointestinal tract are a better demonstration of milder inflammatory processes, such as erosions and small peptic ulcers, and its therapeutic potential.

Endoscopy of the mesenteric portions of the small intestine has shown dramatic advancements in recent years. A variety of endoscopic methods are now available to examine much if not all of the jejunum and ileum; these include push enteroscopy and double-balloon enteroscopy, both of which offer therapeutic options. Capsule endoscopy, in which the patient ingests a pill-sized device containing a photo detector and radio transmitter, takes two images per second, which are transmitted to an external detector and viewed on a computer; this new technology has been shown to be superior to barium small-bowel examination in detecting early Crohn disease, small erosions and polyps, and vascular lesions, such as arteriovenous malformations (AVMs).

Colonoscopy is both a diagnostic and therapeutic modality. Inflammatory and neoplastic diseases of the colon are evaluated accurately. Biopsies can be obtained when needed, and the majority of colonic polyps can be removed through the colonoscope. Despite a steep decline in the use of the barium enema, colonoscopy requires conscious sedation, is more costly, and is associated with more complications, including a small mortality rate. CTC is considered a safer alternative to colonoscopy, but is not as effective in detecting smaller polyps and offers no therapeutic choices.

NORMAL IMAGING

▶ Upper Gastrointestinal Tract

The organs that can be examined in the upper gastrointestinal tract include the pharynx, esophagus, stomach, and duodenum. The pharynx and esophagus may be evaluated separately or as part of more complete examinations of these organs. Various techniques are available to assess the function and structure of the pharynx depending on the indications for the examination. Motion recording (now using mainly digital technology) of pharyngeal function and imaging of pharyngeal structures are often combined for a more thorough examination. Also, materials of variable viscosity can be used in patients to determine aspiration risk and dietary needs; the latter is often called a "modified

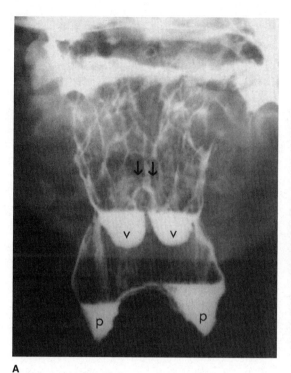
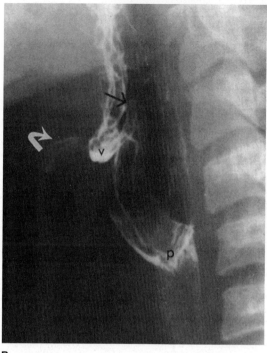

A   **B**

▲ **Figure 10-1.** Frontal (**A**) and lateral (**B**) views of the pharynx. In the frontal position, the paired valleculae (v) and piriform sinuses (p) have a symmetric appearance and are seen separately. On the lateral projections, the valleculae (v) and piriform sinuses (p) are superimposed. The upright epiglottis (arrows both views) lies posterior to the valleculae, which are posterior to the hyoid bone (curved arrow).

barium swallow" and is done in conjunction with a swallowing therapist. An alternate method of assessing swallowing is fiberoptic endoscopic evaluation of swallowing (FEES), which is also performed by a swallowing therapist with training in this technique.

Pharyngeal function is complex and is best evaluated with motion-recording techniques that allow slow-motion review. Imaging of the pharynx is usually done with the patient in the frontal and lateral positions (Figure 10-1). In the frontal view, the paired valleculae and piriform sinuses are separated. The lateral view of the pharynx superimposes these structures, but permits better visualization of the base of the tongue, hyoid bone, and epiglottis anteriorly, and the posterior pharyngeal wall and cervical spine posteriorly.

The esophagus, stomach, and duodenum are usually examined together as part of the upper gastrointestinal series. A variety of radiographic techniques are used and usually combined to optimize the upper gastrointestinal examination; techniques include observation of esophageal motility, filming of the organs with varying amounts of barium suspension, gas, or air, and obtaining views of the mucosal surface (Figures 10-2, 10-3). The upper gastrointestinal tract is best

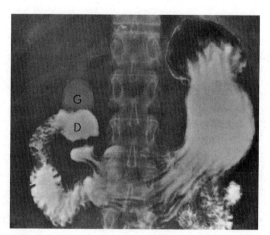

▲ **Figure 10-2.** Prone frontal radiograph of stomach and duodenum from a single-contrast upper gastrointestinal examination. The duodenal bulb (D) is attached to the gastric antrum by the pyloric channel. The gallbladder (G) is also opacified from an oral cholecystogram (OCG; a defunct examination replaced by ultrasound).

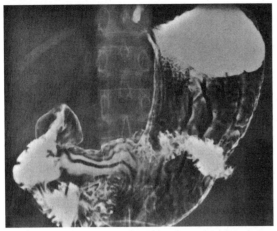

▲ **Figure 10-3.** Supine frontal film of the stomach and duodenum from a double-contrast upper gastrointestinal examination in which a high-density barium suspension and gas crystals (CO_2) are used. Compared to the previous figure, the stomach is better distended, primarily by the generated gas.

examined by luminal contrast studies or endoscopy because mucosal abnormalities are often the cause of disease. CT and MR imaging can also evaluate these organs and detect focal masses, wall thickening, and extrinsic processes, such as an invasive pancreatic malignancy. These modalities can also contribute to the staging of malignancies, especially in the esophagus (Figure 10-4).

The esophagus consists mainly of a tubular portion with a bell-shaped termination called the *esophageal vestibule*. The esophagogastric junction normally lies within or below the esophageal hiatus. When the esophagogastric junction lies above the hiatus, hiatal hernia is present, which is the most common structural abnormality of the upper gastrointestinal tract (Figure 10-5 A). The esophageal mucosal surface has a smooth appearance when distended and shows smooth, thin longitudinal folds when collapsed (Figure 10-5 B). Esophageal peristalsis can be observed by having the patient swallow single volumes of barium suspension.

The stomach has a complex shape and varies considerably depending on the degree of distention (see Figures 10-2, 10-3). When the stomach is collapsed, the rugal folds are seen prominently and may mimic focal or diffuse gastric disorders, whether on luminal contrast or CT studies. With gastric distention, the rugal folds are flattened and the mucosal surface of the stomach is seen more effectively. Barium studies of the upper gastrointestinal tract evaluate gastric function poorly; radionuclide gastric emptying studies are more effective for this purpose.

The duodenum is attached to the stomach at the narrow pylorus and consists of the duodenal bulb and the descending and ascending portions, although a horizontal segment is often added (Figure 10-6; see Figure 10-4 B). The duodenum terminates at the duodenojejunal junction,

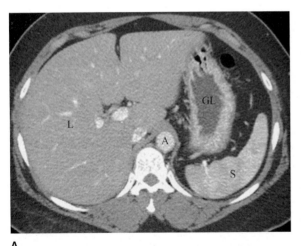

A

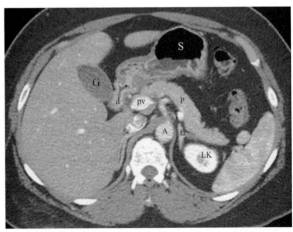

B

▲ **Figure 10-4.** **(A)** Enhanced (ie, intravenous contrast material) CT examination of the upper abdomen showing the stomach (GL, gastric lumen) with an enhancing gastric wall; incomplete distention can mimic gastric wall thickening. L, liver; A, aorta; S, spleen. **(B)** CT section lower in same patient showing the gastroduodenal junction (d, duodenum); note that the anterior stomach (S) wall is now much thinner with gaseous distention of the gastric lumen. G, gallbladder; pv, portal vein; P, pancreas; A, aorta; la, left adrenal gland; LK, top left kidney.

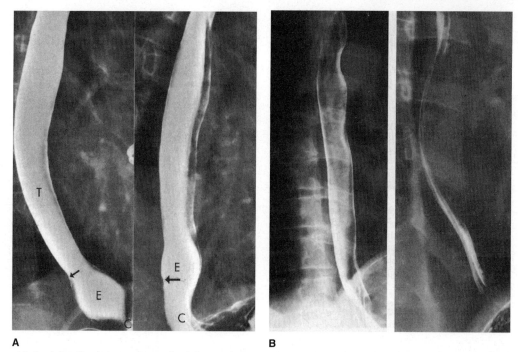

A   **B**

▲ **Figure 10-5.** **(A)** Full-column radiograph of the normal esophagus (left) with the patient drinking barium rapidly in the prone oblique position. The tubular esophagus (T) joins the esophageal vestibule (E) at the tubulovestibular junction (arrow). The lower end of the esophageal vestibule is constricted (C) at the level of the diaphragmatic hiatus. In another patient (right), the esophagogastric junction (arrow) lies above the level of the diaphragmatic hiatus (C), indicating the presence of hiatal hernia. E, esophageal vestibule. **(B)** Double-contrast (left) and mucosal relief (right) views of the esophagus. Multiple radiographic techniques are combined to evaluate the esophagus to optimize the efficacy of the examination.

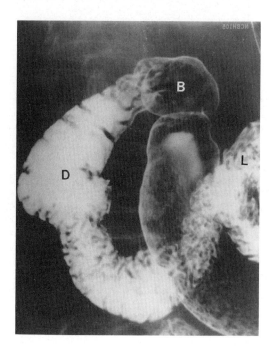

▲ **Figure 10-6.** Radiograph of the duodenum showing the duodenal bulb (B) attached to the gastric antrum. The descending duodenum (D) extends from the apex of the bulb to the inferior duodenal flexure. The horizontal and ascending portions of the duodenum terminate at the duodenojejunal junction (L), which is attached to the ligament of Treitz.

which is attached to the ligament of Treitz. The duodenal bulb has a triangular or heart-shaped appearance normally tapering to the apex of the bulb with its junction to the descending portion. The bulbar mucosal surface is normally smooth. The duodenum assumes a C-shape configuration within the upper abdomen, and the mucosal folds are symmetric. The duodenum is surrounded by many structures, particularly the pancreas, and is often involved secondarily by diseases in other adjacent organs; cross-sectional CT or MR imaging is useful in demonstrating this involvement (see Figure 10-4).

▶ Small Intestine

The radiographic examination of the small bowel evaluates the mesenteric portion of the organ, which consists of the jejunum and ileum. The following luminal contrast methods can be used to examine the small intestine: (1) peroral small-bowel series; (2) enteroclysis; and (3) various retrograde techniques (eg, via an ileostomy). The peroral small-bowel series is often done immediately after an upper gastrointestinal examination and following ingestion of additional barium suspension. Serial images of the abdomen are obtained, and abdominal compression applied to better visualize the small-bowel loops, including the terminal ileum (Figure 10-7). However, the peroral small-bowel study is probably the least effective method of examining this organ; techniques that better distend the small bowel with higher volume are now preferred depending on the indications. These include enteroclysis and CT or MR imaging with volume instillation by oral ingestion or via a tube, that is, CT or MR enterography or CT or MR enteroclysis (Figure 10-8).

Enteroclysis is an intubated examination of the small intestine and can be done by a variety of techniques and using a number of different modalities (as discussed earlier). The small intestine is intubated by a nasal or oral route with a small-bore enteric tube placed with fluoroscopic guidance. A variety of luminal contrast methods exist, but filming is done similarly to the peroral examination. The enteroclysis techniques permit better control of small-bowel distention and more exact visualization of small-bowel loops (Figure 10-9).

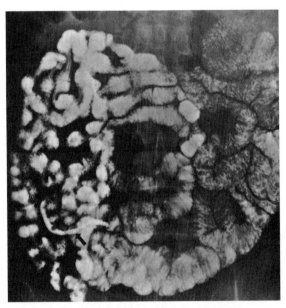 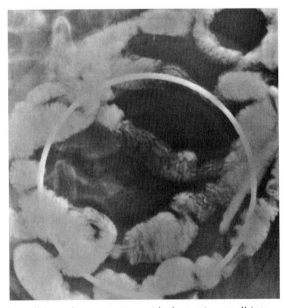

▲ **Figure 10-7. (A)** Large film of the abdomen from a peroral small-bowel examination with the entire small intestine opacified with barium suspension. On the left side of the abdomen, the jejunum shows a more typical "feathery" pattern of the mucosal folds compared to the ileum, which is smaller in caliber and has fewer folds in the right lower abdomen. The appendix (arrow) is also visualized. **(B)** Compression film (balloon paddle is identified by the circular metallic ring) of the small bowel from a peroral examination with separation and clear visualization of the small-bowel loops.

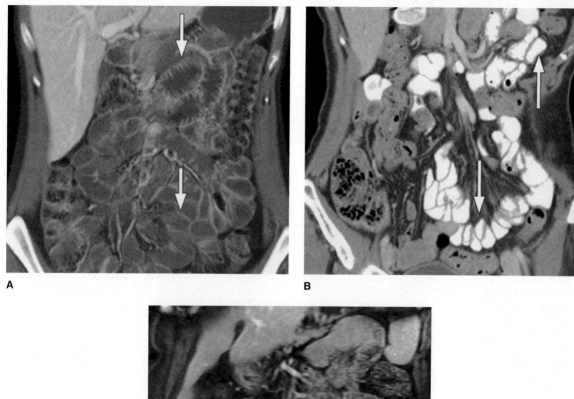

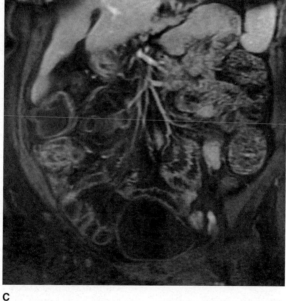

▲ **Figure 10-8.** (**A**) CT enterography. Coronal section of the abdomen with intravenous contrast enhancement and the use of a "neutral" luminal agent (such as water); excellent luminal distention of the small bowel is achieved with the normal thin wall of the small intestine evident (arrows). (**B**) CT enterography using an intravenous contrast agent and positive luminal contrast material, hence, the white appearance of the small bowel. Note that the bowel walls (arrows) are not well seen (both A and B are courtesy of Macari M, Megibow AJ, Balthazar EJ. A pattern approach to the abnormal SB. *Am J Roentgenol,* 2007;188:1344-1355, used with permission). (**C**) Coronal MR image of the abdomen with intravenous contrast enhancement showing the mesenteric vessels and normal small intestine with wall enhancement.

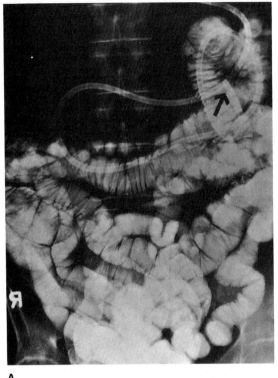
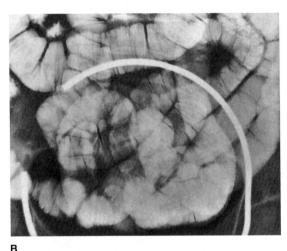

A   **B**

▲ **Figure 10-9.** **(A)** Large film of the abdomen from an enteroclysis examination of the small intestine. The small bowel is intubated with the tip of the tube (arrow) in the jejunum. Compared to the peroral examination, the small-bowel loops are distended more fully, causing the mucosal folds to assume a transverse orientation. **(B)** Compression film (ring of balloon paddle) of the small-bowel loops in the pelvis with the patient in a prone position. Although the loops are overlapped, the "see-through" effect using a dilute barium suspension permits their clear visualization.

Retrograde examination of the small bowel involves filling of the organ from the opposite direction. Various techniques can be used depending on the patient's anatomy. Reflux of the small intestine through the ileocecal valve can be done as part of a barium enema. If the patient has an ileostomy, various devices can be introduced into the ostomy site and a barium suspension instilled directly.

The length of the mesenteric small bowel in adults averages about 20 feet, but varies considerably among individuals. The jejunum comprises just over one-third of the length and the ileum the remainder, although no discrete transition is seen between the two segments. The normally distended small bowel has a caliber of 2 to 3 cm, being slightly larger more orad in the jejunum. Depending on the degree of distention, the mucosal folds (valvulae conniventes) may have a feathery appearance or may be transversely oriented across the intestinal lumen with more complete distention. The mucosal folds are more numer-

ous in the jejunum and gradually decrease in number and size in the ileum.

▶ Large Intestine

The radiographic examination of the large bowel evaluates the entire organ from the rectum to the cecum. Reflux of barium suspension into the ileum and the appendix, if present, occurs commonly. The colon can be evaluated by several techniques, which include single-contrast and double-contrast barium enemas; different types of rectal tips and barium suspensions are used for each examination (Figure 10-10). The single-contrast method simply involves filling the colon with a dilute barium suspension, whereas the double-contrast technique requires a denser, more viscous barium suspension and air. In both methods, large and small compression images of all segments of the colon are obtained. Colonoscopy and CTC have both had a substantial

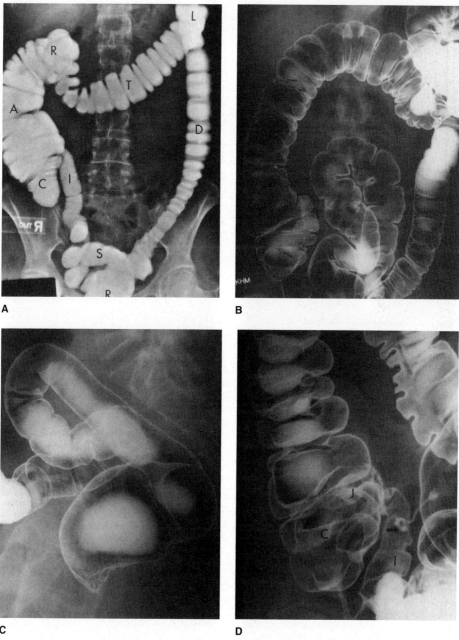

A

B

C

D

▲ **Figure 10-10.** **(A)** Large film of the abdomen from a single-contrast barium enema with the patient in the supine position. The rectum (R), descending colon (D), left colic flexure (L; also known as the splenic flexure), transverse colon (T), right colic flexure (R; also known as the hepatic flexure), ascending colon (A), and cecum (C) are visualized. The sigmoid colon (S) and colic flexures are not seen well in this position and require additional films. The terminal ileum (I) has refluxed from the colon. **(B)** Large film of abdomen from a double-contrast barium enema with the patient in the supine position. The double-contrast effect is produced by coating the mucosal surface of the colon with a moderately dense, viscous barium suspension and distending the organ with air; a specially designed enema tip is needed for the examination. **(C)** Double-contrast film of the rectum and a portion of the sigmoid colon with the patient in a lateral position. **(D)** Double-contrast view of the right side of the colon showing the cecum (C), ileocecal junction (J), refluxed terminal ileum (I), and the appendix (arrow). The multiple haustrations of the colon are seen well and are produced by the teniae coli.

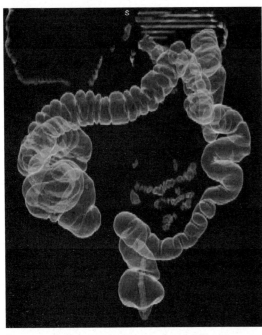

A

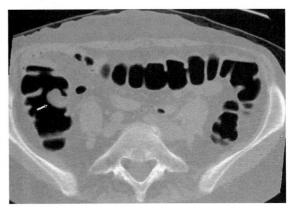

B

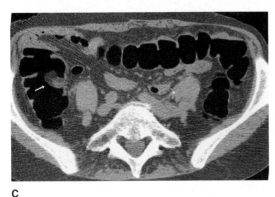

C

▲ **Figure 10-11.** CT colonography (CTC) requires bowel preparation and gaseous distention of the colon. Many display options are available, which include evaluating data as 2-D and 3-D images, endoluminal views (both color and black and white), and "segmented" views of the colon that isolate the organ from other structures. (**A**) Segmented view of the entire colon distended well with gas; this is just one of many ways to manipulate the data acquired during CTC. (**B**) Two-dimensional CTC analysis of a portion of the colon shows a polypoid lesion in the right side (arrow). (**C**) A corresponding CT analysis of the polypoid lesion (same as B) shows low density indicative of fat; colonoscopy showed a prominent ileocecal valve.

impact on the numbers of barium enemas now being performed (Figure 10-11).

The large intestine consists of the rectum, sigmoid colon, descending colon, splenic flexure, transverse colon, hepatic flexure, ascending colon, and cecum (see Figure 10-10). The length of the colon varies considerably, mainly because of differences in length and redundancy of the sigmoid colon and colic flexures. The colon also varies in caliber depending on location and luminal distention achieved. The mucosal surface has a smooth appearance, and the colonic contour is indented by the haustra, which are less numerous in the descending colon. The rectal valves of Houston are often seen,

especially on double-contrast imaging. The ileocecal valve has a variety of appearances and may be large if infiltrated by fat (Figure 10-12).

TECHNIQUE SELECTION

▶ Patient Preparation

Preparation of the patient for examination of the gastrointestinal tract varies depending on the type of examination being performed and the modality used. This discussion emphasizes luminal contrast studies, although for certain modalities,

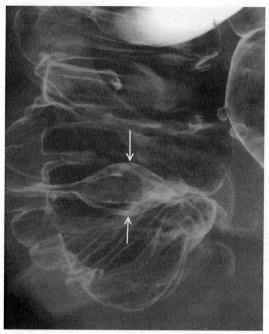

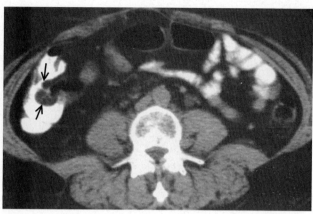

A   B

▲ **Figure 10-12.** (**A**) Double-contrast enema demonstrates a smooth elliptical lesion (arrows) in the right side of the colon felt to represent the ileocecal valve. (**B**) CT examination shows fatty infiltration of the ileocecal valve (arrows); no abnormality was found at the time of colonoscopy.

eg, barium enema versus colonoscopy, preparations will be comparable. The upper gastrointestinal tract and small bowel require minimal preparation; none is needed if only the pharynx and esophagus are being examined.

For an upper gastrointestinal or small-bowel examination, the patient should have nothing orally after midnight or the next morning preceding the radiographic study. Fluid and food in the stomach and small intestine degrade the examination by interfering with good mucosal visualization and causing artifacts that may mimic disease. Also, if patients are to have other imaging examinations that may introduce fluid into the upper gastrointestinal tract, such as an abdominal CT study in which oral contrast material is used, the examinations must be scheduled on separate days. When multiple abdominal radiographic studies are ordered, discussion with the radiologist is appropriate so that the correct sequence can be planned.

Preparation for the barium enema is much more complicated, but must be performed properly to obtain and accurate evaluation of the colon; this is also required for performance of colonoscopy and CT colonography. Various colonic preparations have been recommended and usually combine the use of dietary changes, oral fluids, and several cathartics the day preceding the barium enema examination. At our institution, the standard preparation includes (1) a 24-hour clear liquid diet; (2) oral hydration; (3) a saline cathartic (eg, magnesium citrate) in the afternoon; (4) an irritant cathartic (eg, castor oil) in the early evening; and (5) a tap-water cleansing enema the morning of the radiographic examination (30 to 60 minutes before the barium enema).

▶ Clinical Indications

A variety of radiographic and endoscopic techniques are now available to examine the gastrointestinal tract. Selection of an appropriate technique depends on many factors, including the clinical indications for the examination and the efficacy of the various techniques. The luminal contrast examinations discussed are emphasized relative to the anatomic areas of interest and the presentation of the patient; however, there has been a dramatic drop in the use of these examinations, and other modalities have replaced their evaluation of patients with specific clinical indications. Comments are made regarding this changing status and use of newer techniques.

Upper Gastrointestinal Tract

The main indications for examination of the upper gastrointestinal tract include dysphagia, odynophagia, chest pain, pyrosis, suspicion of esophageal varices, dyspepsia, upper gastrointestinal bleeding, and evaluation of obstruction. Dysphagia may be of oropharyngeal or esophageal origin; a modified examination of the oral cavity and pharynx may be required in some of these patients. The most common diseases causing these symptoms are esophageal and gastric malignancies, reflux esophagitis and peptic stricture, infectious esophagitis, lower esophageal mucosal ring, and peptic ulcers and erosions of the stomach and duodenum. Currently, endoscopy is the most common method for examining the upper gastrointestinal tract, although radiographic evaluation is often indicated for pharyngeal and esophageal complaints.

The diseases most effectively detected by the radiographic examination of the upper gastrointestinal tract include malignancies, peptic stricture, esophageal mucosal ring, more severe forms of reflux and infectious esophagitis, and peptic ulcers larger than 5 mm in size. The limitations of this examination are detection of milder inflammations, such as mild reflux esophagitis or early infectious esophagitis, small gastric and duodenal ulcers, and erosive gastritis and duodenitis.

Small Bowel

The more specific indications for small-bowel examination include gastrointestinal bleeding that is not localized to the upper gastrointestinal tract or colon, diarrhea or more specifically steatorrhea, inflammatory bowel disease, intestinal obstruction, intra-abdominal malignancy, and abdominal fistula involving bowel. The diseases that can cause small-bowel bleeding include Meckel diverticulum, Crohn disease, ischemic or infectious enteritis, erosions or ulcers, vascular malformations, and primary and secondary neoplasms. Small-bowel obstruction is usually due to adhesions, external hernias, or intrinsic or extrinsic neoplasms. The diagnostic approach to patients with these symptoms and potential disorders has changed dramatically. Capsule endoscopy and CT/MR imaging has strongly affected the use of luminal contrast examinations.

The efficacy of the peroral small-bowel examination, especially when not performed well, is poor in evaluation of smaller and more focal disease processes. Enteroclysis is often preferred if a luminal contrast examination is chosen; these examinations are effective in the diagnosis of early inflammatory disease, localization of obstruction, focal structural diseases, and peritoneal adhesions. Capsule endoscopy is most sensitive in detecting small and flat mucosal processes, such as early Crohn disease, erosions, and vascular anomalies. CT and MR enterography (along with enteroclysis) have become increasingly used in the evaluation and staging of various other types of small-bowel disorders, such as Crohn disease.

Colon

The major indications for radiographic examination of the colon are rectal bleeding, suspicion of inflammatory bowel disease, question of neoplastic disease, and evaluation of colonic obstruction. The most common diseases causing colonic bleeding are diverticulosis, idiopathic or ischemic colitis, larger colonic polyps, and carcinoma. Common causes of colonic obstruction include diverticulitis, colonic malignancy, volvulus of the large bowel, and extrinsic disorders, especially pelvic malignancy. Colonoscopy has largely replaced the barium enema for evaluation of many of these disorders, and CT and MR examinations have also had an impact on radiologic imaging of the colon.

The diseases that are detected most effectively by barium enema include diverticular disease and its complications, more severe forms of idiopathic and other types of colitis, larger colonic polyps (ie, greater than 1 cm), and colonic carcinoma. The limitations of the barium enema include diagnosis of small colonic polyps and mild inflammatory bowel disease, especially with use of the single-contrast technique. Also, vascular malformations, which are more common in older patients, are not seen with luminal contrast studies. In particular, CT examination of the colon has become an important means of screening patients with a variety of abdominal complaints, and it often discovers a number of colonic abnormalities, such as various types of colitis, diverticulitis, and colonic obstruction. Presently, CT examination is the preferred method for assessment of diverticulitis.

EXERCISES

In this section, many of the gastrointestinal diseases mentioned previously are illustrated and discussed. Six exercises are presented emphasizing common clinical presentations; these include dysphagia, upper gastrointestinal bleeding, small-bowel bleeding, small-bowel obstruction, colonic bleeding, and colonic obstruction. Luminal contrast studies are the predominant examples for many of these disorders, but other radiologic imaging techniques are also used. It is hoped that this approach will allow a better understanding of how these various radiologic studies can be used in evaluating patients with disorders of the hollow organs of the gastrointestinal tract. Despite the importance of endoscopy in modern gastrointestinal medicine, this modality cannot be discussed fully in this context; however, appropriate comments are added for a better appreciation of the interrelated roles of all of these means of investigating patients with gastrointestinal symptoms.

EXERCISE 10-1. DYSPHAGIA

10-1. What is the most likely cause for the symmetric narrowing at the lower end of the esophagus in Case 10-1 (Figure 10-13; arrows)?
A. Carcinoma of the esophagus
B. Peptic esophageal stricture
C. Lower esophageal mucosal ring
D. Achalasia of the esophagus
E. Esophageal varices.

10-2. What is the most likely etiology of the smooth, tapered narrowing above the hiatal hernia in Case 10-2 (Figure 10-14)?
A. *Candida* esophagitis
B. Reflux esophagitis
C. Herpetic esophagitis
D. Human immunodeficiency virus (HIV) esophagitis
E. Esophageal malignancy

10-3. What is the most likely cause of the focal, irregular esophageal narrowing shown in Case 10-3 (Figure 10-15)?

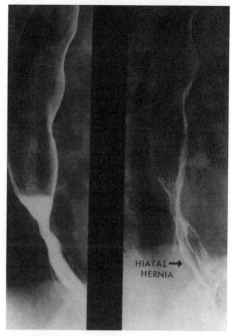

▲ **Figure 10-14.** Case 10-2. A 35-year-old woman with gastroesophageal reflux symptoms presents with more recent onset of dysphagia.

A. Squamous-cell carcinoma
B. Adenocarcinoma
C. Stricture from caustic ingestion
D. Benign peptic stricture
E. Infectious esophageal stricture

10-4. What is the most likely cause of the lower esophageal narrowing (arrow) and the absence of peristalsis noted at fluoroscopy in Case 10-4 (Figure 10-16)?
A. Stricture in Barrett esophagus
B. Stricture in scleroderma
C. Peptic stricture from reflux esophagitis
D. Achalasia of the esophagus
E. Adenocarcinoma of the esophagus

Radiologic Findings

10-1. The thin, annular narrowing at the lower end of the esophagus is a lower esophageal mucosal ring (C is the correct answer to Question 10-1).

10-2. The smooth, tapered narrowing in the lower esophagus in association with a hiatal hernia is typical of a peptic stricture from reflux esophagitis (B is the correct answer to Question 10-2).

10-3. The annular, irregular focal narrowing of the esophagus with abrupt margins is characteristic of a

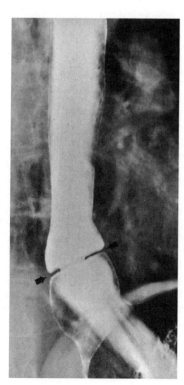

▲ **Figure 10-13.** Case 10-1. A 55-year-old man presents with solid food dysphagia.

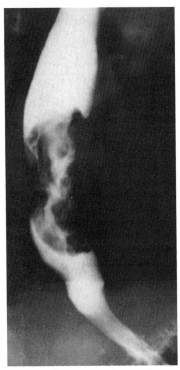

▲ **Figure 10-15.** Case 10-3. A 65-year-old man has weight loss and complains of both dysphagia and odynophagia.

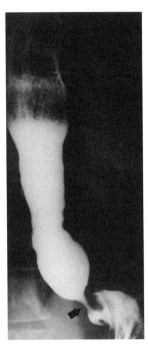

▲ **Figure 10-16.** Case 10-4. A 30-year-old woman presents with dysphagia and regurgitation of undigested food.

squamous-cell carcinoma (A is the correct answer to Question 10-3).

10-4. Esophageal aperistalsis, tapered narrowing at the lower end of the esophagus, and esophageal dilatation are features of idiopathic achalasia (D is the correct answer to Question 10-4).

Discussion

Dysphagia is a frequent indication for radiographic or endoscopic examination of the esophagus. The most common esophageal causes of dysphagia are shown in the case presentations in this exercise.

The lower esophageal mucosal ring is an acquired thin, annular membrane of unknown cause that demarcates the esophagogastric junction and is a sign of hiatal hernia. More importantly, the mucosal ring is probably the most common cause of solid food dysphagia seen in adults (the so-called steakhouse syndrome). Nearly 60 years ago, Schatzki described the association of the mucosal ring, which often bears his name, with dysphagia and determined that the prevalence of dysphagia related to the caliber of the ring. Rings greater that 20 mm in diameter rarely cause symptoms; rings less than 14 mm in caliber are nearly always

symptomatic, whereas mucosal rings 14 to 20 mm in diameter cause dysphagia in about half of patients. The mucosal ring is best detected by radiographic examination, and the use of a solid bolus, such as a portion of a marshmallow, optimizes evaluation of these rings and verifies the structure as a cause of dysphagia (Figure 10-17).

Peptic stricture of the esophagus is a complication of reflux esophagitis and is the second most common benign cause of dysphagia. Reflux strictures typically occur at the esophagogastric junction and are associated with a hiatal hernia in virtually all patients. Peptic strictures show a variety of morphologic appearances from a smooth, tapered narrowing to an annular configuration that may resemble a mucosal ring. Irregularity of the stricture margin may also be seen and must be differentiated from an esophageal malignancy. Barrett esophagus is another complication of gastroesophageal reflux disease and is suggested when a peptic stricture is located above the esophagogastric junction (Figure 10-18); adenocarcinoma is the most serious complication of Barrett esophagus and has increased dramatically in recent decades.

Squamous-cell carcinoma was the predominant primary malignancy of the esophagus in past decades, but the escalating increase in adenocarcinoma of the esophagus has had a dramatic impact on their relative prevalences. The usual

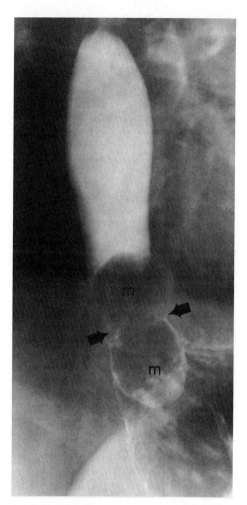

▲ **Figure 10-17.** Patient with solid food dysphagia and a mucosal ring measuring 16 mm in caliber. A one-half portion of a marshmallow (m) impacted at the level of the ring (arrows) and reproduced dysphagia.

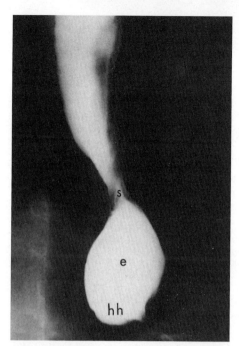

▲ **Figure 10-18.** Peptic stricture (s) above a normal intervening segment of esophagus (e) associated with a small hiatal hernia (hh). The esophagus between the hernia and stricture was lined by columnar epithelium (ie, Barrett esophagus) at endoscopic examination.

appearance of squamous-cell carcinoma is a focal, irregular narrowing with abrupt upper and lower margins, which rarely mimics peptic stricture. This esophageal malignancy occurs in older patients, who often have a history of tobacco and alcohol abuse; squamous-cell carcinomas may also be multifocal and associated with similar lesions in the upper aerodigestive tract. Adenocarcinoma of the esophagus is now seen as frequently as squamous-cell malignancies and is typically found in conjunction with Barrett esophagus (Figure 10-19).

Idiopathic achalasia is a primary motility disorder of the esophagus of unknown cause that presents with dysphagia, regurgitation, and weight loss occasionally. The findings on esophageal manometry include total absence of primary esophageal peristalsis (aperistalsis), and a dysfunctional lower esophageal sphincter (ie, failure of relaxation). The radiographic features mirror the manometric findings; aperistalsis is observed and the lower end of the esophagus has a smooth, tapered or beaklike appearance. In achalasia, hiatal hernia is an uncommon observation, which is usually seen in patients with peptic stricture or scleroderma of the esophagus. An important differential diagnosis is secondary achalasia due to an infiltrative gastric adenocarcinoma (Figure 10-20); patients are usually older and have a more abrupt onset of symptoms, which often include odynophagia.

EXERCISE 10-2. UPPER GASTROINTESTINAL BLEEDING

10-5. What is the most likely cause of the lesser curvature gastric lesion (arrow) shown in Case 10-5 (Figure 10-21)?

A. Malignant gastric ulcer
B. Gastric diverticulum
C. Lymphoma of the stomach
D. Polypoid carcinoma of the stomach
E. Benign gastric ulcer

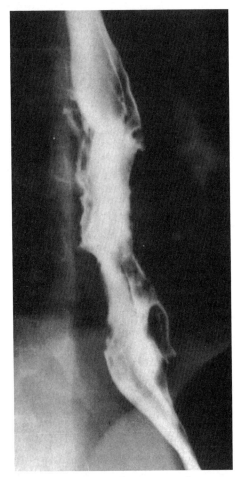

▲ **Figure 10-19.** Patient with Barrett esophagus complicated by an irregular adenocarcinoma, which may be difficult to distinguish from the accompanying changes of esophagitis and stricture. Adenocarcinoma occurs in about 5% to 10% of patients who have Barrett esophagus, and periodic endoscopic surveillance is usually recommended.

10-6. What is the *least* likely cause of the polypoid gastric mass shown in Case 10-6 (Figure 10-22)?
   A. Large gastric adenoma
   B. GIST (gastrointestinal stromal tumor)
   C. Gastric lymphoma
   D. Polypoid gastric carcinoma
   E. Gastric leiomyosarcoma.

10-7. What is the likely diagnosis for the nodular appearance of the duodenal bulb in Case 10-7 (Figure 10-23; p, pylorus)?
   A. Duodenal ulcer
   B. Erosive duodenitis
   C. Brunner gland hyperplasia
   D. Duodenal carcinoma
   E. Swallowed olive pits

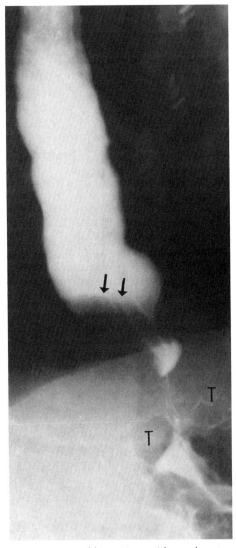

▲ **Figure 10-20.** An older patient with an abrupt onset of dysphagia and odynophagia. Narrowing and mass effect (arrows) are present at the lower end of the esophagus, which was also aperistaltic. These changes mimic idiopathic achalasia, but the tumor mass (T) in the proximal stomach proved to be a gastric adenocarcinoma causing secondary achalasia.

10-8. What is the most likely cause of the barium collection in the duodenal bulb in Case 10-8 (Figure 10-24; patient is prone; d, duodenal diverticulum)?
   A. Benign duodenal ulcer (posterior wall)
   B. Malignant duodenal ulcer
   C. Benign duodenal polyp
   D. Benign duodenal ulcer (anterior wall)
   E. Ulcerated duodenal metastasis

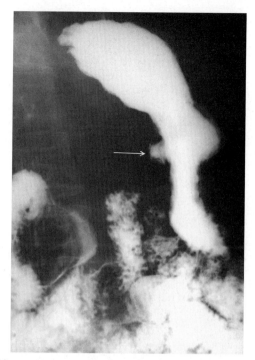

▲ **Figure 10-21.** Case 10-5. A 28-year-old man presents with epigastric pain and occult blood in his stools.

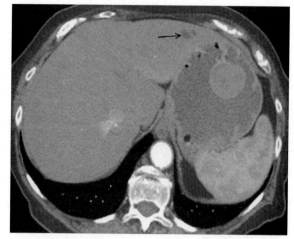

▲ **Figure 10-22.** Case 10-6. A 63-year-old woman presents with epigastric pain, weight loss, and anemia.

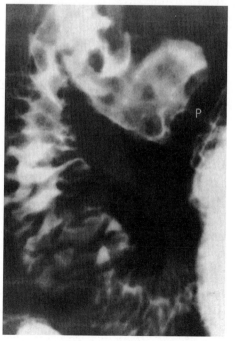

▲ **Figure 10-23.** Case 10-7. A 32-year-old alcoholic man presents with severe epigastric pain and hematemesis.

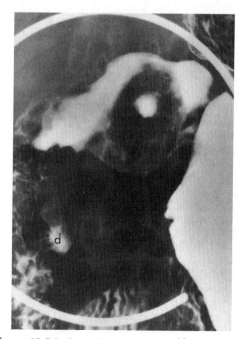

▲ **Figure 10-24.** Case 10-8. A 44-year-old woman presents with occult blood in her stools, and postprandial epigastric pain that is relieved with meals.

Radiologic Findings

10-5. A smooth barium collection projects from the lesser curvature of the stomach and is associated with a lucent "collar" at the neck of the collection, a combination of findings most consistent with benign gastric ulcer (E is the correct answer to Question 10-5).

10-6. A polypoid lesion in the stomach is most likely a gastric neoplasm; the size of the lesion and the presence of a left lobe liver metastasis (arrow) would suggest a malignancy; a GI stromal tumor was diagnosed on pathologic examination (A is the correct answer to Question 10-6).

10-7. Multiple nodules are present in the duodenal bulb, some with central collections of barium, most indicative of duodenal erosions (B is the correct answer to Question 10-7).

10-8. The central collection of barium in the duodenal bulb is located on the anterior wall with the patient prone, thus localizing the lesion; duodenal ulcer with surrounding edema was seen at endoscopy (D is the correct answer to Question 10-8).

Discussion

Many causes of upper gastrointestinal bleeding can be detected on a radiographic examination of this portion of the gastrointestinal tract. As illustrated in the cases of this exercise, the most important causes are gastric or duodenal erosions and ulcers, and neoplasms of the stomach.

The radiographic features that suggest a benign gastric ulcer include (1) projection from the lumen of the stomach; (2) smooth lucent line (Hampton line) or collar (as in this case) at the neck of the ulcer; (3) normal rugal folds that radiate to the edge of the ulcer collection; and (4) complete and permanent healing of the ulcer on repeat radiographic or endoscopic examination of the stomach. If at least two or more of these findings are present, a confident radiographic diagnosis of benign gastric ulcer is possible. A malignant gastric ulcer, which represents a small minority of all ulcers seen in the stomach, is suggested when the collection of barium within the ulcer is irregular and projects within the gastric lumen (ie, ulcerated neoplastic mass), a smooth line or collar at the ulcer margin is not present, or the rugal folds are nodular and terminate abruptly (Figure 10-25). Lack of healing of a gastric ulcer is not a specific sign of malignancy.

Adenocarcinoma remains the most common primary malignancy of the stomach, but its incidence has decreased dramatically in the United States. Gastric adenocarcinoma comprises about 95% of all primary malignancies of the stomach; lymphoma and GI stromal tumors account for most of the remainder. These gastric neoplasms show a wide variety of morphologic forms that include ulcerative, polypoid, infiltrative, or mixed varieties, depending on the type of tumor (Figure 10-26). GIST is the most common mesenchymal

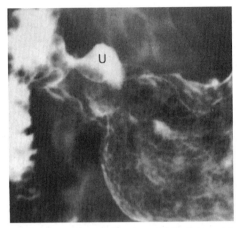

▲ **Figure 10-25.** An irregular ulcer (U) in the gastric antrum that does not project from the lumen or show a smooth ulcer margin. Fixed antral narrowing is present, and the mucosal surface is distorted adjacent to the ulcer. An ulcerated adenocarcinoma of the stomach was found on biopsies from an endoscopic examination.

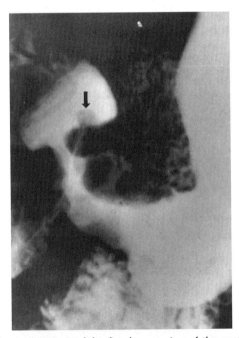

▲ **Figure 10-26.** Nodular fixed narrowing of the gastric antrum associated with a small nodule at the base of the duodenal bulb (arrow). Although gastric carcinoma would be a likely possibility, lymphoma of the stomach was diagnosed at surgery.

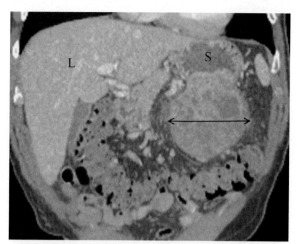

▲ **Figure 10-27.** Coronal CT reconstruction showing a large malignant GIST (interconnected arrows) of the stomach (S); much of the tumor is exophytic with a portion projecting into the gastric lumen at the top margin. L, liver.

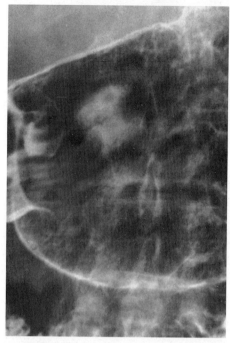

▲ **Figure 10-28.** Close-up double-contrast radiograph of the gastric antrum showing multiple erosions, which appear as small nodular defects with a central punctuate collection of barium. On endoscopic examination, erosions present as reddened nodules with a central yellow exudate at the site of mucosal disruption.

tumor of the stomach and arises from the pacemaker cells of Cajal in the muscularis propria; special stains are used to make a specific diagnosis. GI stromal tumors may be small and polypoid, resembling benign gastric polyps; larger lesions are often ulcerated and reveal malignant features, such as local invasion and metastases. GIST may be endoluminal or exophytic in location (Figure 10-27), although both components may be present ("dumbbell tumors").

Erosions in the stomach and duodenum are a common cause of upper gastrointestinal bleeding. Because these erosions may be few in number and small in size, endoscopic examination of the stomach and duodenum is more sensitive in their detection than radiologic evaluation. The radiographic features of duodenitis depend on the severity of the disease and include thickening and nodularity of the duodenal folds or the presence of erosions, which appear as punctuate collections of barium centered on a nodule. Brunner gland hyperplasia may have an appearance similar to duodenitis, but erosions are not seen, and patients may not be symptomatic. Carcinoma of the duodenal bulb is extremely rare and does not typically enter the differential diagnosis of inflammatory lesions in this anatomic region. Gastric erosions also appear as nodular defects, usually in the antrum of the stomach (Figure 10-28).

Approximately 95% of duodenal ulcers occur within the duodenal bulb and have about an equal distribution on the anterior and posterior walls of the duodenum. The remaining 5% of duodenal ulcers are located near the apex of the bulb. On radiographic examination, a duodenal ulcer is seen as a round or oval collection of barium that should maintain a fixed size and shape on multiple images of the collection;

inconsistent collections of barium, often seen in the duodenal fornices or at the apex or in the presence of bulbar deformity, may be mistaken for an active ulcer. Anterior wall duodenal ulcers are best visualized with the patient in the prone position (as in this case), whereas posterior wall ulcers are seen well with the patient supine (Figure 10-29). As with duodenal carcinomas, polyps in the duodenal bulb are rare and would appear as lucent filling defects and not as a collection of barium.

EXERCISE 10-3. SMALL-BOWEL BLEEDING

10-9. What is the most likely explanation for the abnormal small-bowel loop anterior to the bladder (B) on this contrast-enhanced CT examination of the lower abdomen in Case 10-9 (Figure 10-30)?
   A. Crohn disease
   B. Tuberculosis
   C. Whipple disease
   D. Ulcerated lymphoma
   E. Small-bowel metastases

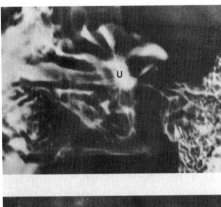

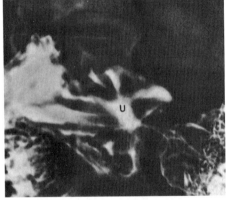

▲ **Figure 10-29.** Two views of the duodenal bulb with the patient in a supine position demonstrating a posterior wall ulcer (u) with radiating folds extending around the circumference of the barium collection.

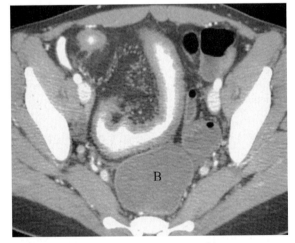

▲ **Figure 10-30.** Case 10-9. A 24-year-old woman presents with intermittent abdominal pain, diarrhea, and anemia.

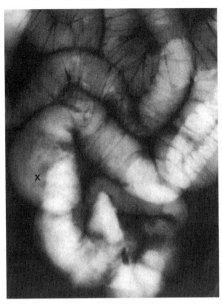

▲ **Figure 10-31.** Case 10-10. A 48-year-old man presents with rectal bleeding but no other symptoms.

10-10. What is the most likely cause of the saccular structure (x) seen in the distal small bowel in Case 10-10 (Figure 10-31)?
   A. Normal loop of small bowel
   B. Large small-bowel ulcer
   C. Meckel diverticulum
   D. Ulcerated primary malignancy
   E. Small-bowel metastases

10-11. What is the least likely etiology of the diffuse fold thickening in the central small bowel in Case 10-11 (Figure 10-32)?
   A. Ischemic enteritis
   B. Small-bowel hemorrhage
   C. Radiation enteritis
   D. Small-bowel edema
   E. Small-bowel malignancy

10-12. What is the least likely possibility to explain the irregular, ulcerated small-bowel lesion in Case 10-12 (Figure 10-33)?
   A. Ulcerated GIST
   B. Lymphoma with ulceration
   C. Metastatic ulcerated mass
   D. Large benign ulcer of small bowel
   E. Adenocarcinoma with ulceration

Radiologic Findings

10-9. The segmental and enhancing wall thickening in the ileum is most consistent with Crohn disease;

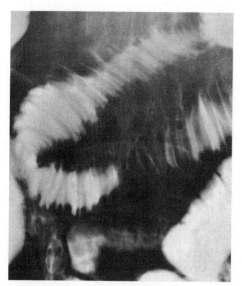

▲ **Figure 10-32.** Case 10-11. A 72-year-old woman presents with sudden onset of abdominal pain and occult rectal bleeding.

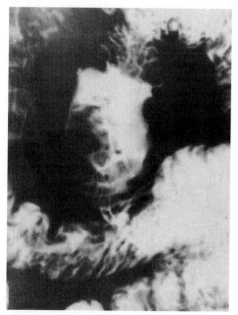

▲ **Figure 10-33.** Case 10-12. A 58-year-old man presents with abdominal pain, anemia, and intermittent rectal bleeding (Used with permission from Chen MYM, Zagoria RJ, Ott DJ, Gelfand DW. *Radiology of the Small Bowel*. New York: Igaku-Shoin; 1992).

tuberculosis might appear similar but is rare, and most neoplasms of the small bowel are focal (A is the correct answer to Question 10-9).

10-10. The smooth, saccular structure of the small bowel proved to be a bleeding Meckel diverticulum; benign ulcers of the small bowel are rare, and ulcerated malignancies are usually irregular in appearance (C is the correct answer to Question 10-10).

10-11. The long segment of small bowel of normal caliber with smooth fold thickening (ie, valvulae conniventes) suggests submucosal infiltration from fluid (eg, edema or blood), which may have many causes but not small-bowel malignancy; ischemic enteritis was the etiology (E is the correct answer to Question 10-11).

10-12. The irregular, ulcerated mass of the small bowel is typical for an ulcerated malignancy of various histologic types, including metastatic neoplasms; the cause was a lymphoma (D is the correct answer to Question 10-12).

Discussion

Small-bowel bleeding and obstruction can be caused by a wide assortment of diseases, some of which may present with both signs. Crohn disease and ischemia of the small bowel are likely the two most common causes in younger and older patients, respectively.

Crohn disease is an inflammatory disorder of the gastrointestinal tract of unknown etiology. The small bowel and the ileocecal region are the most common sites of involvement. Crohn disease may affect a single segment, often the terminal ileum, or multiple areas of the small bowel with normal intervening loops (ie, skip areas). The involved loop(s) is usually narrowed with a nodular mucosal surface due to ulceration; deep ulcers and sinus tracts may progress to fistulas. Mark narrowing of the bowel lumen may relate to active inflammation and spasm with wall thickening or to fibrotic stenosis (Figure 10-34). CT and MR imaging with intravenous contrast enhancement are now commonly used to determine the activity of Crohn disease and to help with clinical management (Figure 10-35).

Meckel diverticulum is one of the most common anomalies of the gastrointestinal tract and occurs in about 2% to 3% of the population. The diverticulum is usually asymptomatic and is found incidentally, but may be a cause of intestinal bleeding if the structure contains ulcerated ectopic gastric mucosa. When shown on radiographic examination of the small bowel, especially using the enteroclysis technique, Meckel diverticulum appears as a changeable saccular outpouching along the antimesenteric border of the bowel within a short distance from the ileocecal junction. A rarer complication of a Meckel diverticulum is inversion into the lumen of the small bowel with subsequent intussusception and obstruction.

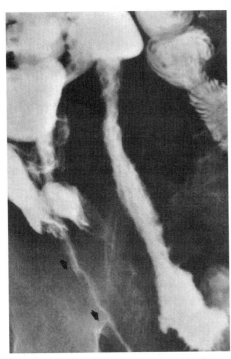

▲ **Figure 10-34.** Another patient with Crohn disease of the distal small bowel with narrowing and irregularity of several segments. The terminal ileum (arrows) is severely narrowed, an appearance called the "string sign," which is often due to spasm.

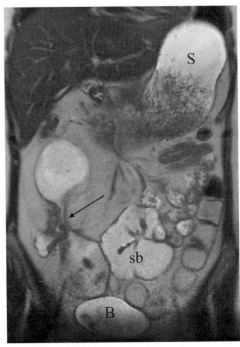

▲ **Figure 10-35.** Coronal MR image of the abdomen in a patient with Crohn disease showing ileocecal stricturing (arrow). S, stomach; B, bladder; sb, dilated small bowel.

Ischemic disease of the small intestine can be caused by nonobstructive hypoperfusion of the organ or result from thrombotic or embolic vascular disease. The radiographic findings are variable depending on the extent and severity of the underlying process and its duration. Small-bowel dilatation from ileus or narrowing due to spasm and submucosal edema and hemorrhage are additional appearances; these changes are also evident on CT and MR imaging, both of which offer further advantages in assessment of the bowel wall, the detection of pneumatosis, and the evaluation of the mesenteric vessels using CTA or MRA (ie, CT or MR angiography). Submucosal infiltration of the small bowel as seen in ischemic enteritis may occur in other disorders and have similar appearances, such as small-bowel hemorrhage related to anticoagulants, trauma, hemophilia, or vasculitis; radiation enteritis is another consideration (Figure 10-36). Small-bowel ischemia may resolve spontaneously or progress to perforation; stricture is a late complication.

Primary small-bowel neoplasms are rare. Benign neoplasms of the small intestine are less often symptomatic compared to malignancies. Adenomas, lipomas, and GISTs/leiomyomas are the most common benign neoplasms but make up only 60% of the benign total because of a large number of miscellaneous rarities. Symptomatic small-bowel neoplasms are usually malignant and nearly all are adenocarcinoma, lymphoma, carcinoid tumor, or malignant GIST. These malignancies, along with metastatic neoplasms of the small bowel, show a wide spectrum of appearances varying from polypoid and ulcerated masses to multifocal and infiltrative processes (Figure 10-37).

EXERCISE 10-4. SMALL-BOWEL OBSTRUCTION

10-13. What is the most likely cause of the lucent band (interconnected arrows) involving the terminal ileum (TI) and causing small-bowel obstruction (arrow; C, cecum) in Case 10-13 (Figure 10-38)?
   A. Ileocolic intussusception
   B. Obstructing adhesions
   C. Meckel diverticulum
   D. Small-bowel volvulus
   E. Polypoid malignancy

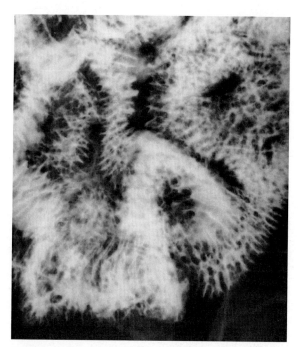

▲ **Figure 10-36.** Patient who had abdominal radiation as a child; peroral small-bowel study shows diffuse fold thickening which is not specific and could be caused by a wide variety of abnormalities, including infections, vasculitis, ischemia, and a number of rare disorders.

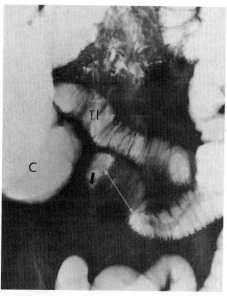

▲ **Figure 10-38.** Case 10-13. A 38-year-old woman with previous abdominal surgery presents with distention of the abdomen and vomiting.

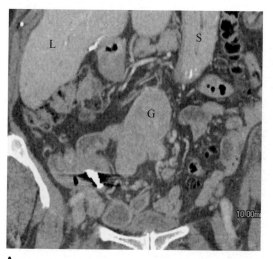

A

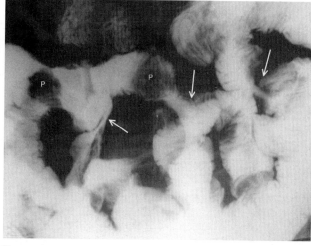

B

▲ **Figure 10-37.** (**A**) Coronal CT image shown a large exophytic (and likely endoluminal) GIST (G) involving the small intestine. L, liver; S, stomach. (**B**) Peroral small-bowel examination in a patient with breast metastases showing bowel angulation (arrows) and polypoid defects (p).

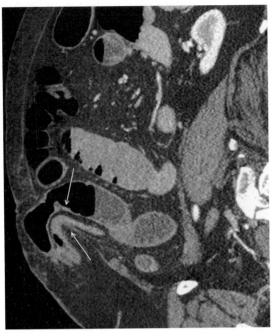

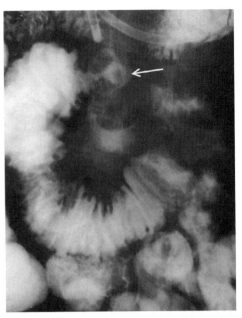

▲ **Figure 10-40.** Case 10-15. A 56-year-old man has epigastric pain and nausea.

▲ **Figure 10-39.** Case 10-14. A 68-year-old man presents with abdominal pain and vomiting, and a mass protruding along the abdominal wall.

10-14. What is the most likely cause of the transition in small-bowel caliber (arrows), which is causing obstruction on this sagittal reformatted CT scan in Case 10-14 (Figure 10-39)?
   A. Meckel diverticulum
   B. Small-bowel volvulus
   C. Adhesions with obstruction
   D. Polypoid small-bowel tumor
   E. Anterior abdominal wall hernia

10-15. What is the least likely cause of the angulated focal narrowing (arrow) seen on the enteroclysis examination in Case 10-15 (Figure 10-40)?
   A. Carcinoid tumor
   B. Metastatic mass
   C. Small-bowel lymphoma
   D. Intussusception due to mass
   E. Small-bowel adenocarcinoma

10-16. What is the most likely cause of the multiple areas of angulation and narrowing (arrows) causing small-bowel obstruction in Case 10-16 (Figure 10-41)?
   A. Peritoneal adhesions
   B. Small-bowel adenocarcinoma
   C. Metastatic disease
   D. Radiation enteritis
   E. Small-bowel intussusception

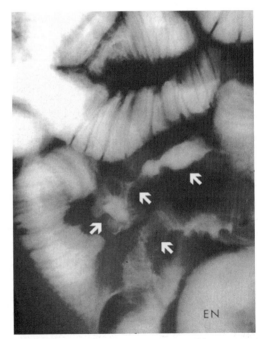

▲ **Figure 10-41.** Case 10-16. A 42-year-old woman with carcinoma of the breast.

Radiologic Findings

10-13. The lucent band is due to adhesions causing a distal small-bowel obstruction (B is the correct answer to Question 10-13).

10-14. A small-bowel loop is contained within an external anterior abdominal wall hernia with narrowing of the lower small-bowel loop (E is the correct answer to Question 10-14).

10-15. The irregular, angulated mass narrowing is likely due to a small-bowel malignancy; a carcinoid tumor was found at surgery. A polypoid mass with intussusception would appear as a focal dilatation of the bowel (D is the correct answer to Question 10-15).

10-16. Multiple sites of narrowing and angulation (arrows) are causing small-bowel obstruction; in a patient with a known malignancy, peritoneal metastasis with serosal bowel involvement is the most likely cause (C is the correct answer to Question 10-16).

Discussion

The most common causes of small-bowel obstruction are adhesions, hernias, and primary or secondary neoplasms of the small intestine. Although barium examinations of the small bowel have been used traditionally to evaluate small-bowel obstruction, more modern imaging using a variety of CT and MR techniques (as discussed previously) is now used more often, particularly in the presence of high-grade bowel obstruction.

Peritoneal adhesions are most often the cause of small-bowel obstruction in adults. Previous abdominal surgery is the usual explanation for development of peritoneal adhesions. Focal small-bowel obstruction is diagnosed on contrast examination and also with cross-sectional imaging (ie, CT or MR) by demonstrating an area of caliber transition from dilated to normal-caliber bowel. If angulated loops are seen at a caliber transition in the absence of a mass effect, adhesions are the likely cause of obstruction; these criteria are useful whether traditional contrast examination or CT imaging is being used for evaluating patients with suspected small-bowel obstruction (Figure 10-42).

Abdominal hernias are now considered the second most common cause of small-bowel obstruction, and their prevalence and location will vary depending on the age and sex of the patient. External hernias are the most common types, with the inguinal canal predominating in the male population; however, hernias may occur in other areas of the abdomen, such as in the umbilical and paraumbilical regions. Hernias can also be seen more laterally (eg, Spigelian type at the lateral margin of the rectus muscle) and may be associated with incisional scars from previous abdominal surgery. CT examination of the abdomen with the ability to reformat in a variety of planes (ie, coronal and sagittal) is an ideal imaging modality for evaluation of abdominal hernias. Internal

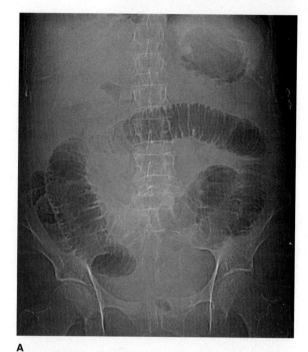

A

B

▲ **Figure 10-42.** (A) Scanogram of the abdomen from a CT examination showing small-bowel distention suggestion obstruction, although the location and etiology remain uncertain. (B) CT examination demonstrates a caliber transition (arrows) without an associated "mass effect" suggesting adhesive small-bowel obstruction. SB, dilated small bowel; AC, ascending colon.

hernias are much less common, but may also be a cause of bowel obstruction.

Small-bowel malignancies were discussed briefly in the previous exercise. Adenocarcinoma of the small bowel occurs most often in the duodenum and jejunum and is much less common in the ileum. The morphologic appearance of adenocarcinomas of the small intestine consists of polypoid, ulcerative, stenosing, and infiltrative forms, which are similar to their counterparts in the stomach and colon. Primary lymphomas of the small bowel are a heterogeneous group of tumors, and controversy persists regarding definition of primary and secondary forms of this neoplasm. Lymphomas may involve any level of the small intestine but are most common in the ileum; the gross pathologic patterns include nodular or polypoid masses, constricting lesions that resemble carcinoma, or a more diffusely nodular or infiltrative process.

Carcinoid tumor and malignant GIST are the other two primary malignancies seen in the small bowel. GIST usually occurs as a single lesion and is most often found in the jejunum and ileum. Pathologically, this tumor typically presents as a polypoid mass with an intraluminal and extramural component; a bulky, irregular mass is common, and ulceration often occurs (Figure 10-43). Special immunohistochemical stains are used to identify the specific tissue types of these neoplasms (ie, c-kit or CD117 positivity). Carcinoid tumors arise from enterochromaffin or similar types of cells, and more than 90% originate in the gastrointestinal tract. Most carcinoid tumors of the small bowel are located in the ileum. Their radiologic appearances reflect their broad pathologic morphology, and they may present as single or multiple polypoid lesions or as focal stenosis leading to partial obstruction; angulation and kinking of bowel loops may occur with a desmoplastic

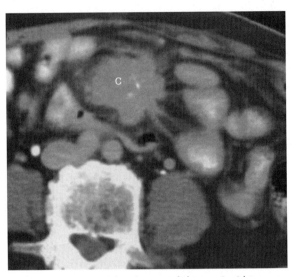

▲ **Figure 10-44.** Axial CT image of the carcinoid tumor (c) in Case 10-15; the mass is better appreciated on the cross-sectional imaging, and the stellate desmoplastic response is evident.

reaction and cause a mass that is best appreciated on cross-sectional imaging (Figure 10-44).

Secondary malignancies involving the small bowel are much more common than the primary types. The three routes of secondary malignancy that can spread to the small intestine include (1) hematogenous metastases, with carcinoma of the breast, lung, and melanoma being the most common; (2) intraperitoneal seeding of tumor from elsewhere within the abdomen; and (3) direct contiguous invasion of bowel (most often seen with pancreatic carcinoma and pelvic malignancies). Carcinoma of the cervix, endometrium, and ovary often affects the distal small bowel by intraperitoneal seeding or direct invasion; the colon may also be involved, and radiographic evaluation of these patients may be best performed with a barium enema, with one goal being reflux into the ileum (Figure 10-45). Presently, CT and MR imaging of the abdomen and pelvis have emerged as the usual modalities for assessing and following patients with intra-abdominal malignancies.

EXERCISE 10-5. COLONIC BLEEDING

10-17. What is the most likely cause of the large polypoid lesion (arrows) in the sigmoid colon in Case 10-17 (Figure 10-46)?
   A. Annular carcinoma
   B. Benign lipoma
   C. Polypoid carcinoma
   D. Pedunculated benign adenoma
   E. Hyperplastic polyp

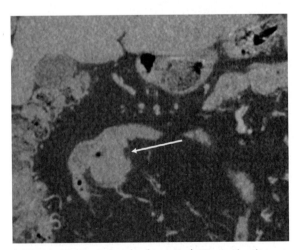

▲ **Figure 10-43.** Coronal reformatted CT examination shows a GIST (arrow); note that the tumor is predominantly exophytic, although an intraluminal component is likely present next to the small amount of gas within the lumen.

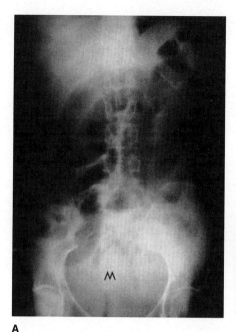
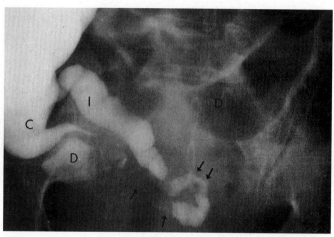

A   **B**

▲ **Figure 10-45.** **(A)** A 55-year-old woman with advanced ovarian carcinoma presents with a large pelvic mass (M) and small-bowel distention on plain film of the abdomen. **(B)** Barium enema in the patient did not show colonic involvement, but reflux into a normal-caliber terminal ileum (I) demonstrated angulated obstruction (arrows) of the small bowel due to the pelvic malignancy with more proximal dilated (D) bowel loops (C, cecum).

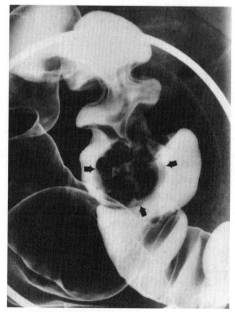

▲ **Figure 10-46.** Case 10-17. A 52-year-old woman presents with intermittent bright red rectal bleeding.

10-18. What is the etiology of the irregular, focal narrowing in the ascending colon in Case 10-18 (Figure 10-47)?
   A. Polypoid carcinoma
   B. Annular carcinoma
   C. Inflammatory stricture
   D. Surgical anastomosis
   E. Ischemic stricture

10-19. What is the most likely explanation of the diffuse rectosigmoid mucosal abnormality on double-contrast barium enema in Case 10-19 (Figure 10-48)?
   A. Ischemic colitis
   B. Pseudomembranous colitis
   C. Lymphogranuloma venereum
   D. Crohn colitis
   E. Ulcerative colitis

10-20. What is the *least* likely cause of the diffuse wall thickening of the sigmoid colon seen on the CT image in Case 10-20 (Figure 10-49)?
   A. Annular carcinoma
   B. Pseudomembranous colitis
   C. Diverticular disease
   D. Crohn colitis
   E. Radiation rectosigmoiditis

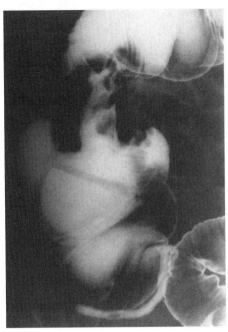

▲ **Figure 10-47.** Case 10-18. A 64-year-old man presents with melena and right-sided abdominal pain.

Radiologic Findings

10-17. The large, lobulated (ie, irregular surface) polypoid mass in the sigmoid colon was a polypoid carcinoma (C is the correct answer to Question 10-17).

10-18. The circumferential, irregular narrowing of the ascending colon was an annular carcinoma (B is the correct answer to Question 10-18).

10-19. The diffuse and continuous mucosal granularity seen in the rectosigmoid colon is most consistent

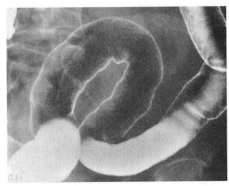

▲ **Figure 10-48.** Case 10-19. A 34-year-old woman presents with bloody diarrhea and tenesmus.

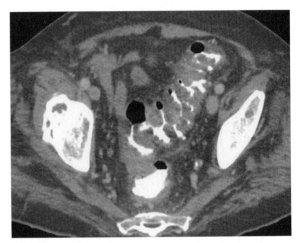

▲ **Figure 10-49.** Case 10-20. A 74-year-old man presents with severe diarrhea with some bleeding after being treated for a febrile urinary tract infection.

with ulcerative colitis (E is the correct answer to Question 10-19).

10-20. The diffuse wall thickening of the sigmoid colon likely is due to an inflammatory (colitis) disorder or diverticular disease; a pseudomembranous colitis was the cause in this patient (A is the correct answer to Question 10-20).

Discussion

Rectal bleeding can result from a multitude of abnormalities throughout the gastrointestinal tract. In this exercise, the more important colonic cause of rectal bleeding are illustrated. Another common cause of rectal bleeding is diverticular disease of the colon, which is readily shown on barium enema and CT examination. In older patients, ischemic colitis and vascular malformations (eg, angiodysplasia) of the right side of the colon are increasingly important causes. In general, contrast studies of the gastrointestinal tract can detect many abnormalities that may be a source of bleeding but cannot determine whether the lesion is bleeding actively; cross-sectional imaging (with and without vascular contrast material), nuclear medicine, and angiography can demonstrate active bleeding, which can also be treated by interventional radiology or endoscopy.

The two most common polypoid lesions of the colon are the hyperplastic and neoplastic polyp. Most hyperplastic polyps are less than 5 mm in diameter, are sessile and smooth, and may resemble small neoplastic polyps of similar size. Neoplastic polyps have a broad pathologic spectrum, which includes: (1) benign adenomas (tubular, tubulovillous, and villous types); (2) adenomas with focal carcinoma; and

(3) polypoid carcinoma. Consequently, the radiologic appearances of neoplastic colonic polyps are varied, and benign and malignant neoplasms may appear similar. Neoplastic polyps can be sessile or pedunculated and smooth or lobulated (Figure 10-50). Size is an important radiologic criterion to estimate the risk of malignancy in a sessile colonic polyp; a polyp less than 1 cm in size has only a 1% chance of malignancy, with the risk increasing to 10% for 1- to 2-cm polyps and 25% or more for polyps over 2 cm. The finding of a pedicle is important because invasion of a cancer, if present, to the adjacent colonic wall is rare. Imaging of the large bowel for colon cancer screening has changed in recent years, with the barium enema assuming a minor role; colonoscopy is now most often performed both for detection of neoplastic lesions and for their removal, which is possible in most patients. CT colonography may become more important as a screening modality, but its efficacy is under intense investigation presently.

Adenocarcinoma of the colon is the second most common malignancy that affects both sexes. About 95% of colonic carcinomas occur in patients older than 40 years, with a peak in the later seventh decade. As with adenocarcinomas elsewhere in the gastrointestinal tract, a variety of morphologic forms are seen, including polypoid carcinoma (malignant potential discussed previously), ulcerative and

infiltrative types, and the annular carcinoma; the last is also called the "apple-core" lesion. In the colon of an adult patient, an irregular constricting lesion having an abrupt transition with the normal colonic wall is nearly always an adenocarcinoma (Figure 10-51). Inflammatory strictures and surgical anastomosis typically have a smooth and often tapered appearance.

Ulcerative and Crohn colitis are the two common idiopathic inflammatory diseases of the colon. Other causes of colitis include infections of various types, drug-related types (ie, pseudomembranous colitis), radiation-induced colitis (usually proctitis), ischemic colitis, and miscellaneous disorders. These other disorders may mimic idiopathic colitis, and clinical correlation and exclusion of infection are important. Radiographic differentiation between ulcerative and Crohn colitis is usually possible in most patients; of course, cross-sectional imaging, endoscopy, and pathologic evaluation have important roles. The features most suggestive of ulcerative colitis are continuous disease with rectal involvement, ahaustral shortening of the colon, and a finely ulcerated or granular mucosal surface. The more

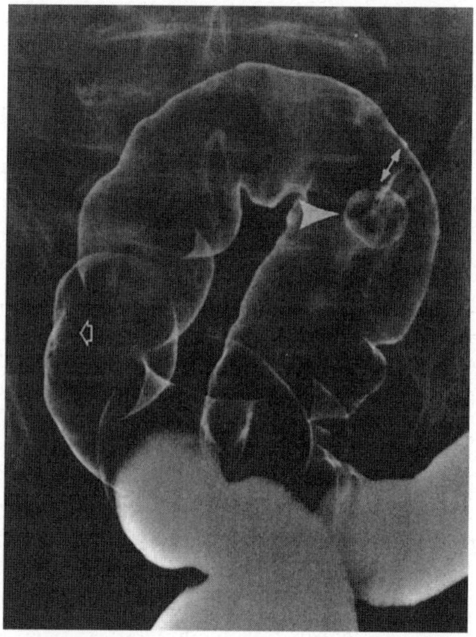

▲ **Figure 10-50.** Double-contrast radiograph of the rectosigmoid region shows a small, smooth, sessile adenoma (arrow) and a larger pedunculated (interconnected arrows) adenoma (arrowhead) more proximally.

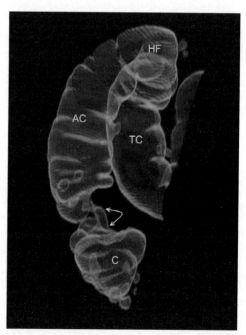

▲ **Figure 10-51.** Segmented CTC image of the right side of the colon showing an annular carcinoma (arrows) arising near the junction of the ascending colon (AC) and the cecum (C); the multiple round structures are mostly diverticula, although retained stool and polyps might appear similar on this modality. HF, hepatic flexure; TC, transverse colon.

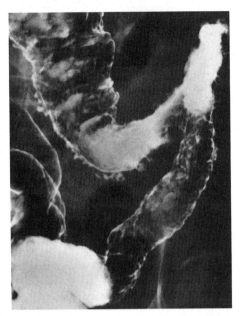

▲ **Figure 10-52.** Segmental Crohn disease of the transverse and descending portions of the colon, showing multiple deep ulcers projecting from the margins of the affected colon and small "aphthoid" ulcers appearing like erosions seen in the upper gastrointestinal tract.

specific findings of Crohn colitis include discontinuous disease (ie, skip areas) with ileitis, eccentric wall involvement, discrete (ie, aphthoid ulcers) or deep ulceration, intramural fissuring, and formation of fistula to adjacent organs (Figure 10-52). Complications that may occur in idiopathic colitis include toxic megacolon, carcinoma, sclerosing cholangitis, and abnormalities of the eyes, skin, and joints. Toxic megacolon and complicating carcinoma are more common in ulcerative colitis.

Pseudomembranous colitis has emerged as a common inflammatory condition of the large bowel in recent decades, especially in hospitalized patients. Although a number of risk factors have been identified, the vast majority of cases are associated with antibiotic exposure. These drugs alter the intestinal flora, resulting in an overgrowth of *Clostridium difficile*, which releases a toxin(s) that produces the inflammatory pseudomembranes and other pathologic changes. Imaging findings, often best seen on CT examination, include wall thickening that may be segmental or pancolonic, fold thickening causing an "accordion sign," and mucosal irregularity due to the pseudomembranous changes; these abnormalities are often nonspecific, and other diagnostic tests (eg, sigmoidoscopy) need to be performed. Ischemic colitis is common in older patients and warrants further discussion. As in the small bowel, a variety of vascular changes may cause colonic

ischemia. The most common site of involvement is in the watershed area of the main mesenteric vessels, that is, the splenic flexure and descending colon, although other areas and diffuse involvement of the colon may be seen. In the severest form, colonic infarction and perforation may occur; however, the most common appearances relate to submucosal hemorrhage, which causes narrowing of the affected colon associated with irregular, smooth margins often called "thumbprinting"; complete healing and return to normal may occur (Figure 10-53), or progression to a smooth, tapered stricture can result.

EXERCISE 10-6. COLONIC OBSTRUCTION

10-21. What is the most likely primary cause of the findings seen on the pelvic CT examination in Case 10-21 (Figure 10-54)?
A. Annular carcinoma of descending colon
B. Ischemic colitis
C. Small-bowel neoplasm involving colon
D. Sigmoid diverticulitis
E. Peritoneal metastases

10-22. What is the most likely cause of the irregular, annular narrowing (arrow) in the lower rectum in Case 10-22 (Figure 10-55)?
A. Rectal carcinoma
B. Lymphoma of rectum
C. Crohn proctitis
D. Infectious proctitis
E. Invasive cervical cancer

10-23. What is the most likely explanation of the two adjacent loops of distended colon (arrows) in Case 10-23 (Figure 10-56)?
A. Right colon volvulus
B. Sigmoid volvulus
C. Ileocecal intussusception
D. Functional colonic ileus
E. Internal colonic hernia

10-24. What is the most likely etiology of the smooth mass (arrows) partially obstructing the anterior rectosigmoid region in Case 10-24 (Figure 10-57)?
A. Annular rectosigmoid carcinoma
B. Rectosigmoid diverticulitis
C. Pelvic endometriosis
D. Invasive endometrial carcinoma
E. Cul-de-sac metastases

Radiologic Findings

10-21. Sigmoid colon narrowing with adjacent air (Figure 10-58 A, arrows) is present along with secondary small-bowel obstruction related to diverticulitis (D is the correct answer to Question 10-21).

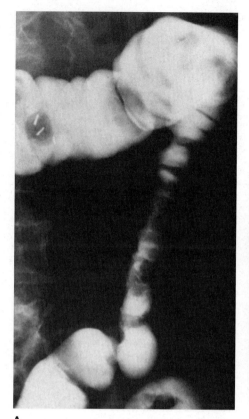 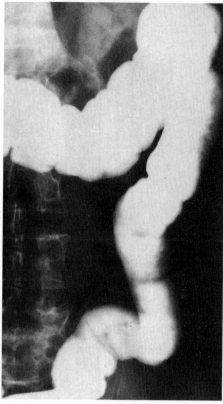

A   B

▲ Figure 10-53. (A) Single-contrast barium enema showing narrowing of the descending colon with a scalloped appearance, that is, "thumbprinting"; patient was elderly and presented with an abrupt onset of hematochezia, suggesting ischemic colitis. (B) Repeat examination in the same patient 6 weeks later now showing complete resolution of the ischemic process and a return to a normal-appearing descending colon.

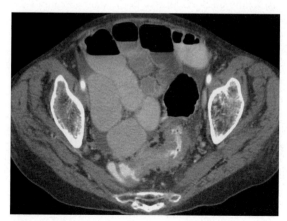

▲ Figure 10-54. Case 10-21. A 47-year-old man presents with left lower abdominal pain and change in bowel habits.

10-22. An annular rectal carcinoma causing distal colonic obstruction is present; rectal lymphoma is rare, and the other possibilities listed do not cause circumferential narrowing of the rectum (A is the correct answer to Question 10-22).

10-23. A sigmoid volvulus is present, which is the most common colonic volvulus; note the colonic loops pointing into the sigmoid colon (B is the correct answer to Question 10-23).

10-24. Pelvic endometriosis is involving the anterior rectosigmoid junction; diverticulitis is rare in this location, and the patient is young for the other options offered (C is the correct answer to Question 10-24).

Discussion

Colonic obstruction when seen in adults is usually caused by diverticulitis or carcinoma of the colon. Volvulus of the colon

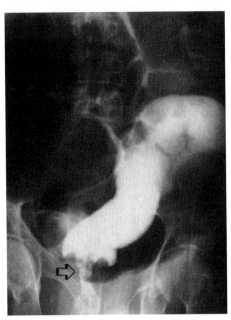

▲ **Figure 10-55.** Case 10-22. A 69-year-old woman presents with rectal bleeding and obstipation.

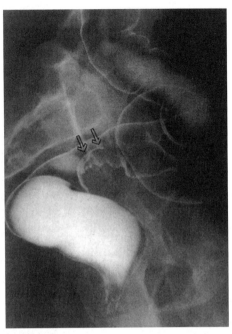

▲ **Figure 10-57.** Case 10-24. A 33-year-old woman presents with cyclic lower abdominal pain, change in bowel habits, and rectal bleeding.

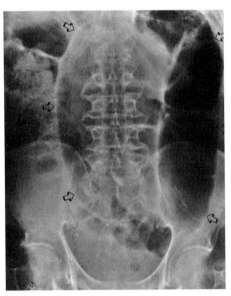

▲ **Figure 10-56.** Case 10-23. A 70-year-old man presents with acute abdominal distention and obstipation (From Ott DJ, Chen MYM. Specific acute colonic disorders. *Radiol Clin North Am.* 1994;32:871-884, used with permission).

is much less common. However, extrinsic involvement of the rectum or sigmoid colon from pelvic malignancies is an important consideration in the middle-aged or older patient.

Diverticulitis is always a differential consideration in the adult patient with a suspected obstruction of the distal colon. Diverticulitis is usually due to perforation of a single diverticulum, with subsequent formation of a paracolic abscess, and typically is located in the sigmoid colon (likely 90% of cases). The radiographic findings suggesting diverticulitis on contrast enema of the colon include (1) extravasation into an abscess (the most definitive finding); (2) eccentric or circumferential narrowing of the colon; and (3) transverse or longitudinal sinus tracts (also seen in Crohn disease) (Figure 10-58 B). Complications of sigmoid diverticulitis are obstruction, fistula formation (especially to the bladder), and development of a stricture. CT examination of the pelvis has become the preferred means of evaluating patients suspected of having this disease; the extramural findings are evident, complications can be identified, and percutaneous drainage of an abscess can be performed using CT guidance, if deemed useful clinically.

Adenocarcinoma of the colon was discussed in the previous exercise as a common source of rectal bleeding but is also an important cause of colonic obstruction. The location and morphologic type of colonic carcinoma will affect the clinical presentation of the patient. Carcinomas of the right side of

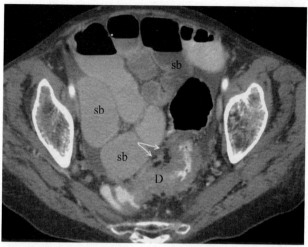

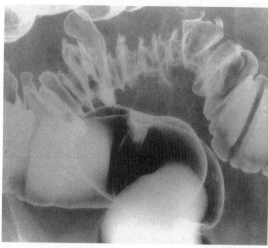

A

B

▲ **Figure 10-58. (A)** Same image as Case 10-21. Diverticulitis (D) is causing luminal narrowing of the sigmoid colon with wall thickening; air (arrows) related to a paracolic diverticular abscess is present, which is causing a secondary small-bowel obstruction with multiple dilated loops (sb). **(B)** Double-contrast barium enema of rectosigmoid colon showing diverticular disease and focal, irregular narrowing at the top of the image due to diverticulitis. Contrast enemas do not depict the extraluminal findings that are often appreciated on CT examination.

the colon are often polypoid, may grow to a large size, and more often present clinically with localized pain, palpable mass, and melena. In the left side of the colon, carcinomas usually present at an earlier stage because obstructive symptoms are more common, often due to an annular carcinoma (Figure 10-59). Cross-sectional imaging and CT colonography

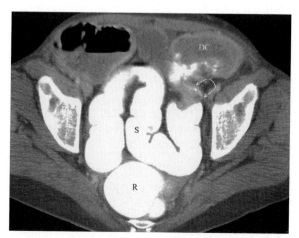

▲ **Figure 10-59.** CT axial image of pelvis showing an annular carcinoma (arrows) near the junction of the sigmoid (S) and descending portions (DC) of the colon; the descending colon is dilated from obstruction (R, rectum).

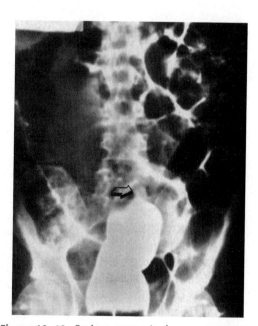

▲ **Figure 10-60.** Barium enema in the same patient as in Case 10-23 (Figure 10-56) showing obstruction at the rectosigmoid junction (arrow) due to sigmoid volvulus (From Ott DJ, Chen MYM. Specific acute colonic disorders. *Radiol Clin North Am.* 1994;32:871-884, used with permission).

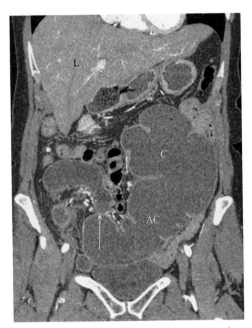

▲ **Figure 10-61.** Coronal CT image showing a right colon volvulus with the twist in the ascending colon (arrow) causing marked distention of a portion of the ascending colon (AC) and the cecum (C). L, liver.

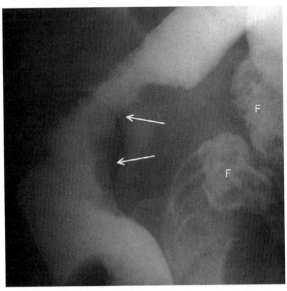

▲ **Figure 10-62.** Lateral view of the rectosigmoid colon from a single-contrast barium enema showing narrowing and irregularity of the rectosigmoid junction (arrows) due to an invasive carcinoma of the cervix. F, calcified uterine fibroids.

have assumed a more important imaging role in the detection of colonic carcinoma, and also in preoperative staging and postoperative evaluation of patients, especially those with recurrent masses; also, percutaneous biopsy of suspicious areas for possible recurrence can be performed.

Sigmoid volvulus is a closed-loop colonic obstruction due to twisting along the mesenteric or long axis of the bowel. Although colonic volvulus is not common, about 90% of cases occur in the sigmoid colon. On plain abdominal films, the sigmoid volvulus forms an inverted U-shaped structure with the twisted sigmoid loops lying adjacent and having an oval appearance called the "coffee bean" sign. On barium enema examination, tapered obstruction of the sigmoid colon is found (Figure 10-60). Cecal volvulus results from a twisting obstruction of the right side of the colon and rarely involves the cecum only (*right colon volvulus* is a better term). The dilated proximal colon may be seen as an oval structure in the midabdomen or the left upper quadrant, but rarely points into the pelvis (Figure 10-61). Contrast enemas or CT examination are used to evaluate patients with potential volvulus of uncertain location; as with high-grade small-bowel obstruction, CT examination is often used initially in patients with possible colonic obstruction.

The anterior wall of the rectosigmoid colon is a common site for involvement of the colon by extrinsic inflammatory or neoplastic diseases. Inflammatory processes may spread into the posterior cul-de-sac and secondarily involve the colon; endometriosis can arise in the same area, implant on the colonic serosa, and invade into the colonic wall. However, pelvic malignancies related to the uterine cervix, endometrium, ovary, bladder, and prostate are the most common neoplastic processes that can affect the rectosigmoid colon. Circumferential narrowing may occur with these extrinsic malignances and mimic a primary carcinoma of the colon (Figure 10-62).

Acknowledgments *Special thanks to my colleagues, Drs. John Leyendecker, Michael Oliphant, and James Perumpillichira, for providing me with nearly all of the CT, MR, and CTC images used in this chapter.*

SUGGESTED READING

1. Gore RM, Levine MS, eds. *Textbook of Gastrointestinal Radiology.* 3rd ed., Vol. 1. Philadelphia: Saunders; 2008.
2. Gore RM, Levine MS, eds. *Textbook of Gastrointestinal Radiology.* 3rd ed., Vol. 2. Philadelphia: Saunders; 2008.
3. Halpert, RD. *Gastrointestinal Imaging: The Requisites.* 3rd ed. Philadelphia: Mosby Elsevier; 2006.
4. Ott DJ, Gelfand DW, Chen MYM. *Manual of Gastrointestinal Fluoroscopy.* Springfield, Ill: Charles C. Thomas; 1996.

Liver, Biliary Tract, and Pancreas

Melanie P. Caserta, MD

Fakhra Chaudhry, MD

Robert E. Bechtold, MD

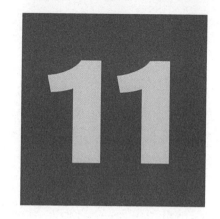

The diagnosis of diseases of the liver, biliary tract, and pancreas optimally depends on using both clinical and radiographic data. Understanding the proper use of these data and ordering radiographic studies in the optimal sequence are helpful for making the diagnosis most efficiently. Frequently, the clinical presentation and associated laboratory work provide most of the clues for diagnosis. Physical examination, history, and pertinent laboratory values are often helpful in making the diagnosis or at least in providing clues for selecting the optimal radiographic studies. If clinical information is insufficient or if radiographic confirmation is necessary, plain films and contrast studies may be performed. Upright and supine plain radiographs are helpful for the detection of free air, calcifications, and other abnormalities. Contrast studies such as endoscopic retrograde cholangiopancreatography (ERCP), magnetic resonance cholangiopancreatography (MRCP) and percutaneous transhepatic cholangiography (PTC) are often helpful in analyzing diseases of the liver, biliary tree, and pancreas. For instance, pancreatic or biliary ductal systems, fistulae from these ductal systems, and associated abnormalities such as encasing tumors can be diagnosed by cholangiography.

Digital cross-sectional imaging, nuclear medicine (NM) and an important form of NM called positron emission tomography (PET), and angiography have provided considerable information in analyzing diseases of these organs, which cannot be directly visualized with plain radiography, even using traditional contrast material, that is, barium. Cross-sectional techniques consist of ultrasound (US), computed tomography (CT), and magnetic resonance (MR) imaging. This chapter reviews the use of cross-sectional imaging and, where pertinent, nuclear medicine and angiography to evaluate abnormalities of the liver, biliary tract, and pancreas.

TECHNIQUES AND NORMAL ANATOMY

Several modalities such as US, nuclear medicine, CT, and MR imaging are commonly used in diagnosing diseases of liver, pancreatic, or biliary ductal system. The detail of each technique has been described in Chapter 1, "Scope of Diagnostic Imaging."

With US, normal organs are displayed as structures of different echogenicity. In general, fluid is anechoic (has no

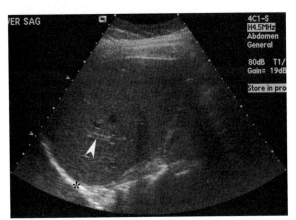

▲ **Figure 11-1.** Longitudinal US image of the normal liver, showing homogeneous parenchymal detail, the hyperechoic hemidiaphragmatic surface (*), and portal triad (arrowhead).

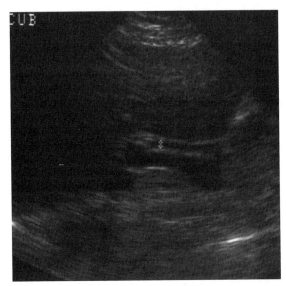

▲ **Figure 11-3.** Longitudinal US image of the normal biliary duct, showing the narrow caliber and the thin, uniform ductal walls (cursors denote the internal walls of the duct).

echoes). Soft tissue has echoes of mild to moderate intensity. Bone has extremely strong echoes. Abnormal organs are displayed as areas of diffuse inhomogeneity or as focal regions of decreased or increased echogenicity within the organ. The normal appearances of the liver, biliary system, and pancreas have been well established. Echogenicity of the organs in the abdomen is evaluated in relation to other nearby organs. The pancreas is typically the most echogenic organ in the upper abdomen, followed by the liver. The liver typically has homogeneous parenchymal detail (Figure 11-1). Numerous intrahepatic vessels including portal veins and hepatic veins are easily seen within the liver. The gallbladder appears as an anechoic pear-shaped structure along the inferior aspect of the liver (Figure 11-2). It normally has a thin, homogeneous wall less than 3 mm in thickness. The degree of distention of

the gallbladder varies with postprandial intervals. As is expected, it contracts after a meal and distends in the fasting state. The biliary ducts are thin tubes, the walls of which are 1.5 mm or less (essentially unmeasurable). The ducts increase in caliber as they extend from the liver to the sphincter of Oddi (Figure 11-3). The upper limit in caliber of the extrahepatic biliary ducts increases with age. When measured at the level where it crosses the right hepatic artery, 6 mm is usually used as the cutoff diameter. The pancreas is homogeneous, comma-shaped, and parallel to the splenic vein and extends from the left upper quadrant caudally and to the right (Figure 11-4). In anteroposterior dimension the pancreatic head is approximately 3 cm, the body 2.5 cm, and the tail 2 cm. The pancreas can sometimes be difficult to image with ultrasound because of its relatively posterior position and overlying bowel gas. The normal pancreatic duct, if seen, should be 3 mm or less.

With NM, normal organs are displayed as regions of homogeneous activity conforming to the general shape of the organ. Abnormal organs are displayed as diffuse inhomogeneity or as focal areas of reduced or increased activity. In the past, the liver was most commonly studied with NM with technetium-labeled sulfur colloid. However, this technique has largely been replaced by CT, US, and MR imaging. The most common NM study of the liver today utilizes technetium-labeled red blood cells to evaluate for cavernous hemangioma. Evaluation of the biliary system is a common application for NM studies. Technetium-labeled hepatobiliary

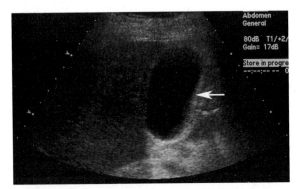

▲ **Figure 11-2.** Longitudinal US image of the normal gallbladder (arrow) showing the anechoic lumen and smooth, thin walls of the gallbladder.

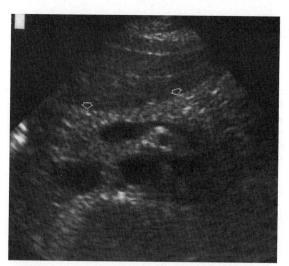

▲ **Figure 11-4.** Transverse US image of the normal pancreas, showing the homogeneous, echogenic pancreatic head, body, and tail (open arrows) lying in front of the splenic and superior mesenteric veins.

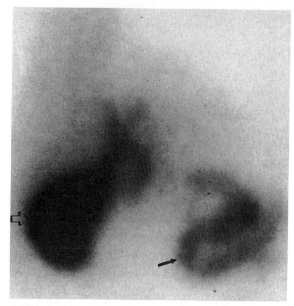

▲ **Figure 11-5.** Hepatobiliary NM scan, showing the presence of radiopharmaceutical within the gallbladder lumen (open arrow) and duodenum (closed arrow), demonstrating the patency of both cystic and common bile duct.

imaging iminodiacetic acid derivatives for hepatobiliary imaging, especially disofenin and mebrofenin, are taken up by the liver, excreted into the bile, carried to the biliary tree and gallbladder, and from there travel to the bowel through the extrahepatic ducts (Figure 11-5). Depending on the exact agent used, these are termed hepatic iminodiacetic acid, HIDA scans. Currently, no practical imaging of the pancreas is done by means of NM techniques.

With CT, normal organs are displayed as regions of differing attenuation. Abnormal organs are displayed as diffuse inhomogeneity or as focal areas of decreased or increased attenuation. The liver, biliary system, and pancreas are well demonstrated by CT (Figure 11-6). Intravenous contrast aids in their evaluation. The liver is the most dense organ in the abdomen. The normal liver parenchyma appears homogeneous, just as in US. The portal and hepatic vessels and the biliary ductal system are likewise easy to identify. Overall measurements of wall thickness and biliary duct caliber are the same as for US. The pancreas is easily identified on CT, and the pancreatic duct is frequently well seen.

At angiography, normal organs enhance to variable extents. Abnormal organs either inhomogeneously enhance or have focal areas of decreased or increased enhancement. Although the parenchyma of the normal organs is rarely demonstrated, the blood vessels of these organs are seen in exquisite detail (Figure 11-7). In the liver, both the hepatic artery and all of its branches can be seen. Delayed studies through the liver in the venous phase demonstrate the portal vein. The cystic artery and any collateral vessels can be angiographically demonstrated. Angiographic studies of the pancreas can demonstrate major pancreatic branches, as well as encasement, displacement, stenosis, or occlusion.

On MR imaging, normal organs have homogeneous signal intensity or well-recognized variations in signal intensity. Abnormal organs have inhomogeneous signal intensity or areas of increased or decreased signal intensity. The normal

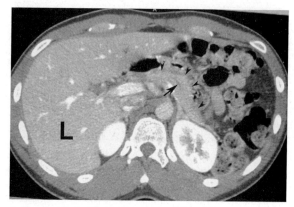

▲ **Figure 11-6.** CT showing normal liver (L) and pancreas (arrowheads) with normal-caliber pancreatic duct (arrow).

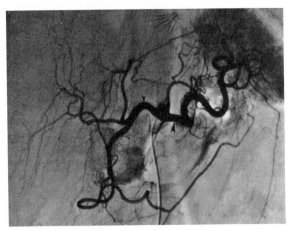

▲ **Figure 11-7.** Celiac arteriogram, showing normal distribution of the splenic (large arrowhead) and hepatic (small arrowhead) arteries, and the normal homogeneous stain of the spleen in the left upper quadrant.

liver, biliary system, and pancreas are well demonstrated on MR imaging (Figure 11-8). The liver has a homogeneous signal intensity which is usually higher than that of muscle and lower than that of the spleen. The biliary system is normally demonstrated as an area of low signal intensity on T1-weighted images and high signal intensity on T2-weighted images. This appearance reflects the fluid bile

within the gallbladder and biliary tree. Magnetic resonance cholangiopancreatography, or MRCP, demonstrates the biliary system as very high signal intensity structures against a very low signal intensity background of surrounding solid tissues (Figure 11-9). The pancreas is of intermediate signal on both T1- and T2-weighted images and may be hard to differentiate from bowel if no oral contrast agent is administered to the patient. As in CT and US, the normal fatty change within the pancreas that occurs with age is visible. Newer hepatocyte-specific contrast agents, such as gadoxetate disodium, are offering new ways of evaluating the liver and biliary system.

TECHNIQUE SELECTION

Diseases of the liver, biliary system, and pancreas can be conveniently, if arbitrarily, separated into the following categories to help illustrate the optimal sequences of imaging techniques: diffuse hepatocellular disease, focal hepatic diseases, abdominal trauma, inflammatory disease of the biliary tract, and pancreatic inflammation or neoplasm.

▶ Diffuse Hepatocellular Disease

In diffuse hepatocellular disease, CT is probably the first study used to survey the liver because it is moderately sensitive to liver lesions and is also helpful for evaluating surrounding organs. Ultrasound may have an application unless

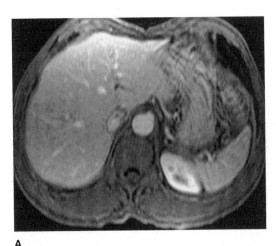

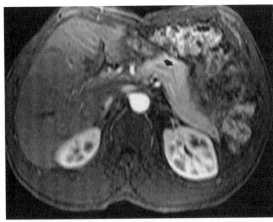

A   B

▲ **Figure 11-8.** **(A)** Dynamic gadolinium-enhanced T1-weighted gradient echo image of the upper abdomen, taken at the level of the mid-liver, demonstrating homogeneous liver, with interspersed intrahepatic vessels, and spleen. **(B)** Dynamic gadolinium-enhanced T1-weighted gradient echo image of the upper abdomen, taken at the level of the pancreas and kidneys, demonstrating the homogeneous pancreatic body and tail with pancreatic duct (arrow), and the corticomedullary differentiation in the kidneys.

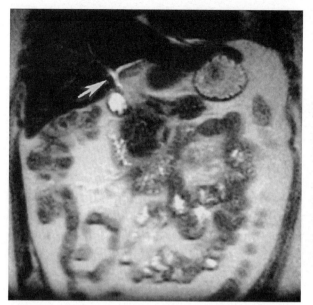
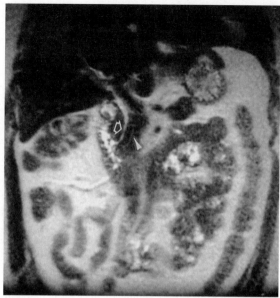

A   **B**

▲ **Figure 11-9.** **(A)** Magnetic resonance cholangiopancreatography (MRCP) of the normal biliary ducts, taken at the level of the porta hepatis, demonstrating the branching proximal intrahepatic ducts (arrow). **(B)** MRCP of the normal biliary ducts, taken at the level of the distal extrahepatic bile duct, demonstrating the intrapancreatic passage of the biliary (arrow) and pancreatic (arrowhead) ducts, entering the duodenum.

fatty liver is present, because fat attenuates the US beam. NM has only infrequent applications. MR imaging may be the most sensitive modality for detecting and characterizing diffuse diseases of the liver, including cirrhosis and he-mochromatosis, especially when combined with contrast agents. Angiography may be used to study collateral forma-tion in cirrhosis.

▶ Focal Hepatic Diseases

In focal diseases of the liver, US is often used first, because it utilizes no radiation, is relatively inexpensive, is widely avail-able, and is moderately sensitive to localized lesions in the ab-sence of preexisting diffuse diseases, such as cirrhosis. It is, however, of limited value in obese patients and whenever air is present, for example when air-filled bowel obscures the liver. CT is a pivotal examination, often employed after US. It is used as a survey of the entire body, is easy to compare in serial stud-ies, and is sensitive to disease. Air and bone do not interfere with CT examinations. Contrast-enhanced MDCT (multide-tector CT) scanners can be used to perform CT angiography, or CTA, which is a noninvasive means of producing images depicting vessels much like conventional angiography. NM techniques may be used to analyze a focal lesion within the liver for possible cavernous hemangioma. MR imaging is used

frequently to characterize focal lesions within the liver, espe-cially those discovered during survey techniques such as US or CT. NM and MR imaging are considered the optimal means for evaluating the liver for cavernous hemangioma, and both are highly accurate (approximately 95%) in evaluating the liver for cavernous hemangioma. In the opinion of some au-thorities, newer MR pulse sequences, contrast agents, and fast scanning techniques arguably make MR imaging the optimal means for both detection and characterization of focal liver le-sions of all types. Gadoxetate disodium is a newer hepatocyte-specific contrast agent that is taken up by functioning hepatocytes. This can be helpful in evaluating indeterminate liver lesions. Angiography is primarily used to provide a vas-cular road map in planning surgery for focal liver lesions. It can also be used in treatment of cancer, such as with chemoembolization.

▶ Abdominal Trauma

CT is the only commonly accepted means for analyzing ab-dominal trauma, particularly of the liver. CT is reasonably accurate in the detection of trauma-related abnormalities of the liver, biliary system, and pancreas. US may be useful if CT is not available or to quickly identify intraperitoneal hem-orrhage in patients who are in the emergency department and are going directly to the operating room. However, it is insensitive for directly identifying solid-organ lacerations. Angiography may be useful to embolize persistently bleeding arteries in the liver or spleen when surgery is not possible. Currently, NM and MR imaging have no application in studying the liver, biliary tract, or pancreas in acute trauma. However, they may have some application if there is clinical concern for a bile leak.

Pancreatic Inflammation or Neoplasm

CT is often the initial means to study pancreatic inflammation or neoplasm. It is effective in evaluating the pancreas. Ultrasound may be limited due to bowel gas or patient habitus. It is notoriously difficult to evaluate the pancreatic tail with ultrasound. NM has no major current application in studying the pancreas. MR imaging may be useful to study tumors of the pancreas. It is insensitive for small calcifications, as in chronic pancreatitis. Recent advances in MR imaging, especially MRCP, have brought MR imaging further to the forefront of pancreatic and biliary duct evaluation. This latter technique highlights fluid-containing structures such as biliary or pancreatic ducts and voids nearly all signal intensity from background solid structures. Angiography is useful to identify bleeding arteries as a source of hemorrhagic pancreatitis but is occasionally used to identify encasement of arteries in a pancreatic neoplasm.

Patient Preparation for Radiographic Techniques

Generally, these radiographic techniques require little patient preparation. This is convenient, especially in evaluation of trauma. Ideally, a patient should fast after midnight before an US examination. As a minimum, the patient should fast for 6 hours, especially when evaluating the gallbladder. Patients ideally should fast before CT examinations as well, but this requirement is not crucial. Dilute oral contrast medium for CT is administered at least 2 hours in advance and again just before the examination begins. Intravenous contrast material is often given as a bolus by a power injector immediately prior to the study. Proper laboratory evaluation of renal function, including serum creatinine below 1.5 mg/dL, is usually required before administering iodinated intravenous contrast material because it can be nephrotoxic. Ideally, NM is also performed after fasting. Preparation for angiography again requires fasting and laboratory evaluation of renal function and possible coagulopathy. Proper preparation of patients for MR imaging is controversial. However, some authorities advise administering an iron-containing oral contrast agent and an agent to relax the bowel, such as glucagon, before scanning. Renal function must be considered when administering gadolinium-based

MRI contrast agents because of nephrogenic systemic fibrosis as previously discussed.

Conflicts among Examinations

These examinations may interfere with each another. No barium should be administered before US or CT. Oral contrast agents may generate bowel gas, decompress the gallbladder, and hinder US. The oral contrast agent administered prior to a CT examination interferes with angiography by obscuring the abdomen. Intravenous contrast material interferes with any subsequent NM tests studying iodine metabolism such as those involving the thyroid gland because intravenous contrast agents contain iodine. Previous angiography usually requires that a CT examination be postponed for a day or two so that residual contrast material within the kidneys can be excreted. Usually, there are no conflicts between these examinations and NM or MR imaging.

EXERCISE 11-1. DIFFUSE LIVER DISEASE

11-1.   What is the most likely diagnosis in Case 11-1 (Figure 11-10)?
   A. Cirrhosis
   B. Diffuse liver tumor
   C. Budd-Chiari syndrome
   D. Schistosomiasis

11-2.   What is the most likely diagnosis in Case 11-2 (Figure 11-11)?
   A. Cirrhosis
   B. Fatty liver
   C. Hepatic iron overload
   D. Old granulomatous disease

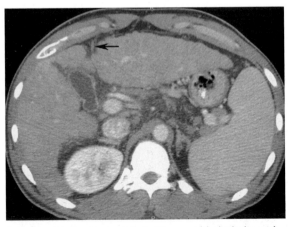

▲ **Figure 11-10.** Case 11-1. A 55-year-old alcoholic with abdominal pain.

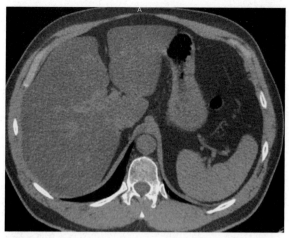

▲ **Figure 11-11.** Case 11-2. A 33-year-old long-time diabetic patient with a large liver mass palpated by physical examination.

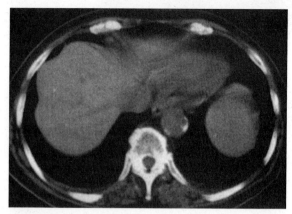

▲ **Figure 11-13.** Case 11-4. A 80-year-old patient without symptoms referable to the abdomen.

11-3. What is the most likely diagnosis in Case 11-3 (Figure 11-12)?
A. Cirrhosis
B. Thorotrast-induced liver disease
C. Hepatitis
D. Hepatic iron overload

11-4. What is the most likely diagnosis in Case 11-4 (Figure 11-13)?
A. Cirrhosis
B. Old granulomatous disease
C. Fatty liver
D. Osler-Weber-Rendu disease

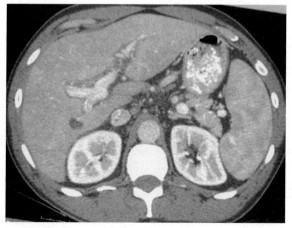

▲ **Figure 11-12.** Case 11-3. A 65-year-old patient with fever and increased liver function tests.

Radiologic Findings

11-1. In this case, the overall size of the liver is small. The contour of the liver is nodular, which is characteristic of cirrhosis. Also note the recanalized paraumbilical vein (arrow), which indicates portal hypertension (A is the correct answer to Question 11-1).

11-2. In this case, the liver is enlarged, there is marked low density throughout the liver when compared with the spleen, and there is no mass effect on the vessels. These are findings of fatty liver (hepatic steatosis) (B is the correct answer to Question 11-2).

11-3. In this case, the liver size is enlarged and the liver demonstrates heterogeneous attenuation throughout. No focal mass is seen. These findings are consistent with hepatitis in this clinical setting (C is the correct answer to Question 11-3).

11-4. In this case, multiple small, highly attenuating, punctuate lesions are scattered throughout liver and spleen, characteristic of calcifications from old granulomatous disease, without any other predominant finding (B is the correct answer to Question 11-4).

Discussion

Differentiation of liver disease into diffuse or focal disease is an artificial but convenient way to analyze liver disorders radiographically. Diffuse hepatocellular diseases are a common diagnostic problem. Although historical, physical, and laboratory testing are the first means for identifying these diseases, imaging may be required as a part of the overall assessment of the patient.

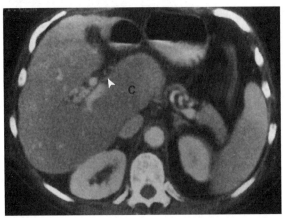

▲ **Figure 11-14.** CT in cirrhosis showing the disproportionate enlargement of the caudate lobe (C), as well as multiple collateral venous channels in the porta hepatis (arrowhead).

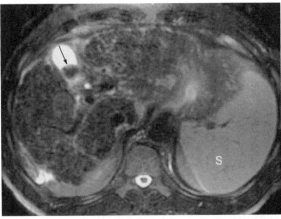

▲ **Figure 11-15.** T2-weighted MR imaging demonstrating cirrhosis, consisting of diffuse heterogeneity due to innumerable tiny low signal intensity nodules, regenerative nodules containing fibrous tissue and iron. Also note cholelithiasis (arrow) and splenomegaly (S).

Cirrhosis is a chronic disease of the liver. It is characterized by injury and regeneration of hepatic parenchymal cells and is accompanied by formation of connective tissue within the liver. In the United States, the most common cause of cirrhosis is alcoholism, whereas in Asia, the most common cause is viral hepatitis. Cirrhosis results in disproportionate diminution of the right lobe compared to the left lobe and caudate lobe of the liver (Figure 11-14). Nodular regeneration of the liver results in a nodular edge of the liver and inhomogeneity of the parenchyma. The process is accompanied by, first, increased resistance to normal hepatopetal (toward the liver) flow and, finally, the development of hepatofugal (away from the liver) flow. The increased resistance in the portal vein secondarily enlarges the spleen. This process also creates enlarged collateral venous channels to reroute blood around the liver (Figure 11-10). These portosystemic collaterals are visible frequently on cross-sectional imaging studies, most commonly in paraumbilical veins, coronary veins, and even spontaneous splenorenal shunts. Ascites is nearly always present. Most authorities are increasingly convinced that MR imaging is the most sensitive imaging modality for examination of the liver in cirrhosis and other diffuse diseases of the liver. MR imaging can demonstrate not only the contour changes and collateral formation visible with CT, but also the more subtle intraparenchymal nodular changes consequent to formation of regenerative and dysplastic nodules characteristic of cirrhosis within the complex fibrotic and inflamed host hepatic tissue (Figure 11-15). Importantly, MR imaging is considered to be a sensitive imaging means in the diagnosis of tumors such as

hepatocellular carcinoma superimposed on a background of cirrhosis (Figure 11-16).

Diffuse tumor in the liver can occur in patients with certain primary malignancies (Figure 11-17), particularly breast carcinoma. It is usually distributed randomly throughout the left and caudate lobes. Collateral veins normally are not found. Portal venous or intrahepatic biliary radicles may be compromised or displaced, although portal vein thrombosis is uncommon.

Budd-Chiari syndrome is a condition involving obstruction of the hepatic veins or the intrahepatic inferior vena cava. It is due to hypercoagulable states that produce thrombosis; tumors of the liver, kidneys, adrenal glands, or inferior vena cava (IVC); trauma (the "three Ts," ie, thrombosis, tumors, trauma); pregnancy; and even webs or membranes in the lumen of the inferior vena cava. This syndrome produces a marked congestion of the liver resulting from resistance to flow out of the liver, which consequently enlarges and becomes edematous. The liver has a mottled appearance on CT that is due to the interstitial edema, especially after administration of intravenous contrast material (Figure 11-18).

Schistosomiasis is one of the world's most common parasitic diseases and is rarely seen in persons living outside the endemic areas of China, Japan, the Middle East, and Africa; it does occur in immigrants to the United States. The larvae are hosts that enter the human gastrointestinal system, pass into lymphatic channels, migrate into mesenteric veins and portal veins, and, as adult worms, deposit ova that embolize to the portal system. This process leads to a granulomatous

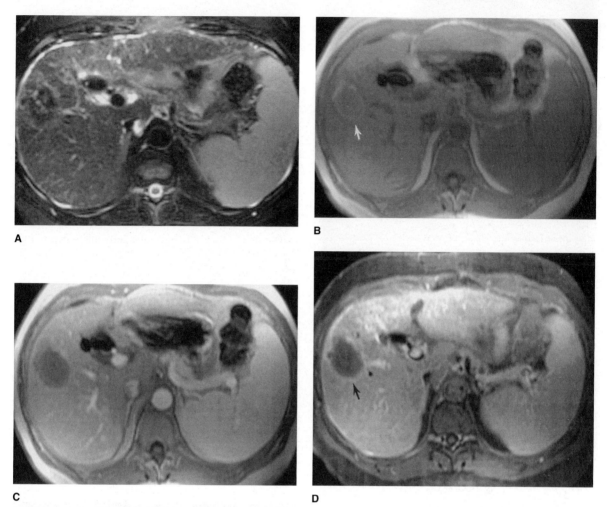

▲ **Figure 11-16.** (**A**) T2-weighted scan showing heterogeneous parenchyma, with superimposed focal mass in the right hepatic lobe. Splenomegaly is present, and small amounts of ascites surround the liver. (**B**) Preinfusion T1-weighted MR imaging showing background of cirrhosis and the high signal intensity of the periphery of the lesion (arrow) before contrast administration. (**C**) Immediate postinfused T1-weighted MR imaging showing the absence of contrast enhancement in the lesion, including the absence of puddling of contrast. (**D**) Delayed postinfused T1-weighted MR imaging showing the lack of centripetal contrast accumulation of contrast within the lesion (arrow), meaning that the lesion is not a cavernous hemangioma; it is compatible with a hepatocellular carcinoma.

inflammation, periportal fibrosis, portal vein occlusion, varices, and splenomegaly. Imaging studies demonstrate periportal fibrosis. The fibrosis enhances on CT after contrast material administration and appears on US as increased echogenicity of the periportal sheath surrounding the portal veins.

Fatty liver, or steatosis, is a common disorder. It is found in up to 50% of diabetic and alcoholic patients and has been found in up to 25% of nonalcoholic, healthy adults who die accidentally. The many causes of fatty liver,

besides diabetes and alcoholism, include (1) obesity, (2) chronic illness, (3) corticosteroid excess, (4) parenteral nutrition, and (5) hepatotoxins, including chemotherapy. Fatty liver may be distributed evenly or focally. When distributed uniformly, fatty liver is recognizable as a pattern of homogeneous increased echogenicity on US, decreased attenuation on CT (Figure 11-11), or increased signal intensity on T1-weighted MR images. On ultrasound, the echogenicity of the liver is compared to the right kidney, whereas on CT, the density of the liver is compared to the

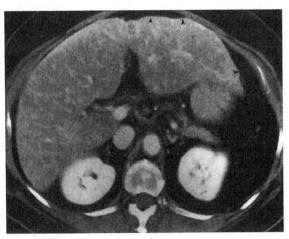

▲ **Figure 11-17.** CT in diffuse tumor showing diffuse, coarse inhomogeneity of the liver parenchyma, with a nodular border (arrowheads). Note absence of caudate lobe hypertrophy.

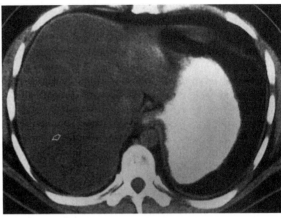

▲ **Figure 11-19.** CT in geographic fatty infiltration of the liver showing well-marginated, focal, low-density portion of the liver posteriorly (arrowhead).

spleen. When distributed nonuniformly, it resembles focal disease of the liver in that normal islands of liver tissue are seen against the background of lower-density fatty liver (Figure 11-19). Specialized MR imaging scans such as chemical shift imaging, NM studies, or biopsy may be required to differentiate among the possibilities.

Hepatic iron overload can be due to deposition in hepatocytes or reticuloendothelial cells. Parenchymal iron deposition occurs in primary idiopathic hemochromatosis, secondary hemochromatosis, cirrhosis, or intravascular hemolysis; the iron overload in these conditions is generally referred to as hemochromatosis. Reticuloendothelial iron deposition occurs in transfusional iron overload or rhabdomyolysis; the iron overload in these conditions is referred to as hemosiderosis. The liver, including the right lobe, is enlarged greatly unless cirrhosis is present. On CT, the density of the liver is very high (Figure 11-20), and on MR imaging the liver has extremely low signal on both T1- and

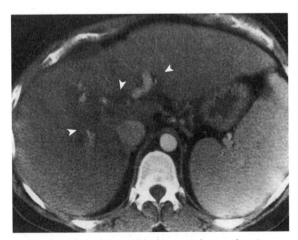

▲ **Figure 11-18.** CT in Budd-Chiari syndrome showing subtle, diffuse mottled appearance of liver (arrowheads).

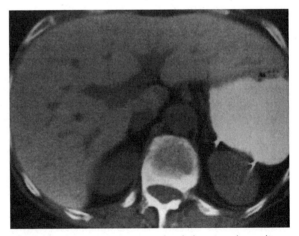

▲ **Figure 11-20.** CT in iron overload showing dense liver in relationship to the lower density intrahepatic portal vessels.

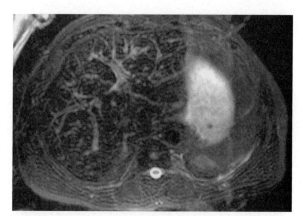

▲ **Figure 11-21.** T2-weighted MR imaging showing almost completely "black" liver, due to the deposition of intrahepatic iron. Note that the liver, which usually has a higher signal intensity than muscle, is isointense to paraspinous muscle.

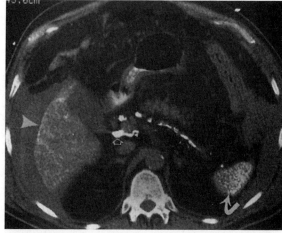

▲ **Figure 11-22.** CT in thorotrast administration showing the presence of high density. Thorotrast in the liver (arrowhead), lymph nodes (open arrow), and spleen (curved arrow).

T2-weighted images (Figure 11-21). Patients with hepatic iron overload may develop hepatocellular carcinoma.

Old granulomatous disease is a disorder in which prior granulomatous inflammation, usually caused by *Histoplasma capsulatum*, involves the liver. Other granulomatous inflammatory conditions that could be involved include sarcoidosis, Wegener's granulomatosis, and certain toxins. The granuloma tends to undergo necrosis, and dystrophic calcification forms within the lesion. This gives the lesion its most characteristic form, multiple punctate calcifications. The granuloma is visible on US as focal, extremely hyperechoic, shadowing lesions, and on CT as extremely high-density punctuate lesions (Figure 11-13). When large enough to be seen on MR, the calcification is seen as a signal void.

Thorotrast, a thorium-containing contrast agent, was used in the early 20th century for angiography and other purposes. Unfortunately, thorotrast emits alpha and beta radiation and has a biologic half-life of 400 years because it is not excreted; it therefore has been responsible for the development of several malignancies of the liver and spleen, including angiosarcoma and hepatocellular carcinoma. The particles are taken up by liver, spleen, lymphatics, and bone marrow. They appear on CT studies as large, dense particles in the liver, spleen, and peripancreatic and periportal lymph nodes (Figure 11-22). US shows typical calcifications.

Hepatitis is a diffuse inflammation of the liver, occurring as either acute or chronic disease. Patients with acute hepatitis have hepatocellular necrosis. In chronic cases, periportal inflammation and even fibrosis may occur. In acute hepatitis, the echogenicity of the parenchyma is decreased as a result of the edema, and the portal radicles are more evident; this has been termed the "starry sky" appearance. In chronic hepatitis, the texture of the liver is coarsened as a result of the fibrotic change in the periportal space, and this may decrease the visibility of the portal vein radicles. Findings on CT include hepatomegaly and decreased density (Figure 11-12). Most commonly, no important findings except hepatomegaly occur on CT in hepatitis. On MR imaging, the liver has low signal intensity on T1-weighted images and high signal intensity on T2-weighted images because of the edema and inflammation.

Osler-Weber-Rendu disease, or hereditary hemorrhagic telangiectasia, affects many organs and is seen predominantly, but not exclusively, in skin and the gastrointestinal tract. In the liver, it produces telangiectasias, cirrhosis, or both. Multiple small aneurysms may be present, and hematomas may occur if the aneurysms bleed. These aneurysms and any consequent hematomas from aneurysmal rupture can be visible on both US and CT. Angiography can demonstrate enlarged hepatic arteries and early but not immediate hepatic vein opacification.

EXERCISE 11-2. FOCAL LIVER DISEASES

11-5. What is the most likely diagnosis in Case 11-5 (Figure 11-23)?
   A. Pyogenic liver abscess
   B. Echinococcal disease
   C. Candidiasis
   D. Amoebic abscess

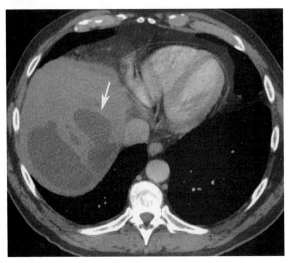

▲ **Figure 11-23.** Case 11-5. A 44-year-old American patient with right upper quadrant pain and fever.

11-6. What is the most likely diagnosis in Case 11-6 (Figure 11-24)?
A. Hemangioma
B. Metastatic disease
C. Angiosarcoma
D. Focal nodular hyperplasia

11-7. What is the most likely diagnosis in Case 11-7 (Figure 11-25)?
A. Hemangioma
B. Hepatocellular carcinoma
C. Metastatic disease
D. Liver cell adenoma

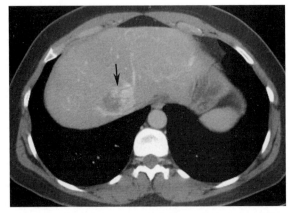

▲ **Figure 11-24.** Case 11-6. A 45-year-old female with an incidentally discovered liver lesion.

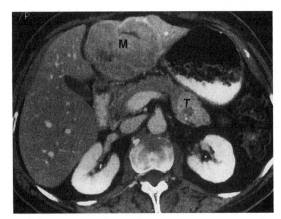

▲ **Figure 11-25.** Case 11-7. A 65-year-old female with long history of a pancreatic mass.

11-8. What is the most likely diagnosis in Case 11-8 (Figure 11-26)?
A. Metastatic disease
B. Hepatocellular carcinoma
C. Liver cell adenoma
D. Abscess

Radiologic Findings

11-5. In this case, CT shows a large, fluid attenuation mass in the posterior dome of the liver with rim enhancement and irregular margins (arrow). In this patient from the United States with fever, the most likely diagnosis is pyogenic abscess. If this patient were from another country or had an appropriate travel history, then amoebic or echinococcal abscess could also be considered (A is the correct answer to Question 11-5).

11-6. In this case, CT shows a focal lesion in the central liver that demonstrates peripheral, nodular, discontinuous enhancement (arrow). Delayed imaging (not shown) would demonstrate centripetal accumulation ("fill in") of contrast. These features are characteristic of cavernous hemangioma (A is the correct answer to Question 11-6).

11-7. In this case, there is a focal lesion occupying the left lobe of the liver (M), and there is a focal enhancing mass in the pancreatic tail (T), representing a pancreatic neoplasm metastatic to the liver (C is the correct answer to Question 11-7).

11-8. In this case, CT shows a hypervascular mass (arrow) on arterial phase CT (Figure 11-26 A). This demonstrates typical washout on portal venous phase imaging (Figure 11-26 B) with an enhancing "pseudocapsule" (arrows) of compressed adjacent hepatic tissue. Both are typical features of HCC (B is the correct answer to Question 11-8).

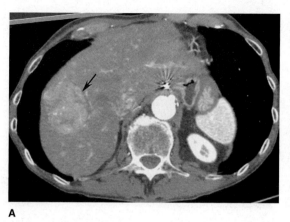 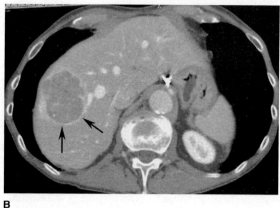

A   B

▲ **Figure 11-26.** Case 11-8. A 61-year-old male with upper abdominal pain.

Discussion

Recognition of the focal or diffuse nature of liver disease is helpful for sorting out the possible causes. The two can overlap, especially because one may lead to another: for example, cirrhosis can cause hepatocellular carcinoma.

Pyogenic liver abscesses are relatively common focal inflammatory lesions of the liver most commonly caused by bacteria. These lesions have high morbidity and mortality, if undiscovered. They are multiple in many cases, involving both hepatic lobes. These abscesses create a severe leukocytosis and can lead to sepsis. Pyogenic abscesses occur when collections of leukocytes undergo necrosis and become walled off. The imaging studies, although not definitive, have helpful findings. On US, these lesions often are well demarcated, may be multiloculated, and have fluid centers and irregular walls. Gas within an abscess creates an echogenic structure with "dirty" shadowing. On CT, the abscess appears as a low-density lesion. Intra-abscess gas occurs in approximately 50% of abscesses (Figure 11-27), and enhancement of the border of the lesion after intravenous contrast infusion also occurs in approximately 50% of abscesses. Low-density edema may surround the abscess (Figure 11-23). Rapid enhancement of the edge of an abscess after bolus injection of contrast material may be helpful. On technetium-99m sulfur colloid scans, the abscess appears as a defect within the liver. MR imaging demonstrates signs of an irregular, fluid-containing lesion, that is, low signal intensity on T1-weighted examinations and high signal intensity on T2-weighted examinations. Edema may be visible surrounding the lesion on T2-weighted images. Pus demonstrates restricted diffusion on MR.

Echinococcal disease is a parasitic infestation that involves multiple organs, most commonly the liver. It is endemic in several regions around the world. The most common form is due to *Echinococcus granulosus*, which, after being ingested by humans, is carried into the gut, transmitted to the portal circula-

tion, and eventually deposited in the liver, where it develops into large, occasionally multiloculated, cysts, which may calcify. On US, these lesions appear as well-defined cysts with regular borders, which may contain swirling debris and multiple septae. Smaller, "daughter" cysts often surround them. Small calcifications are present. CT shows similar morphologic findings, as well as enhancement of the wall after intravenous contrast material infusion. Calcifications are crescentic, corresponding to the membranes. MR imaging shows a cystic mass with a rimlike periphery of low signal intensity on both T1- and T2-weighted images and with a central matrix of high signal intensity.

Candidiasis is a fungal disease. It affects the liver primarily in renal transplant patients and patients who are immunocompromised by malignancy or chemotherapy for the malignancy. The organism forms multiple microabscesses, which

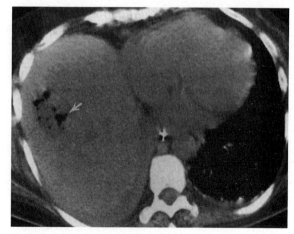

▲ **Figure 11-27.** CT in pyogenic abscess showing the presence of gas within the lesion (arrow).

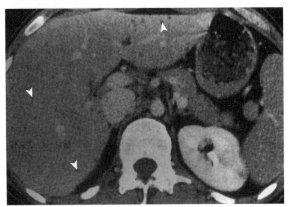

▲ **Figure 11-28.** CT in candidiasis showing multiple small, low-density lesions scattered throughout the liver (arrowheads), representing multifocal fungal abscesses.

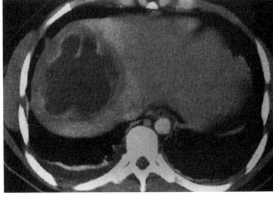

▲ **Figure 11-29.** CT in amoebic abscess showing the presence of an irregular peripherally enhancing lesion within the liver. This is indistinguishable from a pyogenic abscess.

create the characteristic appearance on imaging studies. US shows several patterns, the most common being multiple small hypoechoic structures containing a hyperechoic central spot, the "bull's-eye" lesion. Other patterns may occur. CT shows similar multiple small abscesses (Figure 11-28), including the bull's-eye lesion.

Amebic abscesses are caused by a parasite, *Entamoeba histolytica*, and the liver is the most commonly involved organ. The leukocytosis is much less severe than with a pyogenic abscess. Unlike pyogenic abscesses, which require drainage, amebic abscesses can often be cured by medical treatment. Like echinococcal abscesses, amebic abscesses start when organisms reach the liver through the portal circulation from the

bowel. The abscesses may rupture into the peritoneal cavity or even into the thorax. Imaging studies, including NM, US, and CT, are usually nonspecific and demonstrate focal defects within the liver (Figure 11-29). The lesions can resemble echinococcal abscesses. One helpful finding is intraperitoneal or intrathoracic fluid, if rupture has occurred.

Hemangioma is the most common benign tumor of the liver and is second only to metastases as the most common tumor overall within the liver. Hemangiomas are often peripherally located in the liver, less than 2 cm in diameter, and not associated with abnormalities in liver function tests. They are most commonly single. On US, they are usually homogeneous and hyperechoic (Figure 11-30 A), but an important

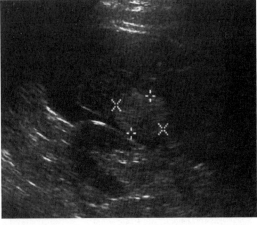

A

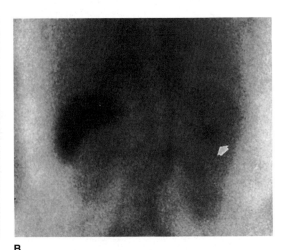

B

▲ **Figure 11-30.** **(A)** Transverse US in cavernous hemangiorna showing a hyperechoic, well-defined, homogeneous lesion at the posterior edge of the liver (cursors). **(B)** Tagged red blood cell NM scan showing the presence of a region of increased activity within the liver (arrowhead). Note that the image was obtained over the posterior aspect of the patient, so the liver is on the left side of the image.

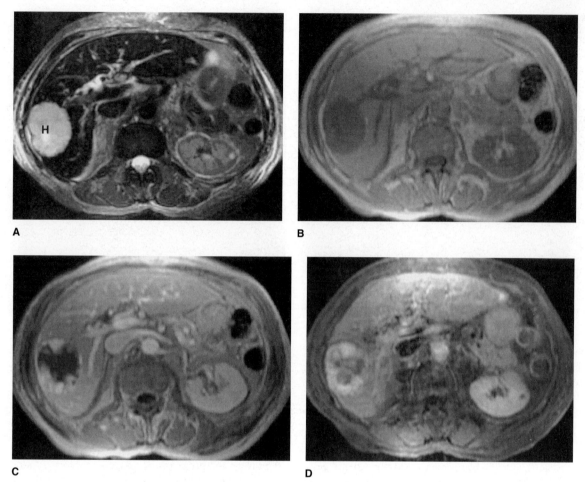

▲ Figure 11-31. (**A**) T2-weighted scan demonstrating the markedly high signal intensity and well-circumscribed margin of a cavernous hemangioma (H). (**B**) Preinfusion T1-weighted MR imaging of cavernous hemangioma, showing the dark signal of the lesion. (**C**) Immediate postinfused T1-weighted MR imaging showing the peripheral nodular "puddling" of intravenous contrast material. (**D**) Delayed postinfused T1-weighted MR imaging showing the centripetal filling in toward the center of the lesion.

variant is the isoechoic mass with hyperechoic periphery. They are often peripheral, with posterior acoustic enhancement. Some large lesions have central scars. CT shows homogeneous, low-attenuation lesions, which enhance after intravenous contrast material administration, have discontinuous peripheral nodular enhancement (called "puddling" of contrast material), and accumulate contrast material centripetally over a period of several minutes (Figure 11-24). This finding is most useful when the patient has no known primary tumor; otherwise, this pattern is more likely due to a metastasis. Technetium-99m labeled red blood cell scans are diagnostic for hemangioma when early vascular-phase images show decreased activity and delayed blood-pool scans demonstrate increased activity at the lesion site (Figure 11-30 B).

MR imaging demonstrates lesions with low signal intensity on T1-weighted scans, which is typical for most lesions. However, T2-weighted MR imaging demonstrates high signal intensity similar to that of fluid, which is considered diagnostic of hemangioma or cyst. Intravenous Gd "puddles" in cavernous hemangioma and gradually migrates centripetally toward the center of the lesion (Figure 11-31), analogous to the distribution of iodinated contrast material in cavernous hemangioma on CT, and likewise is considered diagnostic of cavernous hemangioma. This puddling in cavernous hemangioma is different from the more curvilinear or heterogeneous distribution of contrast accumulation seen in malignant tumor. Angiography can be very helpful, as it shows punctuate collections of contrast material shortly after

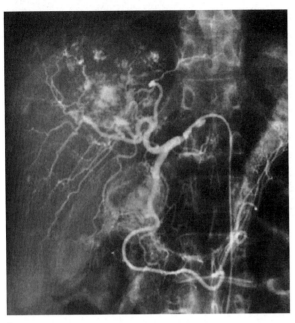

A

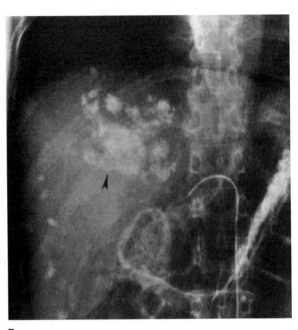

B

▲ **Figure 11-32.** Capillary (**A**) and venous (**B**) phase hepatic arteriogram in cavernous hemangioma showing the dense and persistent stain of the lesions (arrowhead).

injection, analogous to the puddling seen in CT or MR imaging (Figure 11-32 A). These collections become denser, usually within a minute, because contrast puddles in the vascular spaces of the tumor (Figure 11-32 B). On all modalities with intravenous contrast, hemangiomas usually enhance early and retain contrast.

Although typically diffuse, steatosis of the liver can present as focal deposits of fat. Furthermore, sometimes steatosis can present as the reverse, namely, residual focal islands of hepatic tissue unaffected by fatty deposition. Both of these conditions can be confusing because they may resemble focal solid masses including tumor on CT or US. MR imaging is the most accurate means to identify sites of focal fat or focal fatty sparing. In particular, a pulse sequence called "out-of-phase" T1-weighted imaging, which emphasizes the presence of fat intermixed with any host water-containing tissue, is very sensitive in the detection of the presence or absence of fat within focal fat or focal fatty sparing, respectively. Wherever fat is intermixed with water-containing parenchyma, there is loss of signal intensity on out-of-phase images. Therefore, focal fatty infiltration appears as sites of relative signal loss, whereas focal fatty sparing appears as sites of relative signal gain (Figure 11-33). This imaging technique is the most sensitive and specific cross-sectional modality for characterizing focal fatty distribution, a very common condition.

The liver is a common and important site for metastatic disease. As many as 25% to 50% of cancer patients have liver metastases at autopsy. Most tumors metastasize to the liver, and metastasis to the liver strongly affects the stage of the tumor and prognosis of the patient. Most metastases are multiple, diffusely distributed, variable in size, and solid. They may be necrotic and appear more cystic. Liver metastases may be present even when both general and specific serum markers for tumor, such as liver function tests and carcinoembryonic antigen, are normal. Metastases may be poorly vascularized or highly vascular, a difference that affects their appearance after intravenous contrast administration. Metastases from renal cell carcinoma, thyroid carcinoma, carcinoids, and neuroendocrine tumors are classically hypervascular. Mucin-producing carcinomas, such as breast and colon carcinoma, frequently produce calcification, which can be detected with imaging studies. Metastases are almost always evaluated with cross-sectional imaging studies. However, more recently, PET has been used to detect certain malignancies, including liver metastases. Because the liver physiologically takes up the radiopharmaceutical used in PET, metastatic lesions can be obscured. Although US can evaluate for liver metastases when used by skilled operators, it is limited by relative insensitivity to subtle lesions, especially against the background of preexisting liver disease. On US, metastases

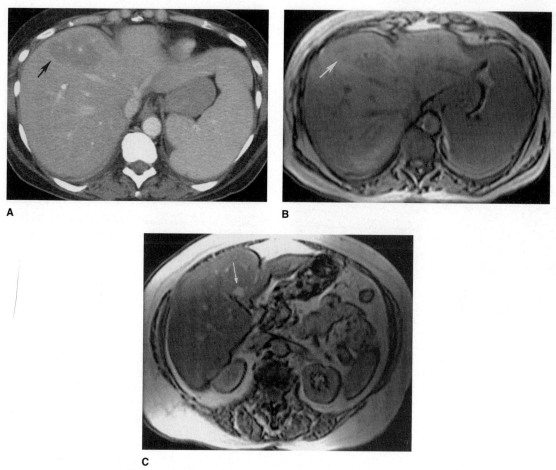

▲ **Figure 11-33.** (**A**) CT scan demonstrating a "mass" (arrow) in the liver. (**B**) Out-of-phase MR imaging scan demonstrating "mass" (arrow) has decreased signal intensity, signifying focal fatty infiltration. (**C**) Out-of-phase MR imaging scan in a different patient with diffuse fatty infiltration and a "mass" on CT (not shown), demonstrating diffuse low signal intensity and a site of higher signal intensity (arrow) along the main fissure of the liver, representing focal fatty sparing.

are usually hypoechoic, poorly defined, and hypovascular, and they may have a peripheral halo (Figure 11-34). Some types, such as breast cancer, may be diffusely distributed in minute form. In most institutions, CT is used to survey and monitor patients for liver metastases, because CT can detect metastases and is probably the most useful technique for evaluating extrahepatic disease. On CT, metastases are usually multifocal, of low attenuation, and often better shown after administration of intravenous contrast material when compared to preinfusion scans (Figure 11-35). Again, some forms present as diffuse inhomogeneity. Because of its sensitivity and potential for characterizing some lesions specifically, MR imaging may become the pre-

ferred technique for detecting and characterizing liver metastases. Lesions have low signal intensity on T1-weighted images and higher signal intensity (but never as high as in cavernous hemangioma) on T2-weighted studies (Figure 11-36). Certain lesions, such as melanoma, carcinoid, and endocrine tumors of the pancreas, have very high signal with strongly T2-weighted scans. Hepatocyte-specific contrast agents, such as gadoxetate disodium, are also being used to detect metastases. Because metastatic lesions do not have normal hepatocytic function, they do not retain the contrast, making them conspicuous as areas of relatively decreased enhancement compared to the normal surrounding liver.

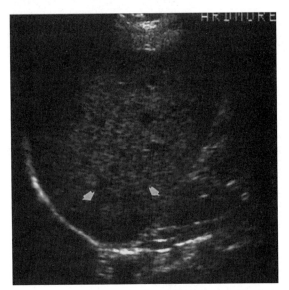

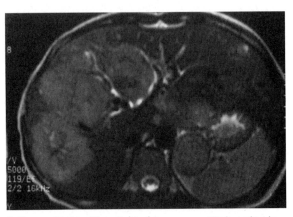

▲ **Figure 11-36.** T2-weighted transverse MR imaging in liver metastasis showing the presence of intermediately high-signal-intensity liver lesions.

▲ **Figure 11-34.** Longitudinal US in liver metastasis showing a lesion in the posterior aspect of the liver, including a peripheral halo of decreased echogenicity (arrowheads).

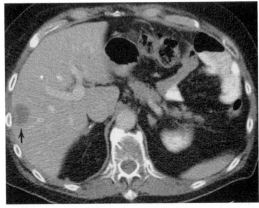

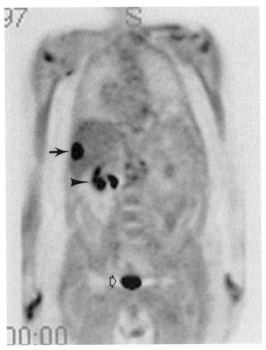

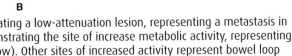

A   B

▲ **Figure 11-35.** (**A**) Contrast-enhanced CT scan demonstrating a low-attenuation lesion, representing a metastasis in the lateral aspect of the liver (arrow). (**B**) PET scan, demonstrating the site of increase metabolic activity, representing the metastatic lesion in the lateral aspect of the liver (arrow). Other sites of increased activity represent bowel loop (arrowhead) and bladder (open arrow) activity.

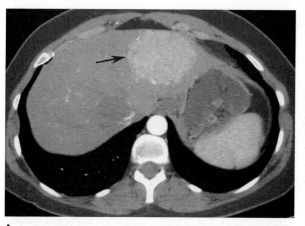 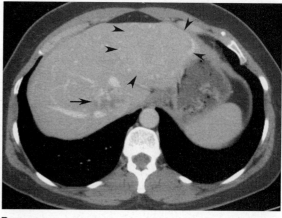

A   **B**

▲ **Figure 11-37.** (**A**) CT of FNH during the arterial phase demonstrates early, uniform enhancement of a mass in the left lobe of the liver (arrow). The central scar is not well seen. (**B**) On the portal venous phase, the FNH becomes isodense to the liver and is difficult to detect (arrowheads). Note that the hemangioma adjacent to the FNH (same patient as in Figure 11-24) shows peripheral nodular discontinuous enhancement (arrow) on portal venous phase imaging. Note that there is also a hemangioma that is hypodense to the liver on arterial-phase imaging and does not show enhancement in this phase.

Angiosarcoma is a rare, highly vascular tumor of the liver. It is seen in patients who have had an occupational exposure to certain chemicals, particularly polyvinyl chloride or thorotrast. If lesions rupture, they may produce serious hemorrhagic sequelae. On US, angiosarcoma is usually hypoechoic. Sometimes the attendant fibrosis so obscures the tumor that it is impossible to identify. On CT, the lesions have low attenuation, may enhance markedly, and, if arising in the presence of thorotrast, can displace and distort the thorotrast collections.

Focal nodular hyperplasia (FNH) and liver cell adenoma are easily confused. Both are histologically benign liver disorders that produce single or multiple lesions. Both processes can occur in young adults. On imaging studies, they can resemble primary or metastatic liver tumors. However, some important differences pertain. FNH is probably a hamartoma of the liver, that is, a localized overgrowth of mature cells that are identical to the types constituting the liver and contain fibrous tissue, blood vessels, bile ducts, and occasional well-differentiated hepatocytes. Adenoma is a true benign tumor composed of one tissue element of the liver, the hepatocyte. FNH often contains a central fibrotic scar. Adenoma is associated with the use of oral contraceptives, whereas FNH probably is not. Adenoma, unlike FNH, tends to undergo hemorrhage, and thus to present as acute abdominal pain. US is nonspecific in studying FNH. Adenoma is usually hyperechoic but heterogeneous. On CT, FNH is transiently but markedly and uniformly hypervascular, and the central scar may be seen (Figure 11-37). Ade-

noma usually shows low density, may demonstrate hemorrhage as high-density collections on preinfusion scans, and enhances variably. On Tc-sulfur colloid NM scans, FNH can show increased, decreased, or normal activity compared to that of liver. Adenoma usually shows no increased uptake in NM studies, but this varies. FNH has low signal intensity on T1-weighted MR imaging and slightly high signal intensity on T2-weighted images. As on CT, it shows uniformly early enhancement and the central scar (Figure 11-38). If the

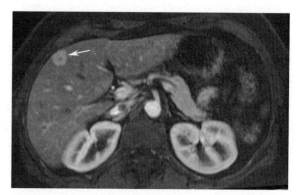

▲ **Figure 11-38.** Postcontrast, axial T1-weighted, fat-suppressed MR sequence demonstrates an avidly, uniformly enhancing mass (arrow) in the right liver with central scar. This is consistent with FNH.

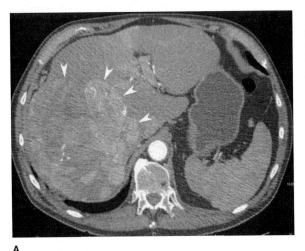 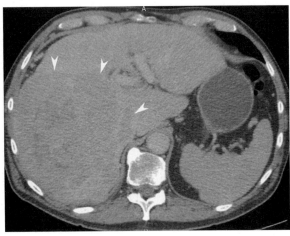

A   B

▲ **Figure 11-39.** **(A)** CT of HCC during arterial phase shows heterogeneous enhancement (bright areas) in a large mass (arrowheads) in the right liver. **(B)** On portal venous phase of CT, the mass demonstrates washout of contrast and an enhancing "pseudocapsule" (arrowheads) becomes apparent.

central scar is present, it may exhibit high signal intensity on T2-weighted images. Adenoma, like many lesions, has a nonspecific appearance of low signal intensity on T1-weighted examinations and slightly high signal intensity on T2-weighted examinations. Hemorrhage is recognizable as high signal intensity on T1-weighted images. Angiographically, FNH is hypervascular with radiating branches that produce a "spoke-wheel" appearance. Adenoma has a variable angiographic appearance but is generally less vascular than FNH.

Hepatocellular carcinoma (HCC), or hepatoma, is a primary malignancy of the liver. It is found in older cirrhotic patients in the United States and in younger patients in areas of the Far East and Africa, where it is endemic. Chronic hepatitis B and C infection and exposure to aflatoxin predispose to formation of hepatocellular carcinoma. On imaging studies, hepatocellular carcinoma appears as (1) a single predominant lesion (most common form), (2) a predominant lesion with multiple, smaller, surrounding daughter lesions, or (3) diffuse tumor. Portal vein invasion by the tumor in any form is relatively common and can aid in distinguishing hepatocellular carcinoma from other lesions. On US, hepatocellular carcinoma is most commonly a discrete lesion with increased, similar, or decreased echogenicity in comparison to that of liver. On CT, lesions are most commonly of low density and may enhance if fast scans in the arterial phase are performed after contrast material administration (Figure 11-39). Portal venous thrombosis can be seen, and preexisting cirrhosis or thorotrast can be demonstrated. MR imaging findings are similar to those of CT, but as with CT, the lesion is inhomogeneous.

EXERCISE 11-3. UPPER ABDOMINAL TRAUMA

11-9. What is the most likely diagnosis in Case 11-9 (Figure 11-40)?
 A. Hepatic contusion
 B. Hepatic laceration
 C. Uncomplicated ascites
 D. Hemoperitoneum

11-10. What is the most likely diagnosis in Case 11-10 (Figure 11-41)?
 A. Pancreatic trauma
 B. Bowel injury
 C. Mesenteric injury
 D. Hepatic laceration

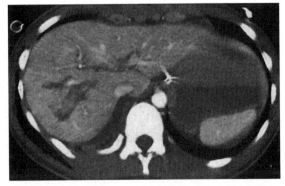

▲ **Figure 11-40.** Case 11-9. A 45-year-old motor vehicle accident victim with upper abdominal pain.

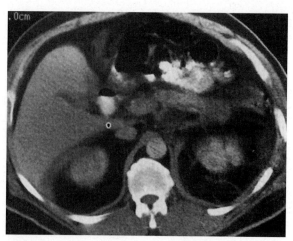

▲ **Figure 11-41.** Case 11-10. A 57-year-old man who was beaten in the abdomen with a baseball bat.

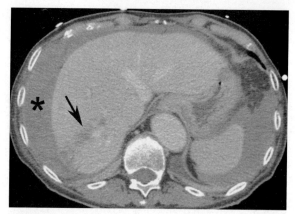

▲ **Figure 11-42.** CT of liver laceration shows an ill-defined low-density defect in the liver extending to the capsule (arrow) with high-attenuation fluid (∗) consistent with blood surrounding the liver.

Radiographic Findings

11-9. In this case, the liver has an irregularly linear lesion in its central aspect, representing a liver laceration (B is the correct answer to Question 11-9).

11-10. In this case, there is a low-density bulbous enlargement of the pancreatic tail, representing a pancreatic injury (A is the correct answer to Question 11-10).

Discussion

Hepatic injury is common after blunt trauma. Hepatic injuries may be life-threatening as a result of bleeding and shock, but more often surgery is not required. Observation and systemic support may be the only treatment necessary. Like trauma to any other organ, injury to the liver varies from mild to severe. A mild injury of the liver produces a localized collection of traumatized liver tissue and an interstitial hematoma, like a bruise, which is termed a contusion.

More severe injuries that involve complete disruption of the tissue into fracture planes, perhaps involving the hepatic veins, inferior vena cava, or portal veins, are called lacerations.

Most blunt abdominal trauma in the United States is radiographically evaluated with CT. Angiography is used to a lesser extent. US, NM, and MR imaging are of little or no value in a general survey of abdominal trauma. On CT, hepatic contusion is seen as a low-attenuation lesion, perhaps with mass effect on surrounding hepatic vessels. Associated hemoperitoneum is not usually seen. On CT, hepatic laceration appears as an irregular, stellate, or linear lesion through the liver parenchyma (Figure 11-40), sometimes extending to the porta hepatis, liver capsule, or IVC (Figure 11-42). A hallmark of severe trauma to upper abdominal organs is accompanying hemoperitoneum,

which appears as a collection of high-density material at the site of bleeding and is termed the sentinel clot. Acute blood that has migrated away from the site of active bleeding, or old hemoperitoneum at any site, often has the attenuation of simple or near-simple fluid and can resemble intraperitoneal fluid, or ascites, from a number of causes. NM hepatobiliary scans, also called HIDA (hepatobiliary iminodiacetic acid) scans, can be used to assess for a bile leak if that is suspected.

Ascites is a nonspecific reaction of the peritoneal space to a variety of causes, including tumor, inflammation, trauma, increased systemic venous resistance (eg, congestive heart failure), renal or hepatic insufficiency, and many other conditions. It is characterized by the production of intraperitoneal fluid. This fluid can be simple, a transudate, in which case it has fluid density (Figure 11-43) and is free to move to

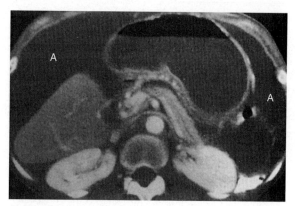

▲ **Figure 11-43.** CT in ascites showing fluid diffusely distributed throughout the abdomen (A).

the dependent portion of the abdominal or pelvic cavity with patient movement. Alternatively, it can be complex, an exudate, in which case it is denser than simple fluid, is accompanied by solid tissue (eg, tumor deposits in peritoneal metastases) or layered material (eg, blood from trauma or inflammatory cellular debris in peritonitis), and often is loculated, or unable to move freely throughout the intraperitoneal cavity (eg, abscess).

Pancreatic injury is uncommon, but potentially serious. Mortality from pancreatic injuries is nearly 20%. Being crushed against the spine probably accounts for the frequency of injury to the body of the pancreas. Pancreatic trauma may or may not be associated with increased amylase. Usually caused by blunt trauma, pancreatic trauma is often associated with injuries to other organs, such as liver and bowel. These injuries produce intraperitoneal blood and fluid and interstitial mesenteric edema, which can be confusing. As with hepatic trauma, CT with intravenous contrast is usually the modality of choice to evaluate pancreatic trauma, but even on CT, the diagnosis can be difficult. On CT, the pancreas may be ill defined, enlarged, or even disrupted, that is, fractured.

Bowel and mesenteric injuries are found in approximately 5% of all patients undergoing laparotomy after motor vehicle accidents. Injuries of the bowel and mesentery frequently accompany injury to the liver or pancreas. These injuries can result in massive intraperitoneal bleeding from disruption of mesenteric vessels, or peritonitis from bowel perforation. As elsewhere, CT is the modality of choice to evaluate patients for possible bowel or mesenteric injuries, but these injuries, like those to the pancreas, can be difficult to detect. On CT, injuries of the bowel and mesentery include free air with the intraperitoneal or retroperitoneal spaces, free intra-abdominal fluid, circumferential or eccentric bowel wall thickening, enhancement of the bowel wall, streaky soft-tissue infiltration of the mesenteric fat, free mesenteric hematoma (Figure 11-44), and especially

sentinel clot. Angiography may demonstrate free extravasation of contrast material in injuries of the mesenteric vessels, and percutaneous embolization may stop bleeding when surgery is not possible.

EXERCISE 11-4. BILIARY INFLAMMATION

11-11. What is the most likely diagnosis in Case 11-11 (Figure 11-45)?
  A. Acute cholecystitis
  B. Uncomplicated cholelithiasis
  C. Chronic cholecystitis
  D. Porcelain gallbladder

11-12. What is the most likely diagnosis in Case 11-12 (Figure 11-46)?
  A. Oriental cholangiohepatitis
  B. Acquired immunodeficiency syndrome (AIDS)-associated cholangiopathy
  C. Choledocholithiasis
  D. Porcelain gallbladder

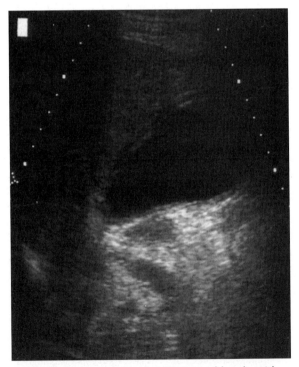

▲ **Figure 11-45.** Case 11-11. A 53-year-old male with acute right upper quadrant pain, fever, pain on palpation over the gallbladder, and elevated liver function tests.

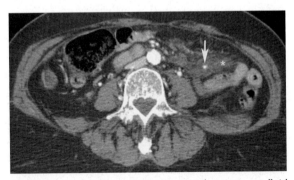

▲ **Figure 11-44.** CT of mesenteric injury demonstrates fluid and hematoma (∗) in the jejunal mesentery with active extravasation of contrast material (arrow) into the mesentery.

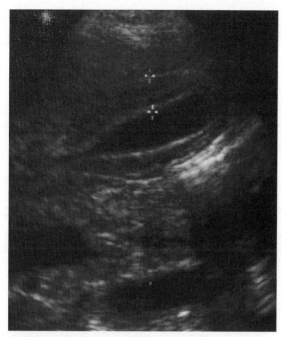

▲ **Figure 11-46.** Case 11-12. A 22-year-old HIV-positive female with debilitating and chronic illness with vague right upper quadrant pain, but no tenderness on palpation over the gallbladder.

11-13. What is the most likely diagnosis in Case 11-13 (Figure 11-47)?
   A. Acute cholecystitis
   B. Emphysematous cholecystitis
   C. Porcelain gallbladder
   D. Hydrops of gallbladder

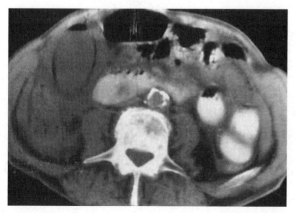

▲ **Figure 11-47.** Case 11-13. A 84-year-old male with right upper quadrant pain, marked fever, and suspicion of sepsis.

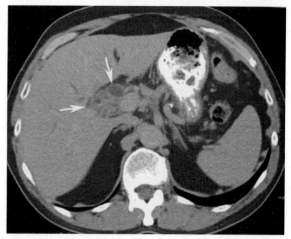

▲ **Figure 11-48.** Case 11-14. A 53-year-old male with history of cholecystectomy, upper abdominal pain, jaundice, and fever.

11-14. What is the most likely diagnosis in Case 11-14 (Figure 11-48)?
   A. Choledocholithiasis
   B. Ascending cholangitis
   C. Acute cholecystitis
   D. Emphysematous cholecystitis

Radiographic Findings

11-11. In this case, the gallbladder is distended and the wall is thickened, measuring more than 5 mm, and has multiple lamina, indicating gallbladder wall inflammation from acute cholecystitis (A is the correct answer to Question 11-11).

11-12. In this case, the gallbladder wall is markedly thickened, measuring over 1 cm, with multiple lamina, but is not tender to palpation, findings often seen with AIDS cholangiopathy (B is the correct answer to Question 11-12).

11-13. In this case, gas within the gallbladder wall and lumen is the primary abnormality, indicating emphysematous cholecystitis (B is the correct answer to Question 11-13).

11-14. In this case, CT demonstrates dilatation of the biliary ducts with enhancement and thickening of the wall (arrows). In the clinical setting of fever and jaundice, this most strongly suggests cholangitis (B is the correct answer to Question 11-14).

Discussion

Calculi are a common problem in the gallbladder and biliary ducts. Cholelithiasis is one of the most common abdominal disorders overall and is the most common cause of cholecystitis, as well as the most common indication for abdominal surgery. Gallstones develop when the composition of bile, which includes bile salts, lecithin, and cholesterol, varies from normal and creates supersaturation of cholesterol, which then precipitates. Historically, patients thought to be harboring gallstones on the basis of clinical criteria were examined by oral cholecystography, which shows filling defects in the gallbladder lumen opacified by orally ingested iodinated contrast material. However, this examination has been largely replaced by sonography, occasionally supported by other imaging information. On US, gallstones usually appear as mobile, intraluminal, echogenic foci that cast a well-defined acoustic shadow (Figure 11-49). Two other possible appearances are echogenic foci in the gallbladder fossa without visible surrounding bile when the gallbladder is contracted, and small, mobile, echogenic foci that do not cast a shadow. On CT, gallstones appear as dense, well-defined, intraluminal structures (Figure 11-50), but their density can vary from fat density to near bone density, depending on the relative concentration of calcium and cholesterol. Because of their varying density, they can sometimes be difficult to see on CT. MR imaging of the biliary system, especially MRCP, has become more important in biliary imaging, including the detection of calculi of the gallbladder and biliary tree. Although US remains the primary and initial means of identifying biliary calculi, MRCP can be used as a supplementary technique, especially in ductal calculi, because imaging of the biliary tree

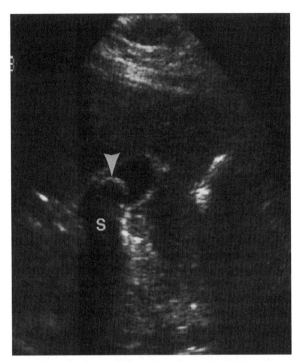

▲ **Figure 11-49.** Transverse US in cholelithiasis showing an echogenic structure (arrowhead) casting an acoustic shadow (S).

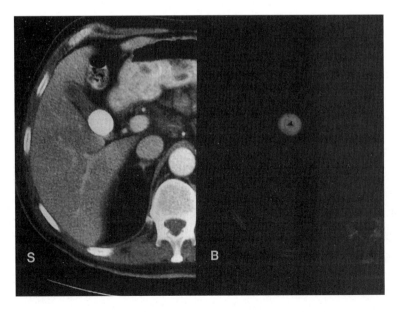

▲ **Figure 11-50.** CT in cholelithiasis using both soft-tissue windows (S) and bone windows (B) showing an extremely dense structure lying in the gallbladder. Note the laminated architecture of the gallstone on the bone windows (arrowhead).

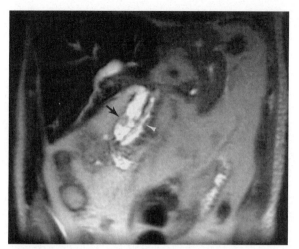

▲ **Figure 11-51.** Coronal MRCP demonstrating choledo-cholithiasis, appearing as filling defects (arrow) in the distal bile duct. Note the parallel pancreatic duct (arrowhead).

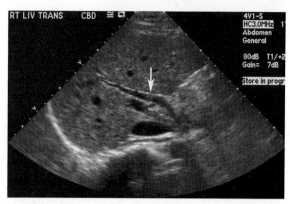

▲ **Figure 11-52.** Transverse US in patient with choledo-cholithiasis shows the presence of an intraductal stone (arrow). Note that unlike gallbladder stones, it does not cast an acoustic shadow; this is typical of intraductal stones.

by US may be suboptimal when obscured by bowel gas. MRCP can depict the biliary system, filling defects within the biliary tree (Figure 11-51), and congenital variants of the biliary ducts and is about as accurate as ERCP in displaying a biliary "road map." It can also be used to evaluate the biliary ducts when ERCP is impossible to perform, such as when the patient has undergone a Billroth procedure, interrupting the continuity of the upper gastrointestinal tract. NM and angiography have no major role at this time in assessment of gallstones.

Choledocholithiasis occurs when calculi pass from the gallbladder into the biliary ducts or when calculi develop originally within the ductal system. Regardless of origin, they may obstruct the biliary ducts, cause biliary colic, and lead to cholangitis. Common duct stones can be evaluated with US, CT, and MRI, or by direct visualization with ERCP. On US, choledocholithiasis appears as echogenic foci within the lumen of the biliary duct. Sonographically, common duct stones are detected less readily than gallbladder stones, and meticulous technique is required. The entire course of the common bile duct may be technically difficult or impossible to follow. Choledocholithiasis can cause acoustic shadows, but for technical reasons these stones are detected less frequently than cholelithiasis (Figure 11-52). On CT, choledocholithiasis appears as intraluminal biliary ductal foci, which, like gallbladder stones, may vary in density from hypodense to isodense to hyperdense to bile, depending on their composition (Figure 11-53). On MRCP, choledocholithiasis is seen as a filling defect in the duct.

Cholecystitis is inflammation of the gallbladder that is almost always caused by obstruction of the cystic duct, usually by an impacted calculus. The inflammation may be acute or

chronic, uncomplicated or complicated, calculous or acalculous. As the gallbladder continues to accumulate bile, intraluminal pressure increases and vascular insufficiency of the wall occurs, causing ischemia, necrosis, and often supervening inflammation. The gallbladder distends, the gallbladder wall thickens from edema, and the patient is tender to palpation over the gallbladder (positive Murphy's sign).

Both ultrasound and hepatobiliary NM studies are the modalities of choice to evaluate possible cholecystitis. Sonographic signs of acute cholecystitis include cholelithiasis, gallbladder wall thickening (greater than 3 mm), irregular or

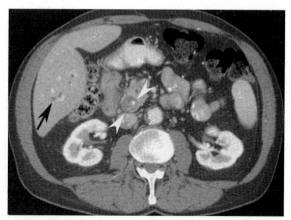

▲ **Figure 11-53.** CT in choledocholithiasis showing the presence of a stone within the common bile duct (arrowheads), which is dilated and inflamed around the dense stone. Note the associated intrahepatic biliary ductal dilatation (arrow).

linear hypoechoic structures within the gallbladder wall, a positive sonographic Murphy's sign, and marked gallbladder distention (Figure 11-54). A combination of these signs is a good positive predictor of acute cholecystitis. In marked chronic cholecystitis, US shows persistent gallbladder wall thickening or sludge, stones, and contraction of the gallbladder. However, in the presence of cholelithiasis, the gallbladder almost always shows signs of chronic inflammation histologically, even without symptoms or sonographic findings.

Hepatobiliary NM HIDA scans depict acute cholecystitis as an absence of filling of the gallbladder with the radionuclide once it is excreted by the liver into the biliary ducts; this absence of filling is due to the obstruction of the cystic duct lumen by inflammatory edema of the cystic duct wall (Figure 11-55). Sufficient time must be given to fill the gallbladder. This time interval depends upon whether or not morphine is administered. Morphine increases the tone of the sphincter of Oddi and increases intraluminal common bile duct pressure to overcome the resistance to bile flow into the gallbladder in chronic cholecystitis, but not in acute cholecystitis when a stone obstructs the duct. Acute cholecystitis is diagnosed when absence of activity is noted either 45 minutes after morphine augmentation or after 4 hours without morphine

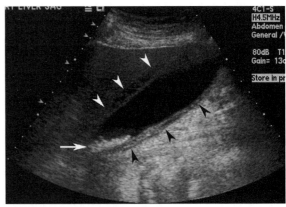

▲ **Figure 11-54.** Longitudinal US in acute cholecystitis showing a thickened GB wall with linear, hypoechoic fluid/edema in the wall (arrowheads). Note the numerous rounded echogenic foci with shadowing in the neck of the GB representing gallstones (arrow). These findings, in conjunction with tenderness to palpation by the transducer over the GB (sonographic Murphy's sign), strongly suggest acute cholecystitis.

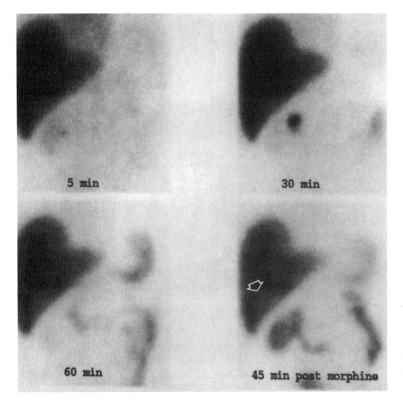

▲ **Figure 11-55.** NM hepatobiliary scan in acute cholecystitis showing the absence of gallbladder activity in the gallbladder fossa (arrowhead), 60 minutes following administration of the agent and even after administration of morphine.

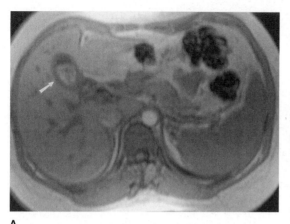 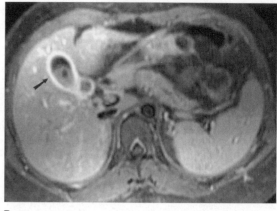

A   **B**

▲ **Figure 11-56.** (**A**) Preinfused T1-weighted MR imaging scan showing cholelithiasis and a low signal intensity gallbladder wall (arrow). (**B**) Postinfused T1-weighted MR imaging scan demonstrating gallbladder wall enhancement (arrow), reflecting the hyperemia of inflammation, signifying acute cholecystitis.

augmentation. Delayed gallbladder visualization after 1 hour usually reflects chronic cholecystitis. On CT, the morphologic findings in patients with acute cholecystitis are similar to the US findings, including gallstones and thickened and inhomogeneous gallbladder wall. However, CT is not as sensitive as US or NM either to the presence of gallstones or to acute cholecystitis. MR imaging can depict the presence of gallbladder wall inflammation in the absence of wall thickening by demonstrating wall enhancement following Gd infusion (Figure 11-56). The exact role of MR imaging in cholecystitis

has not yet been completely evaluated. Angiography has no role in the diagnosis of cholecystitis.

Many potential complications and conditions are associated with cholecystitis. These include hydrops, porcelain gallbladder, milk-of-calcium bile, and emphysematous cholecystitis.

Hydrops refers to the marked distention of the gallbladder by clear, sterile mucus, usually under conditions of chronic, complete cystic duct obstruction. On imaging studies, the primary finding is enlargement of the gallbladder (Figure 11-57).

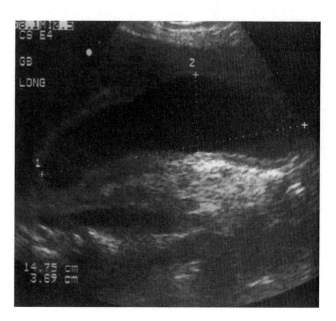

▲ **Figure 11-57.** Longitudinal US in hydrops showing a massively enlarged gallbladder due to complete obstruction of the cystic duct and accumulation of clear mucus.

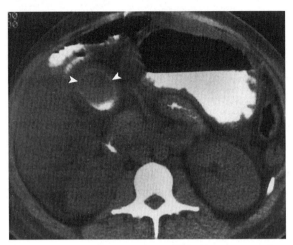

▲ **Figure 11-58.** CT in porcelain gallbladder showing the calcification of the gallbladder wall (arrowheads) and the dependent accumulation of calcified material in the gallbladder lumen.

Porcelain gallbladder refers to calcification of the gallbladder wall, as a result of chronic inflammation causing dystrophic calcification and often associated with recurrent acute cholecystitis. Gallbladder stones are usually present, and there is a higher incidence (approximately 10% to 20%) of gallbladder carcinoma. On imaging studies, complete or incomplete circular wall calcification is present and is seen as a curvilinear, highly echogenic wall on US or as a curvilinear, high-attenuation wall on CT (Figure 11-58).

Milk-of-calcium bile refers to a precipitation of calcified material within the lumen of the gallbladder, usually associated with chronic cholecystitis. US shows echogenic sludgelike material, possibly with gallstones. CT demonstrates the distinctive appearance of a horizontal bile-calcium level.

Emphysematous cholecystitis is a distinctive condition and should be treated as a medical/surgical emergency. Like acute cholecystitis, it is marked by intense gallbladder wall inflammation, but unlike acute cholecystitis, it is not necessarily associated with gallstones. It may be related to ischemia of the gallbladder wall from small-vessel disease, and it affects an older age group than does acute cholecystitis. The most common group affected is older diabetic men. Gas is released by bacterial invasion and accumulates in the gallbladder wall, lumen, or both. On US, gas is seen as an echogenic focus producing poorly defined or "dirty" shadowing behind it. The wall is thickened, perhaps focally, with gas. On CT, air-density gas is seen within the lumen or wall (Figure 11-47). MR imaging

and angiography have no current role in evaluation of these complications.

Like inflammation of the gallbladder, inflammation of the biliary ducts, or cholangitis, is an important clinical condition. It is less common than cholecystitis. AIDS-associated cholangiopathy, ascending cholangitis, and oriental cholangiohepatitis are three important forms of cholangitis.

AIDS-associated cholangiopathy is marked by the frequent isolation of opportunistic organisms, including *Cryptosporidium* and cytomegalovirus from the bile, and by considerable inflammation of the bile duct wall. On US or CT, the gallbladder or biliary duct walls may be markedly thickened (greater than 4 mm) (Figure 11-46) and may contain irregular lamina. Inflammation is present, but stones may or may not be present. Cholangiography shows irregular strictures, papillary stenosis, or both.

Ascending cholangitis is a bacterial inflammation of both walls and lumina of the biliary system, including the gallbladder. It is almost always due to obstruction of the biliary tract, especially when caused by choledocholithiasis and distal bile-duct stenosis. The presence of grossly purulent material within the duct indicates suppurative cholangitis. Cross-sectional imaging studies are used to define the level and cause of obstruction. Cholangiography can show the abnormal biliary ducts directly. The purulent material of suppurative cholangitis may be seen as echogenic material on US, high-density material on CT, or filling defects on cholangiography.

Oriental cholangiohepatitis is a common illness in endemic areas of Asia and can be seen in Asian immigrants in this country. It may be caused by bile duct wall injury from the parasitic infestation. Ductal stones commonly form, and the ducts are dilated. A characteristic finding is the presence of intraductal (especially intrahepatic ductal) calculi. These findings are readily demonstrated with US, CT, and cholangiography.

EXERCISE 11-5. PANCREATIC INFLAMMATION

11-15. What is the most likely diagnosis in Case 11-15 (Figure 11-59)?
  A. Acute edematous pancreatitis
  B. Pancreatic abscess
  C. Pancreatic phlegmon
  D. Hemorrhagic pancreatitis

11-16. What is the most likely diagnosis in Case 11-16 (Figure 11-60)?
  A. Acute edematous pancreatitis
  B. Hemorrhagic pancreatitis
  C. Gastroduodenal artery pseudoaneurysm
  D. Pancreatic abscess

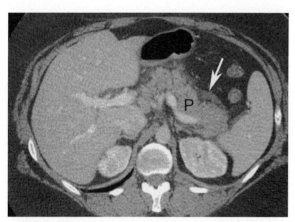

▲ **Figure 11-59.** Case 11-15. A 54-year-old alcoholic male with marked epigastric pain and increased amylase.

11-17. What is the most likely diagnosis in Case 11-17 (Figure 11-61)?
  A. Acute edematous pancreatitis
  B. Chronic pancreatitis
  C. Pancreatic phlegmon
  D. Hemorrhagic pancreatitis

Radiographic Findings

11-15. In this case, the overall size of the pancreas (P) is enlarged, and the tissue around the pancreas is edematous with associated fluid (arrow). All are findings of

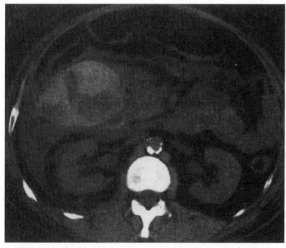

▲ **Figure 11-60.** Case 11-16. A 45-year-old male with marked epigastric pain and falling hematocrit, who is "crashing."

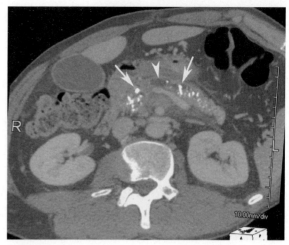

▲ **Figure 11-61.** Case 11-17. A 65-year-old male with chronic epigastric pain.

acute edematous pancreatitis (A is the correct answer to Question 11-15).

11-16. In this case, peripancreatic inflammatory changes and a high-density collection are seen adjacent to the pancreatic head, representing a collection of blood created by hemorrhagic pancreatitis (B is the correct answer to Question 11-16).

11-17. In this case, multiple calcifications are distributed throughout the pancreas (arrows) and there is enlargement of the pancreatic duct (arrowhead) with atrophy of the parenchyma. All are findings of chronic calcific pancreatitis (B is the correct answer to Question 11-17).

Discussion

Pancreatitis, an inflammatory condition of the pancreas, has a number of causes including alcohol abuse, trauma, cholelithiasis, peptic ulcer, hyperlipoproteinemia, hypercalcemia, and infection. Pancreatic inflammation may be acute or chronic. Acute pancreatitis and chronic pancreatitis may not represent different stages of the same disease.

Acute pancreatitis can occur once or repetitively and usually has the potential for healing. It can be associated with mild to severe inflammatory edema (edematous or interstitial pancreatitis) or with hemorrhage (hemorrhagic or necrotizing pancreatitis). These two forms of acute pancreatitis may be distinguishable only by the severity and time course of the disease. Edematous pancreatitis resolves within 2 to 3 days with appropriate therapy, whereas hemorrhagic pancreatitis requires much longer to resolve. The

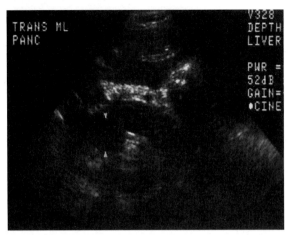

▲ **Figure 11-62.** Transverse US in acute pancreatitis showing a diffusely hypoechoic pancreas with more pronounced hypoechogenicity in the pancreatic head (arrowheads).

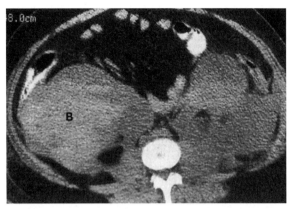

▲ **Figure 11-64.** CT in hemorrhagic pancreatitis showing diffusely distributed pancreatic inflammatory exudate containing high-density blood (B) in the right side of the abdomen.

diagnosis of simple pancreatitis is usually based on medical history, physical examination, and laboratory results. With this information, imaging studies are usually unnecessary, and scans show the pancreas to be normal or only slightly enlarged. The surrounding fat is edematous. The pancreas appears hypoechoic on US (Figure 11-62). On CT the surrounding fat appears as areas of streaky interstitial soft-tissue density in the transverse mesocolon around the pancreas (Figure 11-63).

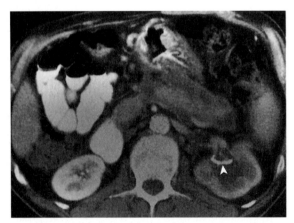

▲ **Figure 11-63.** CT in pancreatitis showing the presence of poorly defined soft tissue planes around the pancreas, obscuring the boundary between the pancreas and the stomach and colon. Note the stent in the renal pelvis (arrowhead) of the left kidney, placed to relieve urinary obstruction.

Clinical criteria to predict the severity or likelihood of complications of pancreatitis correlate well with the presence and extent of extrapancreatic abnormalities on imaging studies. Imaging is useful in acute pancreatitis when assessing potential complications. These complications include hemorrhagic pancreatitis, vascular complications, phlegmon, and abscess.

Hemorrhagic pancreatitis is usually due to erosion of small vessels, is often a serious problem, and indicates an acutely and critically ill patient. It appears as a collection of echogenic material on US. On CT, it appears as a collection of high-density material and can be extremely extensive as it is an aggressive process (Figure 11-64). This material represents the blood.

Large vessels are at risk for developing pseudoaneurysms when the histiolytic enzymes released by the inflamed pancreas erode their walls, leading to a focal, highly vascular structure within the region of the pancreas. The splenic, gastroduodenal, and hepatic arteries are particularly vulnerable. On US and CT, flow within an enlarged rounded vessel can be seen. Angiography establishes the diagnosis by showing a focally enlarged vessel, sometimes with extravasation. However, CTA is also effective for detecting pseudoaneurysms related to pancreatitis.

Phlegmon is an inflammatory, boggy, edematous, soft-tissue mass, distinct from fluid, arising from the pancreas and diffusely spreading away from it. Phlegmon appears as a diffuse soft-tissue echogenicity or density process surrounding the pancreas and contains neither the blood of hemorrhagic pancreatitis nor the fluid of an abscess (Figure 11-65).

Abscesses are a potentially life-threatening complication of pancreatitis. Infection associated with pancreatitis can be

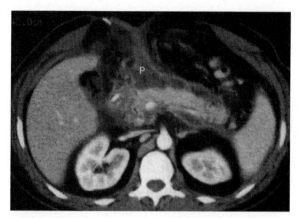

▲ **Figure 11-65.** CT in pancreatic phlegmon showing the presence of poorly defined phlegmonous exudate (P) surrounding the entire pancreas and extending from the pancreas toward the anterior abdominal wall.

thought of as representing infected necrosis (diffuse infection without pus collection) or pancreatic abscess (collection of pus surrounded by a capsule). Infected necrosis is harder to identify on imaging studies than is pancreatic abscess, because it is less distinct and blends into the surrounding edema. On US, abscess appears as a poorly defined anechoic or hypoechoic lesion. It enhances sound posteriorly and may contain debris. Gas appears as a poorly defined echogenic

focus within the nondependent aspect of the lesion and casts a "dirty" shadow. On CT, the lesion is poorly defined and may contain gas collections. After contrast material infusion, the border enhances. If gas is absent, abscess cannot be differentiated from phlegmon or pseudocyst (Figure 11-66). In general, NM and angiography do not have a major role in evaluation of acute pancreatitis.

Unlike acute pancreatitis, chronic pancreatitis is considered to indicate permanent pancreatic damage. Chronic pancreatitis may or may not be preceded by prior attacks of acute pancreatitis. The pancreas will develop calcifications within the ductal system (Figure 11-61). Masslike enlargement of the pancreas can periodically occur, but often the gland eventually atrophies. The pancreatic duct may dilate. These findings are visible on both US and CT. NM and angiography do not have a current major role in evaluation of chronic pancreatitis.

EXERCISE 11-6. PANCREATIC NEOPLASM

11-18. What is the most likely diagnosis in Case 11-18 (Figure 11-67)?
   A. Pancreatic cyst
   B. Ductal pancreatic carcinoma
   C. Pancreatic metastasis
   D. Peripancreatic lymphadenopathy

11-19. What is the most likely diagnosis in Case 11-19 (Figure 11-68)?
   A. Cholangiocarcinorna
   B. Cystic pancreatic neoplasm
   C. Ductal pancreatic carcinoma
   D. Pancreatic cyst

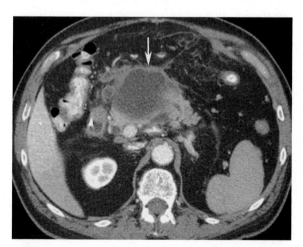

▲ **Figure 11-66.** CT of pancreatic abscess demonstrating a fluid collection with rim enhancement (arrow) and surrounding inflammatory change in the region of the pancreatic head and neck in this patient, who recently underwent resection of a pancreatic tumor. The absence of gas makes this difficult to distinguish from phlegmon or pseudocyst based on imaging alone.

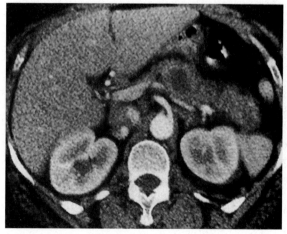

▲ **Figure 11-67.** Case 11-18. A 62-year-old female with vague, deep, and persistent abdominal pain.

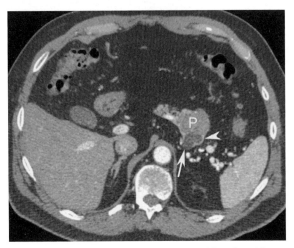

▲ **Figure 11-68.** Case 11-19. A 65-year-old male with midepigastric pain over a long period of time.

11-20. What is the most likely diagnosis in Case 11-20 (Figure 11-69)?
 A. Acute edematous pancreatitis
 B. Pancreatic pseudocyst
 C. Pancreatic cyst
 D. Cystic pancreatic neoplasm

Radiographic Findings

11-18. In this case, there is a low, but not fluid, density lesion in the pancreatic body, expanding the contour of the

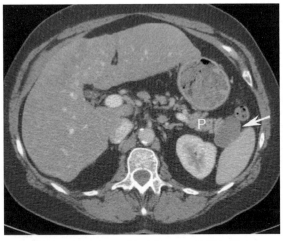

▲ **Figure 11-69.** Case 11-20. A 32-year-old healthy, asymptomatic woman.

pancreas, and not associated with any inflammatory changes in the peripancreatic fat, findings most consistent with a ductal adenocarcinoma (B is the correct answer to Question 11-18).

11-19. In this case, CT demonstrates a fluid density lesion (arrow) in the tail of the pancreas (P). There is enhancement along the rim (arrowhead) that is not associated with surrounding inflammatory change in the peripancreatic fat. Findings are compatible with a cystic neoplasm of the pancreas (B is the correct answer to Question 11-19).

11-20. In this case, CT demonstrates a unilocular fluid attenuation mass (arrow) in the tail of the pancreas (P) without enhancement or nodularity. This is difficult to distinguish from a cystic neoplasm; however, at surgery this was a lymphoepithelial cyst (C is the correct answer to Question 11-20).

Discussion

Pancreatic masses include tumors, tumor-like masses such as cysts and developmental anomalies, and inflammatory lesions. These can overlap in appearance, as when an inflammatory mass simulates a neoplastic mass on imaging studies. They can be causally related, as when a neoplastic mass secondarily causes an inflammatory mass. Therefore, differentiation among them is not entirely possible, either clinically or radiographically. However, the prognostic and management implications of the lesions that create pancreatic masses differ considerably and therefore require extensive and often invasive investigation. Although contrast studies of the gastrointestinal tract can be used to infer the presence of a mass, usually cross-sectional imaging studies are employed to establish the diagnosis.

Tumors of the pancreas are important clinical entities; some have an extremely poor prognosis and some produce serious clinical symptoms. They can be classified according to origin as epithelial tumors, endocrine tumors, and miscellaneous lesions. Epithelial tumors can be solid or cystic. Solid ductal adenocarcinoma is the most common overall and carries the worst prognosis (mean survival 4 months). Cystic tumors can be divided into cystic lesions arising from the pancreatic parenchymal cells, such as cystadenoma or cystadenocarcinoma, and those arising from the pancreatic ductal cells, such as intraductal papillary mucinous tumors. Compared to adenocarcinoma, these tumors have a less serious prognosis. Endocrine, or islet cell, tumors elaborate hormonal substances and can create clinically significant symptoms. The two most common of these are insulinoma, which releases insulin and produces hypoglycemia, and gastrinoma, which releases gastrin and produces Zollinger-Ellison syndrome. There are many other important kinds of hormonally active pancreatic endocrine tumors, and each is designated by the hormone it

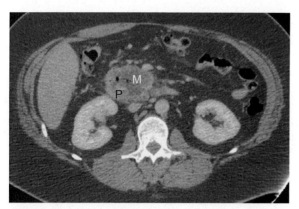

▲ **Figure 11-70.** CT of pancreatic ductal adenocarcinoma demonstrates a mass (M) expanding the head of the pancreas with hypoenhancement relative to the pancreatic parenchyma (P).

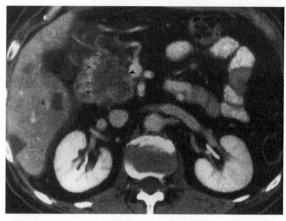

▲ **Figure 11-71.** CT in metastatic pancreatic carcinoma showing a pancreatic mass (arrowheads) and numerous liver metastases.

secretes (eg, glucagonoma, somatostatinoma). Miscellaneous lesions arise from pancreatic parenchymal tissue (eg, metastases, especially from melanoma, and lung or breast cancer) or from tissue other than pancreas (eg, intrapancreatic cholangiocarcinoma or peripancreatic lymph node). These miscellaneous lesions are important because they sometimes strongly simulate true pancreatic neoplasms on imaging studies.

Ductal adenocarcinoma has a variety of appearances on imaging studies. On US, it usually is seen as a focal, hypoechoic, irregular, solid mass. Rarely, it is isoechoic or involves the entire gland. In some pancreatic head masses, the only finding may be that the uncinate process is rounded. The pancreatic or biliary duct may be dilated by the obstructing tumor. Pseudocysts, cystic collections in or around the pancreas, may form because of pancreatic duct dilatation and perforation. On CT, the tumor presents as a solid, low-density, irregular mass, perhaps with ductal dilatation, pseudocyst formation, or both (Figure 11-67). It usually enhances to a lesser extent than the surrounding pancreas (Figure 11-70). Occasionally, the tumors will enhance brightly. The pancreas distal to a ductal adenocarcinoma is often atrophic. Angiography may be used to demonstrate the vascular anatomy and establish definitively whether certain key vessels (eg, the superior mesenteric artery or vein) are encased. If so, the lesion is unresectable. NM currently has no established role in evaluation of pancreatic tumors. Associated metastases in the liver establish the fact that a pancreatic mass cannot be simply inflammatory (Figure 11-71). General pertinent negatives on cross-sectional imaging may help to differentiate adenocarcinoma from other nontumorous masses. Calcification is rarely, if ever, seen in ductal adenocarcinoma, and it is almost never hypervascular.

Ductal adenocarcinoma is simulated by a number of other entities. These include peripancreatic lymphadenopathy, intrapancreatic cholangiocarcinoma, and pancreatic metastases.

Peripancreatic lymphadenopathy from lymphoma, leukemia, or any other primary malignancy can closely resemble a pancreatic mass. On imaging studies it may appear as solid soft tissue in the pancreatic region (Figure 11-72). Keys to

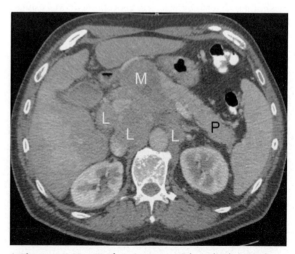

▲ **Figure 11-72.** CT of peripancreatic lymphadenopathy showing the presence of a large hypoenhancing mass (M) abutting the head and neck of the pancreas. The tail of the pancreas is normal (P). There is adjacent enlargement and heterogeneous enhancement of multiple lymph nodes (L).

differentiating lymphadenopathy from a primary solid mass include smooth lobulation and pseudoseptations caused by incomplete coalescence of the lymph nodes. Also, peripancreatic lymphadenopathy is much less likely to obstruct the pancreatic duct, although suprapancreatic lymph nodes obstruct the biliary duct as it passes through the porta hepatis.

Two uncommon neoplastic processes that occur in the pancreas are cholangiocarcinoma and metastases. Cholangiocarcinoma usually does not occur within the pancreas, but when it does, it can exactly mimic a pancreatic head mass to the extent of producing both the pancreatic and common bile duct dilatation. Metastases appear as solid intrapancreatic lesions, but with necrosis, they appear as fluid masses. Because they may be completely indistinguishable from primary tumors, the diagnosis may be inferred only from the clinical history. Pancreatic metastases are quite uncommon, usually arise from melanoma or lung primary lesions, and mimic a focal mass lesion of any neoplastic origin (Figure 11-73).

Pancreatic endocrine tumors may also simulate ductal adenocarcinoma, and in fact, no specific features consistently distinguish the two. Occasionally, however, certain imaging features can be helpful, especially when combined with the history. Many islet cell tumors appear simply as solid masses within the pancreas. However, some (especially in insulinoma) may appear hypervascular when studied with fast bolus or dynamic CT, and they may appear as extremely dense lesions immediately after enhancement with intravenous contrast material. Calcifications, which sometimes are very dense, are more commonly seen with islet-cell tumors. MR imaging may have a role in the evaluation of islet-cell tumors, because these tumors have a characteristic appearance on MR studies.

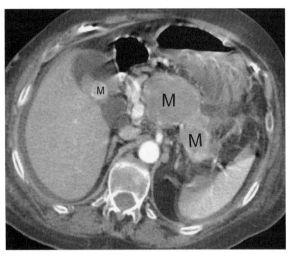

▲ **Figure 11-73.** CT of metastatic melanoma demonstrating multiple masses (M) involving the pancreas and gallbladder.

Islet-cell tumors and their metastases have extremely high signal intensity on T2-weighted MR imaging, which can be used to characterize the origin of the lesion.

Primary cystic pancreatic malignancies and pancreatic cysts are not readily confused with typical ductal adenocarcinoma. Currently, cystic pancreatic masses are classified according to whether they arise from parenchymal cells or ductal cells. Cystic malignancies arising from pancreatic parenchyma

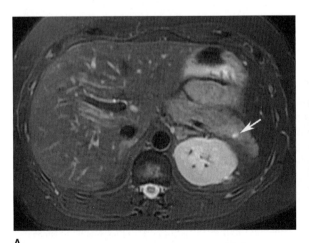

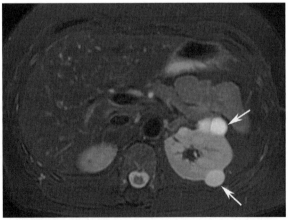

A   B

▲ **Figure 11-74.** (A) Axial T2-weighted fat-suppressed image of a patient with von Hippel-Lindau disease demonstrates a cyst in the tail of the pancreas (arrow). (B) Note the associated multiple kidney cysts (arrows) in the same patient, different image.

are classified as either serous or mucinous cystic neoplasms. This classification is helpful, because the two lesions are distinguishable from each other and from solid lesions on imaging studies. Serous cystadenomas are usually composed of innumerable very small cysts (1 mm to 2 cm). Sometimes they contain highly vascularized fibrous septa and a central stellate fibrotic scar, which may calcify. They are generally benign. Mucinous cystic neoplasms are composed of unilocular or multilocular cysts larger than 5 cm and may have large papillary excrescences. They are considered malignant or premalignant lesions. Both serous cystadenomas and mucinous cystic neoplasms are cystic, but differences in the typical sizes of the cysts can be recognized on US or CT. Cystic malignancies arising from pancreatic ductal epithelial cells are called intraductal papillary mucinous tumors. These tumors contain considerable mucus and therefore exhibit complex appearances on MR imaging. MRCP can be helpful to demonstrate communication with the pancreatic duct. Pancreatic cysts can occur as isolated congenital cysts or as part of a more generalized multiorgan process that includes adult polycystic disease or von Hippel-Lindau disease (Figure 11-74). Regardless, their appearance is similar to that of a cyst in any other organ (Figure 11-69). US and CT depict a uniloculated or multiloc-ulated cyst. A pancreatic cyst can be very difficult to differentiate from a mucinous cystic neoplasm. Management is controversial, and they are often followed even when small.

Acknowledgments *Special thanks to my colleagues Robert Cowan, MD, for providing Figure 11-5; Nat Watson, MD, for providing Figure 11-30; and James Ball, MD, for providing Figure 11-55.*

SUGGESTED READING

1. Gore R, Levine MA. *Textbook of Gastrointestinal Radiology*. 3rd ed. Philadelphia: Saunders; 2007.
2. Semelka RC. *Abdominal-Pelvic MRI*. 2nd ed. Hoboken, NJ: Wiley; 2006.
3. Knowlton JQ, Taylor AJ, Reicheleerfer M, Stang J. Imaging of biliary tract inflammation: an update. *AJR Am J Roentgenol.* 2008; 190:984-992.
4. Parikh T, Drew SJ, Lee VS, et al. Focal liver lesion detection and characterization with diffusion-weighted MR imaging: comparison with standard breath-hold T2-weighted imaging. *Radiology.* 2009;246:812-822.
5. Takahashi N, Fletcher JG, Fidler JL, Hough DM, Kawashima A, Chari ST. Dual-phase CT of autoimmune pancreatitis: a multi-reader study. *AJR Am J Roentgenol.* 2008;190:280-286.

Brain and Its Coverings

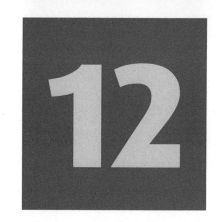

Michael E. Zapadka, DO

Michelle S. Bradbury, MD, PhD

Daniel W. Williams III, MD

Technological advances in radiology during the past 30 years have vastly improved our ability to diagnose neurologic diseases. Prior to the introduction of computed tomography (CT) in 1974, neuroradiologic examinations of the brain consisted primarily of plain films of the skull, cerebral arteriography, pneumoencephalography, and conventional nuclear medicine studies. Unfortunately, these techniques, for the most part, provided only indirect information about suspected intracranial processes, were insensitive in detecting subtle or early brain lesions, or were potentially harmful to the patient. Computed tomography revolutionized the radiologic workup of central nervous system (CNS) abnormalities because for the first time normal and abnormal structures could be directly visualized with minimal risk to the patient.

In the late 1980s, it became apparent that magnetic resonance (MR) imaging would become the procedure of choice for evaluating many neurologic disorders, as well as for demonstrating vascular flow phenomena. Since then, there have been many technological advances associated with this modality. These include improvements in magnet and coil design, decrease in imaging time, and the development of new pulse sequences. In addition to advances in conventional anatomic imaging, there has also been substantial growth of "physiologic" MR imaging including MR spectroscopy (MRS), diffusion-weighted (DW) and perfusion-weighted (PW) MR imaging, and functional MR imaging (fMRI), among others. These imaging modalities provide functional information about the brain and have the potential to greatly extend our understanding of neuropathology beyond structure alone.

Revolutionary breakthroughs in CT scanning technology during the 1990s facilitated the development of advanced CT applications, namely, dynamic contrast-enhanced CT angiography (CTA) and CT perfusion (CTP). These techniques, which allow high spatial resolution imaging of the cervical and intracranial vasculature, are currently being used in the evaluation of the acute stroke patient in many medical centers. Furthermore, recent technologic advances in CT imaging have markedly decreased scan times and have allowed evaluation of very tiny anatomic structures because of improvement in spatial resolution.

Recent advances in nuclear medicine functional imaging techniques, including single photon emission computed tomography (SPECT) and positron emission tomography (PET), improvements in conventional angiographic methods, and expansion of catheter-based therapeutic procedures have provided the neuroradiologist today with an even greater variety of strategies for diagnosing and treating neurologic abnormalities.

The main purpose of this chapter is to acquaint the reader with the major radiologic techniques used currently to evaluate the brain and its coverings. The strengths and weaknesses of these techniques are discussed. Imaging anatomy of the brain and its coverings is briefly reviewed. Basic guidelines pertaining to technique selection for evaluating common neurologic conditions are provided. Finally, examples of common brain abnormalities are presented. It is assumed that readers have a basic understanding of neuroanatomy and neuropathology.

Although this chapter may give some insight into neuroradiologic study interpretation, that is not its primary goal. Rather, readers should expect to become reasonably familiar with the various techniques employed to examine the brain and should gain some idea about the appropriate ordering of examinations in specific clinical situations.

TECHNIQUES

Radiologic modalities useful in evaluating the brain and its coverings can be divided into two major groups: anatomic modalities and functional modalities. Anatomic modalities, which provide information mostly of a structural nature, include plain films of the skull, CT, MR imaging, cerebral arteriography (CA), and ultrasonography (US). On the other hand, SPECT and PET imaging, CT perfusion, DW and PW MR imaging, fMRI, and MRS are primarily functional modalities, which give information about brain perfusion or metabolism. Some techniques provide both anatomic and functional information. For example, cerebral arteriography depicts blood vessels supplying the brain but also allows us to estimate brain circulation time. Ultrasound of the carotid bifurcation is another modality that provides both anatomic and functional information. A routine sonogram of the carotid bifurcation gives anatomic data that, when combined with Doppler data, readily provides information about blood flow.

The following discussion of current neuroradiologic techniques emphasizes relative examination cost and patient risk, along with the advantages and disadvantages of each technique. The normal imaging appearance of the brain and its coverings is also illustrated.

▶ Plain Radiographs

Plain radiographs of the skull are obtained by placing a patient's head between an x-ray source and a recording device (ie, x-ray film). Whereas bones of the skull attenuate a large number of x-rays to create an image, soft tissues such as scalp or brain are poorly visualized, if at all. Another difficulty in plain film interpretation results from the spherical shape of the skull, leading to multiple superimposed structures. The resultant skull radiograph primarily gives information about the bones of the skull, but no direct information about the intracranial contents. Indirect information about intracranial abnormalities can sometimes be obtained from the skull plain radiograph, although this information can be quite subtle, even in the setting of advanced disease. Skull plain radiographs have been largely replaced today by more sensitive techniques such as CT or MR imaging. Even in the setting of suspected skull fracture, plain radiographs are rarely indicated, because CT scans also show the fracture, as well as any intracranial abnormality that might require treatment. Currently, plain radiographs of the skull serve a very limited role in routine neuroimaging and are only briefly discussed.

▶ Computed Tomography

CT scans consist of computer-generated cross-sectional images obtained from a rotating x-ray beam and detector system. Advances in scanning technology now permit simultaneous acquisition of multiple images during a single rotation of the x-ray tube (eg, currently up to 256 slices) during a breath-hold. The resultant images, unlike plain films, exquisitely depict and differentiate between soft tissues, thus allowing direct visualization of intracranial contents and abnormalities associated with neurologic diseases. The contrast or brightness ("window" or "level," respectively) of these images can be adjusted to highlight particular tissues.

Typically, a head CT consists of images adjusted to emphasize soft-tissue detail (soft-tissue windows) as well as images adjusted to visualize bony detail (bone windows) (Figure 12-1). As stated earlier, CT image generation is dependent on variable attenuation of the x-ray beam based on the density of structures it passes through (eg, bones of the skull base are very dense and attenuate a large percentage of the x-ray beam). Therefore, cortical bone appears white (has a high attenuation value or Hounsfield unit), whereas air within the paranasal sinuses appears black (has a low attenuation value)

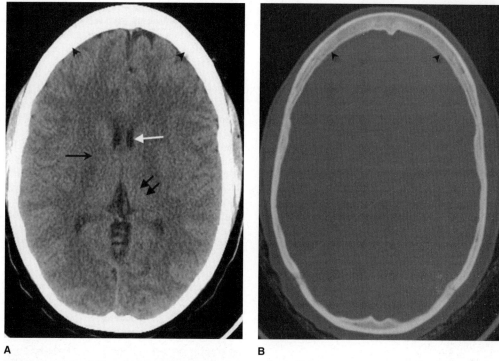

▲ **Figure 12-1.** Normal axial head CT images. Appropriate window selection allows visualization of both intracranial contents (**A**) and bony calvarium (**B**). Note differences in attenuation among gray matter (left thalamus, double black arrows), right internal capsule (single black arrow), cerebrospinal fluid (CSF; frontal horn of the left lateral ventricle, white arrow), and bone (skull, arrowheads).

(Figure 12-1). Cerebral white matter has a slightly lower Hounsfield number than does cerebral gray matter and consequently appears slightly darker than gray matter on a head CT scan (Figure 12-1A). Intracranial pathologic conditions can be either dark (low attenuation) or bright (high attenuation), depending on the particular abnormality. For example, acute intracranial hemorrhage is typically very bright, whereas an acute cerebral infarction demonstrates low attenuation when compared to the surrounding normal brain because of the presence of edema.

The CT technologist can change the slice thickness and angulation, among other technical factors, to alter the way an image appears. Images are typically obtained axially in helical fashion, with acquisition of a volumetric data set. Current scanner technology allows the axial data set to be reformatted in coronal, sagittal, or oblique planes or as a 3-D image, with little, if any, loss of resolution. CT examinations may be performed after intravenous administration of an iodinated contrast agent, especially when MRI is contraindicated or unavailable. These agents "light up" or enhance normal blood vessels and dural sinuses, as well as intracranial structures that lack a blood-brain barrier (BBB), such as the pituitary gland, choroid plexus, or pineal gland. Pathologic conditions that interrupt the BBB (such as neoplasm, infection, or cerebral infarction) also demonstrate enhancement after contrast material administration. For this reason, lesions that may be invisible on a noncontrast study are often obvious on the contrast-enhanced scan.

The intravenous administration of a contrast bolus can be appropriately timed to maximize vascular opacification of the arterial or venous circulation (CTA or CTV, respectively). These high spatial resolution 3-D CTA images (Figure 12-2) of the cervical and intracranial vasculature are routinely employed to quantify vessel stenosis due to atherosclerotic disease, to assess for vascular injury related to trauma, or to detect cerebral aneurysm in the patient with subarachnoid hemorrhage.

In particular, CTA has become a standard component of evaluating the acute stroke patient. CTA accurately identifies the location and extent of large vessel occlusions and can be supplemented by a more detailed, quantitative evaluation of the cerebral microvascular hemodynamics (CT perfusion)

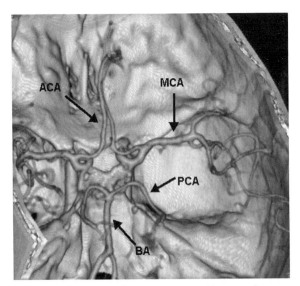

▲ **Figure 12-2.** Normal CT angiogram with 3-D volume rendering. Image is oriented slightly oblique with the superior calvarium cut away. Major vessels demonstrated include the anterior cerebral artery (ACA), middle cerebral artery (MCA), basilar artery (BA), and posterior cerebral artery (PCA).

during the early phase of bolus passage. Software analysis of this tailored CTA data produces maps of capillary-level cerebral perfusion, typically measured by mean transit time (MTT), cerebral blood flow (CBF), and cerebral blood volume (CBV). In the setting of cerebral infarction, these parameters can help interpret the infarct "core" (CBV) versus the ischemic "penumbra" (MTT and CBF). Evaluation of potential mismatch between the infarct core and surrounding penumbra serves as the rationale for instituting various reperfusion techniques.

Another recent application of CTA is in the screening evaluation of blunt cerebrovascular injury, including closed head injuries, seatbelt abrasion (or other soft-tissue injury) of the anterior neck, basilar skull fracture extending through the carotid canal, and cervical vertebral body fracture. It is an accurate technique for detecting internal carotid artery (ICA) dissections and for assessing stenoses, although evaluation is difficult in areas of surrounding dense bone as a result of associated "streak artifact." However, this noninvasive, relatively short imaging procedure rivals conventional angiographic methods, as it requires no patient transfer and can sensitively identify vascular injury in relation to other associated brain insults, cervical spine injury, or facial or basilar skull fractures.

High-resolution data acquisition during the venous phase following intravenous contrast administration (CT venography) can be used to identify dural sinuses and cerebral veins,

evaluate for dural venous sinus thrombosis, and distinguish partial sinus obstruction from venous occlusion in the setting of adjacent brain masses. CT venography can also differentiate slow flow from thrombosis, which may occasionally be difficult with MR techniques.

The major advantages of CT are that it is inexpensive, is widely available, can be used in patients with MR-incompatible hardware, and allows a relatively quick assessment of intracranial contents in the setting of a neurological deficit. The images obtained are very sensitive to the presence of acute hemorrhage and calcification, and images revealing exquisite bony detail of the skull and skull base can be acquired. Because of the configuration of the scanner, patients are reasonably accessible for monitoring during the examination.

CT scanners do have a number of disadvantages, however. Patients are exposed to ionizing radiation and iodine-based contrast agents (although lower doses of contrast are needed with newer multidetector scanners). Imaging artifacts can interfere with accurate interpretation. In particular, images of the brainstem and posterior fossa are often degraded by "streak artifacts" from dense bone (Figure 12-3).

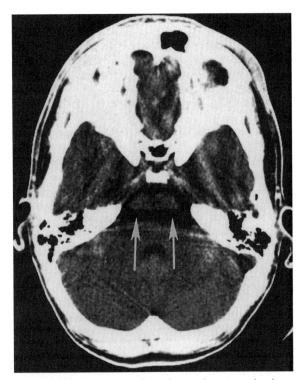

▲ **Figure 12-3.** Streak artifacts (arrows) commonly obscure portions of the brainstem, posterior fossa, and temporal lobes on routine head CT scans.

Streak artifacts from metallic objects (eg, fillings, braces, surgical clips) can also obscure abnormalities. Images can be severely degraded by patient motion. Fortunately, unlike MR scans, individual CT images degraded by motion can be rapidly reacquired.

▶ Magnetic Resonance Imaging

One of the most exciting developments in radiology during the past 30 years has been the growth of magnetic resonance imaging (MRI), which is currently the mainstay of clinical neuroimaging. The concept of nuclear magnetic resonance (NMR), initially used for probing the physiochemical structure of molecules, was first described in the 1930s, but it took more than 40 years before the translation of NMR phenomena could be used for clinical imaging.

MR examinations, like CT scans, consist of computer-reconstructed cross-sectional images (Figure 12-4). In MR imaging, however, unlike CT scans or plain radiographs, the information collected is not x-ray beam attenuation. The MR image is a visual display of NMR data collected principally from nuclei within body tissues—especially hydrogen nuclei within water and fat molecules. Intrinsic tissue relaxation occurs by two major pathways, called longitudinal, or T1, and transverse, or T2, decay. MR imaging sequences that emphasize T1 decay are commonly referred to as T1-weighted; sequences that accentuate T2 relaxation properties are called T2-weighted (Figure 12-4). Most MR scans of the brain use both of these sequences, because certain abnormalities may only be obvious on one or the other. T2-weighted images are usually easy to identify because fluid (eg, cerebrospinal, globe vitreous) is very bright; fluid on a T1-weighted scan is usually dark. Fat is bright on T1-weighted scans, but darker on T2-weighted images. On the other hand, both cortical bone and air are very dark on all imaging sequences. Brain tissue has intermediate intensity; vessels can have almost any signal, depending on the velocity of flowing blood.

The most commonly used clinically approved contrast agent for MR imaging is gadopentetate-dimeglumine or Gd-DTPA, which is very well tolerated and generally safe, although caution must be used in patients with renal impairment because of the associated risk of developing nephrogenic systemic sclerosis (refer to Chapter 1). Its major use in the CNS is to improve lesion detectability by "lighting up" pathologic conditions that either lack a BBB or have a disrupted BBB.

Conventional MR imaging depicts excellent soft-tissue contrast. Traditionally, long image acquisition times, image artifacts related to patient motion, and the increased cost of scanning due to limited patient throughput have hampered the clinical utility of MR imaging. Over the past 15 years, technical advances in gradient technology, coil design, image reconstruction algorithms, contrast adminis-tration protocols, and data acquisition strategies have accelerated the development and implementation of fast imaging methods. These techniques, including fast gradient echo imaging, fast spin echo imaging, FLAIR (fluid-attenuated inversion recovery), and echo planar imaging, have enabled substantial reductions in imaging time. Images may be acquired during a single breath-hold on a clinical scanner, eliminating respiratory and motion artifacts. Vessel conspicuity can be enhanced by application of fat-suppression sequences, which eliminate unwanted signal from background tissues. These improvements have led to a vast range of applications that were previously impractical, including high-resolution MRA, DW and PW MR imaging, MRS, fMRI, and real-time monitoring of interventional procedures.

Since its first clinical application nearly 15 years ago, MRA has proven to be a useful tool for evaluation of the cervical or intracranial carotid vasculature. MRA represents a class of techniques that utilize the MR scanner to noninvasively generate three-dimensional images of the carotid or vertebral-basilar circulations. Although a detailed discussion of these techniques is beyond the scope of this chapter, several comments are noteworthy. These methods permit distinction between blood flow and adjacent soft tissue, with or without administration of intravenous contrast. As noted earlier, revolutionary developments have permitted MRA images to be rapidly acquired with ever-improving temporal and spatial resolution.

Presently, MRA serves as one of the first-line studies for evaluation of arterial occlusive disease and for screening of intracranial aneurysms. These methods have largely replaced conventional arteriographic studies for evaluation of atherosclerotic disease, except in cases of critical stenosis (>70%). In these instances, the degree of luminal narrowing may be overestimated by MRA and may require verification with CTA, catheter-based study, or Doppler ultrasound. Moreover, aneurysms detected on an intracranial MRA typically require a catheter-based study for detailing aneurysm size and orientation, for establishing the location of adjacent vessels and collateral flow, and for confirming suspicious vascular dilatation, as well as for detecting the presence of vasospasm or additional aneurysms that may not be readily apparent on the MRA study. In an increasing number of cases, catheter-based studies will additionally be performed for coil embolization (obliteration) of detected aneurysms, rather than surgical clipping.

Molecular diffusion, the random translational movement of water and other small molecules in tissue, is thermally driven and is referred to as Brownian motion. Over a given time period, these random motions, expressed as molecular displacements, can be detected using specifically designed diffusion-sensitive MR sequences. A common application of diffusion imaging is the detection of early ischemic infarction, where the infarcted tissue "lights up"

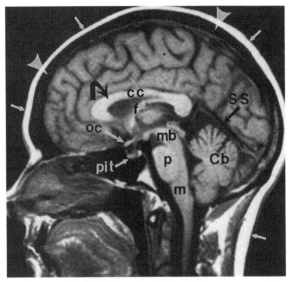

A

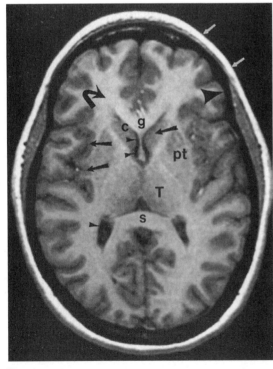

B

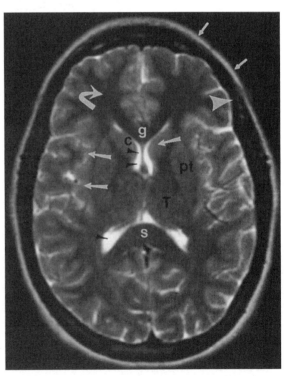

C

▲ **Figure 12-4.** Normal head MR images. Sagittal T1-weighted (**A**), axial T1-weighted (**B**), and axial T2-weighted (**C**) images. Note differences in signal between gray matter (large arrows), white matter (curved arrows), CSF (small arrowheads), fat (small arrows), and cortical bone (large arrowheads) on different pulse sequences. Normal structures include the genu (g) and splenium (s) of the corpus callosum (cc), fornix (f), optic chiasm (oc), pituitary gland (pit), midbrain (mb), pons (p), medulla (m), cerebellar vermis (Cb), straight sinus (SS), caudate head (c), putamen (pt), and thalamus (T).

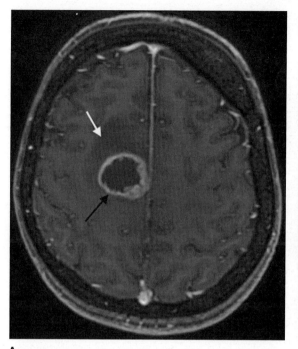 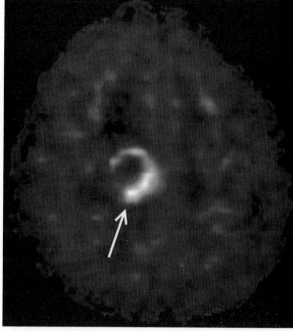

A   B

▲ **Figure 12-5.** MR images of a newly diagnosed high-grade glioma. **(A)** Axial postcontrast T1 image shows a periph-erally enhancing, centrally necrotic mass in the right frontal lobe (black arrow) as well as surrounding hypointense T1 signal consistent with vasogenic edema (white arrow). **(B)** Cerebral blood flow image (pulsed arterial spin labeling technique) shows increased perfusion (arrow) along the peripheral aspect of the mass.

because of a "restricted diffusion" state within the intracellu-lar compartment. Other applications of diffusion-sensitive sequences include differentiating cysts from solid tumors, as well as evaluating inflammatory/infectious conditions (en-cephalitis, abscess) or white matter abnormalities (hypertensive encephalopathy).

Perfusion MR imaging measures cerebral blood flow at the capillary level of an organ or tissue region. Perfusion-weighted MR imaging has applications in the evaluation of a number of disease states, including cerebral ischemia and reperfusion, brain tumors (Figure 12-5), epilepsy, and blood flow deficits in Alzheimer's disease. In addition, the close spa-tial coupling between brain activity and CBF permits the ap-plication of perfusion MR techniques to imaging brain function. MR perfusion imaging is technically complex and requires advanced scanner and postprocessing software for image generation. Various methods can be employed includ-ing contrast bolus technique (analogous to CT perfusion) or arterial spin labeling (ASL). ASL uses a radiofrequency pulse to "label" protons flowing in the cervical arteries and that signal is subsequently imaged as those protons flow into the cerebrum. One of the major advantages of ASL is that it

requires no contrast administration, which is of great benefit in patients with renal impairment.

Functional MR imaging is an important brain mapping technique that uses fast imaging techniques to depict re-gional cortical blood flow changes in space and time during performance of a particular task (eg, flexion of the index fin-ger). The utilization of this technique to localize brain activ-ity is historically based on measurable increases in cerebral blood flow (and blood volume) with increased neural activ-ity, referred to as neurovascular coupling. The hemodynamic response to a stimulus is not instantaneous, but on the order of a few seconds. Consequently, fMRI techniques are consid-ered an indirect approach to imaging brain function, but provide excellent spatial resolution and can be precisely matched with anatomic structures. Changes in blood oxy-genation and perfusion can be imaged using fMRI tech-niques, which has become the most widely used modality for depicting regional brain activation in response to sensorimo-tor or cognitive tasks.

An important clinical application of fMRI is presurgical mapping, whereby eloquent brain cortex can be defined in relation to mass lesions (Figure 12-6). This allows for the

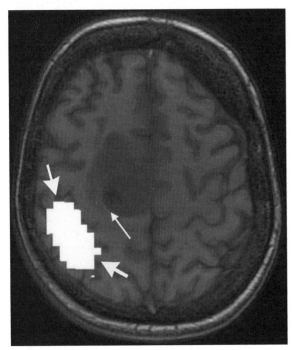

▲ Figure 12-6. Functional MR image for preoperative planning reveals left-hand motor activation (large arrows) adjacent to, but separate from the right frontal lobe mass and surrounding edema (small arrow).

judicious selection of an appropriate management strategy (surgical versus nonsurgical) according to the functional nature of the adjacent brain tissue. A second application involves determination of the cerebral hemisphere responsible for language and memory tasks in a patient with complex partial seizures, prior to undergoing temporal lobectomy. Additionally, several groups have reported successful functional activation studies for lateralizing language preoperatively utilizing fMRI.

MR spectroscopy (MRS) provides qualitative and quantitative information about brain metabolism and tissue composition. This functional analysis is based on detecting variations in the precession frequencies of spinning protons in a magnetic field. One factor influencing the precession or resonance frequency is the chemical environment of the individual proton. Protons in different cerebral metabolites can be sensitively discriminated on this basis, and the position of these metabolites can be displayed as a spectrum. The x-axis position of a given metabolite reflects the degree of "chemical shift" of the metabolite with respect to a designated reference metabolite and is expressed in units of parts per million (or ppm). The area under the peak is determined by the number of protons that contribute to the MR signal.

The major metabolites detected in the CNS are *N*-acetyl aspartate (NAA), a neuronal marker; choline, a marker for cellularity and cell membrane turnover; creatine, a marker for energy metabolism; and lactate, a marker for anaerobic metabolism. In addition to these metabolites, others have been assessed, including alanine, glutamine, myoinositol, and succinate, using various MR strategies. Presently, MRS is being used in clinical practice to provide functional information regarding many CNS abnormalities, and complements the conventional MR imaging study. A common application relates to the pre- and posttreatment evaluation of brain tumors, with MRS playing an important role in assessing for residual or recurrent tumor following surgical resection.

MR imaging offers a number of advantages over CT in the workup of patients with neurologic disease. Its soft-tissue contrast resolution is superior to that of CT, and lesions that may be subtle or invisible on CT are frequently obvious on MR imaging. MR imaging also allows acquisition of multiplanar views in the sagittal, axial, coronal, and oblique projections that may be impossible to obtain with CT. Furthermore, MR imaging gives information about blood flow without the need for a contrast agent, and bony streak artifacts that obscure lesions of the brainstem and cerebellum on CT scans are not present on MR images. Finally, MR imaging does not expose the patient to ionizing radiation.

▶ Cerebral Arteriography

Cerebral arteriography involves the injection of water-soluble contrast material into a carotid or vertebral artery. Contrast material is injected into the desired vessel via a small catheter, which has been introduced into the body through the femoral or brachial artery. Information about the arterial, capillary, or venous circulation of the brain is recorded on serial plain films or, most commonly, digitized for viewing on a monitor or for storage within a computer (Figure 12-7).

Cerebral arteriograms are expensive (two to three times as much as MR examinations) and are relatively more risky procedures than other noninvasive neuroradiologic studies. The major risk of the procedure is stroke, which may occur in one of every 1,000 patients. Stroke during cerebral arteriography occurs either from an embolic event (eg, inadvertent injection of air, thrombus formation on the catheter tip, atherosclerotic plaque dislodged by catheter manipulation) or from catheter-related local vessel trauma (eg, dissections or occlusions).

Although CT angiography has largely replaced catheter angiography for most routine diagnostic evaluations, catheter angiography is invaluable in the workup of vascular

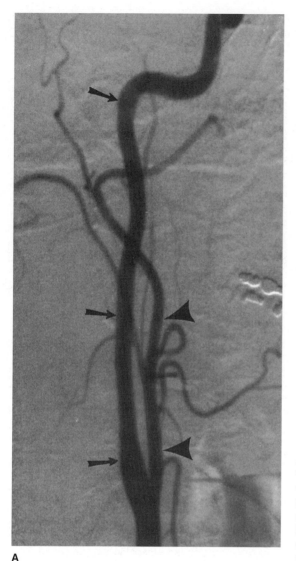

A

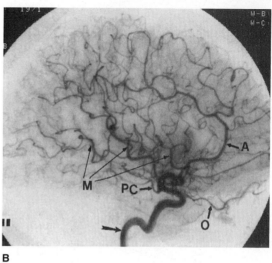

B

▲ **Figure 12-7.** Normal cerebral arteriogram. **(A)** Lateral view of the cervical carotid artery. Catheter is located within the common carotid artery, and contrast material fills internal (arrows) and external (arrowheads) carotid arteries. **(B)** Lateral view of the head after injection of the carotid artery (arrow). Note anterior cerebral (A), ophthalmic (O), posterior communicating (PC), and middle cerebral (M) branches.

diseases affecting the CNS. Specifically, it remains the gold standard for assessing vasculitis and is indispensable in evaluating and treating cerebral aneurysms and certain intracranial vascular malformations or fistulas. It is a useful adjunct to cross-sectional imaging (CTA, MRA, or US) to assess vascular stenosis as well as carotid or vertebral artery integrity after trauma to the neck, especially in the setting of acute neurological deficit. Finally, it is unsurpassed for showing vascular anatomy of the brain and is, therefore, useful as a preoperative road map.

The field of interventional neuroradiology continues to grow and exert considerable impact on the diagnosis and treatment of certain CNS diseases. New catheter designs and materials, recently developed endovascular devices (extracranial/intracranial stents), and an increasing number of trained specialists performing endovascular procedures have led to novel therapeutic applications and approaches for managing previously untreatable conditions. Endovascular diagnostic and therapeutic procedures, based on fundamental cerebral arteriography principles, have gained widespread

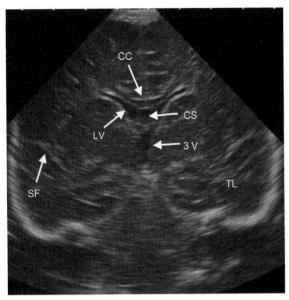
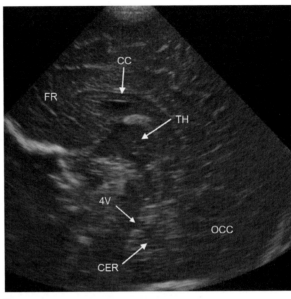

A   B

▲ **Figure 12-8.** Coronal (**A**) and sagittal (**B**) head ultrasound of a neonate. Normal structures include the corpus callosum (CC), lateral ventricle (LV), cavum septum pellucidum (CS), sylvian fissure (SF), third ventricle (3V), fourth ventricle (4V), temporal lobe (TL), frontal lobe (FR), occipital lobe (OCC), cerebellum (CER), and thalamus (TH).

acceptance and, in some cases, rival traditional neurosurgical approaches in terms of complication rates, clinical outcomes, and long-term survival benefit. Although a full discussion of these techniques is beyond the scope of this chapter, they include pharmacologic and mechanical thrombolysis of intracranial clot in the setting of acute infarction or dural sinus thrombosis; embolization (obliteration) of intracranial aneurysms using thrombosing material (ie, coils); carotid artery angioplasty and/or stent placement for critical stenotic narrowing or radiation-induced arterial stricture; preoperative or definitive devascularization of a hypervascular mass or arteriovenous malformation; embolization of small, bleeding external carotid artery branches in epistaxis; balloon occlusion tests of the carotid artery; and endovascular treatment of vasospasm. Embolization materials include particulate emboli, liquid adhesive glues, and various coils.

▶ Ultrasonography

Ultrasonography is the diagnostic application of ultrasound to the human body. Major applications of ultrasonography in CNS disease include gray-scale imaging and Doppler evaluation of carotid artery patency and flow in the setting of atherosclerosis, assessment of vasospasm in the setting of subarachnoid hemorrhage using transcranial Doppler, screening evaluation of intracranial abnormalities in the newborn and young infant (Figure 12-8), and detection of intracranial hemorrhage in premature infants prior to extracorporeal membrane oxygenation therapy. Ultrasound has also been used intraoperatively to demonstrate the spinal cord and surrounding structures during spine surgery and to define tumor and cyst margins during craniotomies.

Transcranial Doppler is a recently developed tool in the evaluation of cerebrovascular disorders. It uses low-frequency sound waves to adequately penetrate the skull and produces spectral waveforms of the major intracranial vessels for evaluation of flow velocity, direction, amplitude, and pulsatility. Present clinical applications include diagnosis of cerebral vasospasm, evaluation of stroke and transient ischemic attack, detection of intracranial emboli, serial monitoring of vasculitis in children with sickle cell disease, and assessment of intracranial pressure and cerebral blood flow changes in patients with head injury or mass lesions.

Ultrasound examinations, although moderately expensive, are virtually risk-free to the patient, involve no ionizing radiation, and are portable (ie, can be performed at the bedside). However, examination quality and therefore diagnostic accuracy are operator-dependent. Also, the heavy reliance of ultrasonography on the presence of an adequate "acoustic window" through which an examination can be performed diminishes its usefulness in examining the brain after the fontanelles close in infancy. Finally, to the untrained eye, anatomic structures and pathologic processes as depicted by US are not as readily apparent as they are on CT or MR images.

Single Photon Emission Computed Tomography

SPECT uses a rotating gamma camera to reconstruct cross-sectional images of the distribution of a radioactive pharmaceutical that has been administered to a patient (usually intravenously). For brain imaging, radioactive iodine (^{123}I) or technetium (^{99m}Tc) is combined with a compound that rapidly crosses the BBB and localizes within brain tissue in proportion to regional blood flow. The rotating gamma camera detects gamma rays emitted by the radiopharmaceutical and produces cross-sectional images of the brain that are really a map of brain perfusion (Figure 12-9). SPECT imaging also gives indirect information about brain metabolism, because perfusion is usually highest to parts of the brain with high metabolic activity and lowest to areas with low metabolic demand. Normal SPECT examinations demonstrate activity concentrated primarily in areas of high perfusion/metabolism, such as the cortical and deep gray matter (Figure 12-9).

SPECT studies are moderately expensive (as much as or more than brain MR imaging), and, as expected, they provide limited anatomic information. SPECT also exposes patients to ionizing radiation. Because patients rarely have allergic reactions to the radiopharmaceuticals used, the examination is of low risk. Although SPECT provides critical information regarding regional cerebral perfusion, particularly in the setting of stroke, this information can be more readily obtained during CTA/CT perfusion or MR perfusion acquisitions. SPECT has also been used with varying degrees of success in the workup of patients with epilepsy or dementia.

Positron Emission Tomography

PET scans consist of computer-generated cross-sectional images of the distribution and local concentration of a radiopharmaceutical. This technique is very similar to SPECT imaging; however, there are differences in the type of camera and radiopharmaceuticals used. PET studies use radiopharmaceuticals labeled with a cyclotron-produced positron emitter, which are very expensive to produce and have a very short half-life (on the order of seconds to minutes). The most widely used radiotracer is ^{18}F-deoxyglucose. PET scanning with this agent gives a measurement of brain glucose metabolism. Areas of high metabolic activity (ie, cerebral cortex, deep gray nuclei) demonstrate greater radiopharmaceutical uptake than do areas of low metabolic activity, such as white matter or cerebrospinal fluid (Figure 12-10). The bones of the skull and scalp soft tissues are, for the most part, invisible. Other agents are useful in assessing regional cerebral blood flow, neuroreceptor function, and the like.

Since the previous edition, PET scans have become much more widely available, although they remain expensive. The expense, in large part, is related to the cost of imaging equipment and in the production or delivery of radiopharmaceuticals. Although patients undergoing PET examinations are exposed to ionizing radiation, the overall risk to the patient is low. Anatomic resolution, although not as good as with CT or MR imaging, is better than with SPECT imaging. The major advantage of PET imaging is that it is extremely versatile, providing in vivo information about brain perfusion, glucose metabolism, receptor density and, ultimately, brain function.

PET provides useful information in the setting of stroke, epilepsy, dementia, and tumors. At present, the two main indications are in the workup of patients with complex partial seizures and in identifying tumor recurrence in patients who have undergone surgery, radiation therapy, or both, for brain tumors.

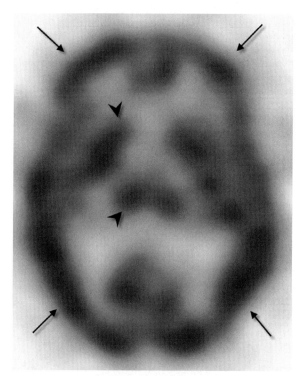

▲ **Figure 12-9.** Axial SPECT image of normal cerebral perfusion. Note that perfusion is greatest to gray matter structures, including the cerebral cortex (arrows) and deep gray nuclei (arrowheads). White matter and ventricles are nearly invisible because of low or no perfusion.

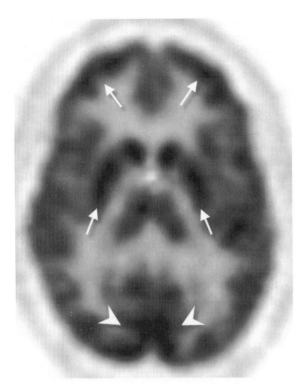

▲ **Figure 12-10.** Normal axial image of brain PET scan. As in the SPECT study (Figure 12-10), areas of high activity correspond to metabolically active gray matter (arrows), especially the visual cortex (arrowheads).

TECHNIQUE SELECTION

The primary goal of a radiologic examination is to provide useful information for disease management. Radiologic studies can provide a diagnosis or can give information about disease extent or response to treatment. In the present medical climate, it has also become imperative that radiologic workups be performed efficiently and in a cost-effective manner. This requirement presents a problem for clinicians trying to decide which test to order in a given clinical situation.

The major strengths and weaknesses of neuroradiologic examinations have been discussed earlier in this chapter. The following brief discussion concerns the appropriate ordering of examinations in clinical situations. Several points should be emphasized. First, although a recommended modality may clearly be superior to another in evaluating a particular neurologic condition, the choice of examination is not always obvious before the diagnosis is established. For example, in patients with nonfocal headache, MR scans are more sensitive than CT scans for detecting most intracranial abnormalities. However, if the headache is produced by subarachnoid

hemorrhage, CT would be a much better examination than MR imaging, because subarachnoid hemorrhage is nearly invisible on MR images. Choice of examinations may also be limited by what is locally available. If MR imaging is unavailable, or if the MR scanner is of poor quality or the interpreting radiologist is inadequately trained in MR image interpretation, then CT would be an excellent examination for evaluating most neurologic disorders.

Next, it is important to realize that the least expensive examination is not always the best first choice, even in this cost-conscious age. For example, most suspected skull fractures should be evaluated with CT scanning and not with plain films, despite the significant cost differential, because what is really important in management decisions is not the fracture itself but the potential underlying brain injury. Some neurologic diseases require multiple radiologic studies for accurate evaluation. Complex partial seizures refractory to medical management frequently require multiple examinations to localize the seizure focus prior to temporal lobectomy. Such a workup normally includes MR imaging and ictal/interictal SPECT and/or PET scanning of the brain, as well as a cerebral arteriogram to identify cerebral dominance.

Finally, certain examinations are contraindicated in certain patients, and an alternative test must suffice. Patients with ferromagnetic cerebral aneurysm clips or pacemakers should not undergo MR imaging. Patients with a strong history of allergic reaction to iodinated contrast media should not routinely undergo contrast-enhanced CT scanning, unless they are pretreated with anti-inflammatory agents (ie, steroids). MR scanning is frequently unsuccessful in claustrophobic or uncooperative patients unless they are sedated.

▶ Congenital Anomalies

Congenital anomalies of the brain are best evaluated by MR imaging. MR imaging is the best examination for demonstrating intracranial anatomy. It provides excellent discrimination between gray matter and white matter, superb views of the posterior fossa and craniocervical junction, and, most importantly, the ability to view the brain in any plane. MR imaging has, for all practical purposes, completely replaced CT for this indication. The one exception is in evaluation of osseous structures including various craniofacial anomalies and in suspected premature fusion of the cranial sutures.

▶ Craniocerebral Trauma

CT is the preferred modality for studying practically all acute head injuries. Examination times are short, intracranial hemorrhage is well demonstrated, and skull fractures are readily apparent. Unstable patients can also be easily monitored. Intravenous administration of contrast agents is unnecessary in the usual trauma setting. CTA and occasionally MRA are utilized with increasing frequency to assess for vascular injury associated with blunt or penetrating trauma. CTA is typically the first-line evaluation for dissection or laceration, particularly when a displaced fracture crosses a vascular foramen or in the case of penetrating vessel injury. Occasionally, cerebral arteriography is performed to look for carotid or vertebral artery injury, particularly when CTA or MRA are inconclusive or when there is an anticipated endovascular treatment of the injured vessel.

Although MR imaging is not routinely performed in the acute trauma setting, it may sometimes be helpful in patients with neurologic deficits unexplained by a head CT examination. For example, traumatic brainstem hemorrhages are often difficult to see on CT scans but are usually quite obvious on MR images. MR imaging is also useful in demonstrating tiny shear lesions within the brain in diffuse axonal injury and in assessing the brain in remote head trauma.

▶ Intracranial Hemorrhage

The best examination to perform in most cases of suspected acute intracranial hemorrhage is a head CT scan. CT scans can be obtained quickly, allowing rapid initiation of treatment, and they are very good at demonstrating all types of intracranial hemorrhage, including subarachnoid blood. Because most nontraumatic subarachnoid hemorrhage (SAH) is secondary to a ruptured cerebral aneurysm, CTA is now performed routinely following a conventional head CT demonstrating SAH. In most cases, the CTA is adequate for aneurysm detection and characterization prior to surgical or endovascular treatment. MR imaging takes much longer to perform in a potentially unstable patient, and subarachnoid hemorrhage may be difficult to see. However, MR imaging is more useful in the subacute or chronic setting, especially because it gives information about when a hemorrhagic event occurred. This information might be useful in such settings as nonaccidental head trauma (eg, child abuse). MR imaging is also very sensitive to petechial hemorrhage that frequently accompanies a cerebral infarction and could potentially help to identify an underlying cause for an intracranial hemorrhage (eg, tumor, arteriovenous malformation, occluded dural sinus). Cerebral arteriography is generally reserved when the etiology of hemorrhage is not discernable by CTA/MRA, when it is necessary to evaluate the flow dynamics of a vascular lesion or for planning endovascular treatment.

▶ Aneurysms

Although cerebral arteriography has traditionally been considered the "gold standard" for cerebral aneurysm evaluation, CTA has supplanted catheter arteriography as the first-line imaging modality for aneurysm detection. The current literature varies slightly; however, CTA is reported to have excellent sensitivity (greater than 95% for aneurysms measuring

4 mm or larger) as well as high specificity. In most cases, CTA is adequate for surgical or endovascular treatment planning. If CTA fails to identify a suspected aneurysm following SAH, cerebral arteriography will typically be performed. Cerebral arteriography not only allows aneurysm identification, but also provides other critical preoperative information such as aneurysm orientation, presence of vasospasm, location of adjacent vessels, and collateral intracranial circulation. Arteriography also helps to determine which aneurysm has bled when more than one aneurysm is present. As mentioned previously, interventional neuroradiologists can treat aneurysms, usually in nonsurgical patients, by placing thrombosing material (ie, coils) within the aneurysm itself via an endovascular approach.

Although most patients with symptomatic cerebral aneurysms present with subarachnoid hemorrhage, some aneurysms act like intracranial masses. These situations usually warrant evaluation by MR imaging as a first examination. The same is sometimes true with posterior communicating artery aneurysms (which can produce symptoms related to the adjacent third cranial nerve) or with aneurysms arising from the internal carotid artery as it courses through the cavernous sinus (which can affect any of the cranial nerves that lie within this structure, including cranial nerves III, IV, V, or VI).

▶ Vascular Malformations

Patients with a vascular malformation (eg, arteriovenous malformation, cavernous angioma, venous angioma, or capillary telangiectasia) often seek medical attention after an intracranial hemorrhage or a seizure. In this setting, the first test that should be performed is either a CT examination (to look for intracranial hemorrhage) or MR imaging. Although an intracranial hemorrhage is usually very obvious on a CT scan, the vascular malformation itself may be difficult, if not impossible, to see unless intravenous contrast material is administered. MR imaging, on the other hand, is quite sensitive for detecting vascular malformations, whether they have bled or not. The choice of the initial examination for evaluation of a vascular malformation can be difficult. Usually, patients undergo noncontrast head CT scanning to look for intracranial hemorrhage when they come to the emergency department. This is usually followed by CTA, particularly if an arteriovenous malformation (AVM) is suspected. Otherwise, the head CT is followed by gadolinium-enhanced MR imaging to further characterize the CT findings. If a true high-flow arteriovenous malformation is suspected, either clinically or from a cross-sectional imaging study, then cerebral arteriography is performed. In contrast to cerebral aneurysms, catheter angiography is still performed routinely to evaluate AVMs. This is done because catheter angiography provides details of flow dynamics within the AVM and demonstrates certain anatomic features that are necessary to elucidate prior to initiation of treatment. As spatial resolution and dynamic sequences improve, CT or MR angiography may someday replace conventional arteriography in the workup of these lesions, as with aneurysms.

▶ Infarction

Today, most patients with suspected cerebral infarction undergo CT scanning in the acute setting, even though infarctions are demonstrated earlier and are more obvious on MR imaging. So why is CT usually performed first? The answer is that clinicians who manage stroke patients are not so interested in seeing the infarct itself. Infarct location is usually suspected from the physical examination, and acute infarcts may not even be visible on CT scans for 12 to 24 hours after onset of stroke symptoms. Clinicians are very interested, though, to know if a stroke is secondary to something besides an infarct (eg, intracranial hemorrhage, brain tumor), or if an infarct is hemorrhagic, because thrombolytic agents would be contraindicated in this setting. CT can quickly answer both of these questions. MR imaging, specifically diffusion-weighted imaging, can sensitively detect acute infarctions and is typically ordered in cases of high clinical suspicion, when the initial CT study is nondiagnostic or when brainstem or posterior fossa infarcts are suspected.

The underlying cause of most cerebral infarctions is thromboembolism related to atherosclerosis. A CT/CTA or MR/MRA (including DW and PW MR imaging) study may provide a positive imaging diagnosis of brain infarction, reveal the extent and location of vessel occlusion, demonstrate the volume and severity of ischemic tissue, and predict final infarct size and clinical prognosis. CT and MR perfusion can identify areas of completed infarct (ie, infarct core) and potentially salvageable surrounding brain parenchyma at risk of infarction (ie, ischemic penumbra). Ultrasonography and cerebral arteriography can also be performed in the setting of stroke or transient ischemic attack to identify vascular stenoses or occlusions; these examinations are usually reserved for patients who might be candidates for carotid endarterectomy. Functional examinations (SPECT and PET) have also been used in patients with strokelike symptoms to identify regions of the brain at risk for infarction. These studies are not widely available and therefore do not enter into the imaging algorithm for most stroke patients.

▶ Brain Tumors and Tumor-like Conditions

The best examination to order in the setting of suspected brain tumor is a contrast-enhanced MR scan. This is true for primary neoplasms as well as for metastatic disease. MR imaging is especially useful in identifying tumors of the pituitary region, brainstem, and posterior fossa, including the cerebellopontine angle.

Although MR imaging is the preferred examination for intracranial neoplasms, it is occasionally supplemented by a CT scan, which can give important pretreatment information not provided by MR images. For example, CT can demonstrate tumor calcification, occasionally a useful factor in differentiating between types of neoplasms. Also, CT is very useful in identifying bone destruction in skull-base lesions.

In most medical centers, MR imaging is performed to assess brain tumor response to treatment. Anatomic imaging is often supplemented with some type of physiologic imaging including MR perfusion, MR spectroscopy, and PET scanning. Perfusion MRI, MRS, and PET scanning can frequently differentiate recurrent tumor from postradiation tissue necrosis, which can mimic tumor on an MR or a CT scan. MR perfusion imaging also provides functional information regarding the vascular density (ie, neovascularity) of a tumor, which may help to predict tumor grade or help guide a potential biopsy site.

Today, cerebral arteriography is rarely performed for brain tumor evaluation except to map the blood supply of very vascular tumors (ie, juvenile angiofibromas, paragangliomas) preoperatively. Such lesions can also be embolized prior to surgery in order to minimize intraoperative blood loss by injecting various materials into feeding vessels to occlude them.

▶ Infection

Intracranial infections are best evaluated by contrast-enhanced MR imaging. Abscesses, cerebritis, subdural empyemas, and other infectious or inflammatory processes are all very well demonstrated. MR imaging is especially useful in assessing patients with acquired immunodeficiency syndrome (AIDS). Not only does it allow identification of secondary infections (eg, toxoplasmosis, cryptococcosis, progressive multifocal leukoencephalopathy), but it is also exquisitely sensitive to the white matter changes produced by the human immunodeficiency virus itself. CT scanning is less sensitive than MR imaging in the detection of intracranial infections and should be reserved for patients in whom MR imaging is contraindicated. Cerebral arteriography is only useful in one particular situation, suspected vasculitis. Involvement of brain arteries and arterioles in this condition requires arteriography for diagnostic confirmation.

▶ Inherited and Acquired Metabolic, White Matter, and Neurodegenerative Diseases

As with suspected intracranial infections, this large and diverse group of diseases is best evaluated with MR imaging, which sensitively detects white matter abnormalities. In fact, one of the very first clear indications for MR imaging was in the workup of suspected multiple sclerosis. Although brain abnormalities in these conditions may be quite obvious on MR imaging, there is one problem: many of these conditions appear very similar, and an exact diagnosis may not be possible.

In patients with dementia and suspected neurodegenerative disease, PET imaging is currently the procedure of choice for diagnostic evaluation.

▶ Seizure and Epilepsy

Seizure is a common clinical indication for imaging the brain, particularly in the emergency setting. CT is the best modality to screen for multiple underlying causes of seizure including hemorrhage, mass lesion, or vascular malformation. CT is also very useful to assess for secondary trauma that may occur during a seizure. MRI is often subsequently performed depending on various factors including the patient's age, clinical presentation, and type of seizure, or in the case of epilepsy. MRI is superior to CT in evaluating fine cerebral anatomy because of its excellent soft-tissue contrast and the absence of beam hardening artifact, as well as its multiplanar capability. Particular MR protocols are utilized to discriminate the hippocampal structures and to detect other epileptogenic foci, including various cortical malformations, neoplasms, and vascular malformations.

In the case of medically refractory epilepsy, patients may pursue surgery for more definitive treatment. During surgical planning, additional functional imaging performed includes ictal SPECT and interictal PET. These studies help confirm a suspected epileptogenic focus, which demonstrates increased activity during or immediately following a seizure (SPECT) versus decreased metabolic activity between seizures (PET). Cerebral arteriography is often performed prior to epilepsy surgery in order to establish cerebral dominance by intracarotid sodium amytal injection (Wada test). Following catheter injection of amytal into the internal carotid artery, function within the corresponding cerebral hemisphere is temporarily depressed, allowing for neurological testing of memory and language in the contralateral hemisphere.

EXERCISE 12-1. CONGENITAL ANOMALIES

12-1. In Case 12-1, what is the major abnormality (Figure 12-11 A, B)?
  A. Enlarged ventricles
  B. Cyst in the posterior fossa
  C. Lack of brain cleavage into two hemispheres
  D. Herniation of intracranial contents through a skull defect
  E. Abnormal migration of gray matter

12-2. In Case 12-2, what is the etiology of the patient's seizures (Figure 12-12 A, B)?
  A. Brain tumor
  B. Gray matter in the wrong place (ie, heterotopic gray matter)
  C. Congenital infection

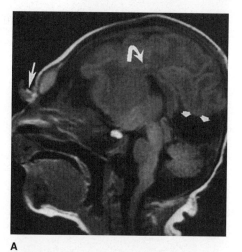

A

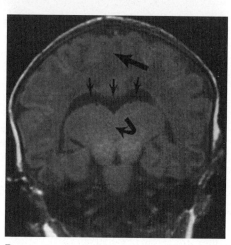

B

▲ **Figure 12-11.** Case 12-1. Sagittal (**A**) and coronal (**B**) T1-weighted MR imaging of the brain in a 2-day-old male infant who presents with multiple craniofacial deformities, including microcephaly and a fleshy mass on the bridge of the nose.

  D. Nodules along ventricles in a patient with tuberous sclerosis
  E. Infarction of periventricular white matter

Radiologic Findings

12-1. In this case, the corpus callosum (curved arrow) is absent on the sagittal T1 MR image (Figure 12-11 A). Also note other midline abnormalities, including abnormal tissue at the bridge of the nose (large arrow) and a posterior cyst (small arrows). Coronal T1-weighted MR image (Figure 12-11 B) demonstrates a

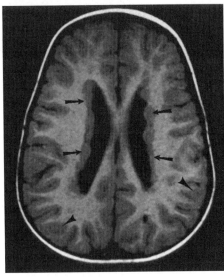 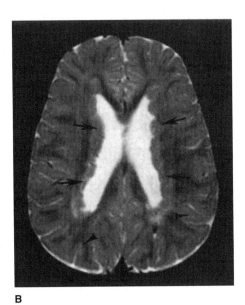

A   **B**

▲ **Figure 12-12. (A, B)** Case 12-2. Axial T1- and T2-weighted MR images in a 15-month-old female infant who presents with new onset of seizures.

monoventricle (small arrows) and thalamic fusion (curved arrow). Also note the lack of separation of the two hemispheres (large arrow) (C is the correct answer to Question 12-1).

12-2. In this case, T1-weighted (Figure 12-12 A) and T2-weighted (Figure 12-12 B) MR images show abnormal tissue lining the lateral ventricle (arrows). Signal of this tissue follows that of normal gray matter (arrowheads) on both T1- and T2-weighted images (B is the correct answer to Question 12-2).

Discussion

Two common reasons for performing MR scans in young infants are illustrated by the cases in this section. Infants with craniofacial anomalies frequently have underlying congenital malformations of the CNS. Seizures, too, may be the first sign of an underlying brain malformation. As discussed in the section on technique selection, whenever a congenital brain anomaly is suspected, MR imaging is the best examination to perform.

Insults to the developing brain lead to predictable alterations of brain morphology. By analyzing patterns of altered brain morphology, we can often determine which stage of CNS development has been disrupted. This analysis, combined with knowledge of neuroembryology, has allowed for the development of systems to classify congenital anomalies of the CNS. One simplified classification system divides congenital malformations into disorders of organogenesis (which include abnormalities of neural tube closure,

diverticulation/cleavage, sulcation/cellular migration, and size, as well as destructive lesions acquired in utero), disorders of histogenesis (ie, neurocutaneous syndromes), and disorders of cytogenesis (ie, congenital neoplasms). Readers are referred to the suggested readings at the end of this chapter for further information on this topic.

The patient in Case 12-1 has alobar holoprosencephaly, a classic example of disordered ventral induction. In this condition, there is complete (alobar) or partial (semilobar, lobar) failure of separation of the forebrain (prosencephalon) into two hemispheres. In alobar holoprosencephaly, the most severe form of this disorder, there is no separation of the two hemispheres at all. The thalami are fused, a central monoventricle is present, and there is no corpus callosum. Infants with this form of holoprosencephaly frequently have severe facial anomalies.

In Case 12-2, the patient has heterotopic gray matter lining the lateral ventricles. This congenital anomaly is one type of disordered cellular migration. Neurons that make up the gray matter of the cerebral cortex actually develop along the edges of the lateral and third ventricles within the so-called germinal matrix zone. They then migrate outward to their final cortical location. If this normal neuronal migration is disrupted, a normal cortex may not develop, and foci of gray matter may be present in abnormal locations along the migration route. Collections of these normal neurons in abnormal locations are called gray matter heterotopias.

Several different types of heterotopias have been described. The case presented in this section demonstrates a focal nodular gray matter heterotopia involving the subependymal region

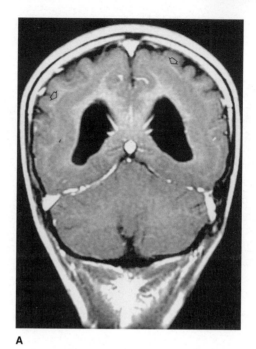

A

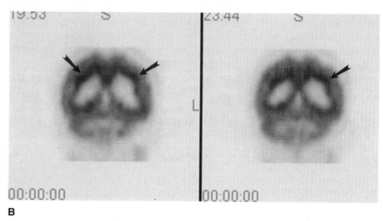

B

▲ **Figure 12-13.** (**A**) Postcontrast coronal T1-weighted images of the brain in a 32-year-old with intractable seizures. An additional circumferential band of gray matter is seen (arrows) deep to the normal gray matter within the occipital region. This finding was noted to be diffusely present throughout the remaining brain parenchyma (not shown). (**B**) The corresponding PET image in the same patient reveals increased activity of the band heterotopia relative to the adjacent normal cortex (arrows), of unclear significance.

at the edge of the lateral ventricles. Seizures frequently occur in patients with this condition, as in the patient in Case 12-2. Because MR imaging usually provides an exact diagnosis of this condition, biopsies of CNS tissue are unnecessary.

In contrast to focal nodular heterotopias, diffuse (or laminar) heterotopias are commonly seen within or adjacent to the cortex, while "band" type heterotopias are located deep to the normal cortex, in a subcortical location, separated by a thin interface of white matter (Figure 12-13). Band-type heterotopias are well defined, with smooth margins, demonstrating signal intensities identical to those of normal gray matter. Mass effect on the underlying white

matter or deep gray structures may be seen, and the sulcation pattern of the brain superficial to the heterotopia may be abnormal. Associated CNS anomalies may be present, such as agenesis of the corpus callosum, holoprosencephaly, or herniation of brain tissue (encephaloceles). Although at first glance the cortex may appear to be markedly thickened, closer examination will reveal an additional band of gray matter in a subcortical location, which may or may not demonstrate increased ^{18}F-FDG activity on a PET scan. This band of heterotopia is known to be associated with intractable seizures, occurring earlier than in the focal type, as well as severe developmental delay.

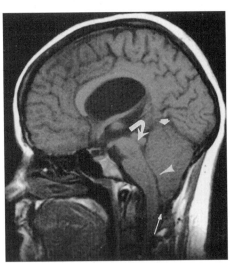
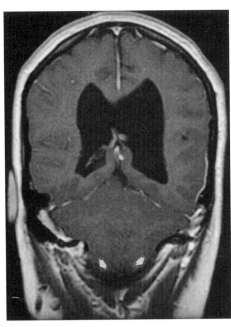

A   **B**

▲ **Figure 12-14.** Uninfused sagittal T1-weighted (**A**) and coronal T1 postcontrast (**B**) imaging in a 30-year-old patient with a Chiari II malformation. (**A**) A small posterior fossa is present, resulting in cerebellar tonsillar ectopia (long arrow), towering of the cerebellum (short arrow), beaking of the tectum (curved arrow), and compression of the fourth ventricle (arrowhead) with resulting hydrocephalus. Partial agenesis of the rostrum and splenium of the corpus callosum is noted. (**B**) Cerebellar tonsillar ectopia into the foramen magnum is demonstrated (arrowheads).

Several types of Chiari malformations were initially described by the German pathologist Hans Chiari, who classified these congenital hindbrain anomalies into three types. In each case, abnormal descent of cerebellar tissue into the cervical canal is demonstrated. A Chiari I malformation is associated with a relatively small posterior fossa and a normal-sized cerebellum. Consequently, elongated peglike cerebellar tonsils extend below the foramen magnum with effacement of the corresponding CSF spaces. There is often dorsal tilting of the dens, which may indent the brainstem. There is no association between Chiari I malformations and neural tube defects; however, the spine should be imaged because of the common coexistence of a syrinx.

In contrast to Chiari I, the Chiari II malformation is very highly associated with myelomeningocele and generally supratentorial abnormalities. The posterior fossa is small with herniation of cerebellar tonsils, vermis, and medulla below the foramen magnum. Because the cervical cord is somewhat fixed in position by the dentate ligaments, this downward displacement results in a characteristic cervicomedullary kink. The fourth ventricle is low-lying and elongated as well, with distortion of the cerebral aqueduct and tectum (so-called tectal beaking), often resulting in hydrocephalus. The superior cerebellum towers superiorly through a widened tentorium incisura, with the remainder of the cerebellum wrapping around the brainstem. Supratentorial abnormalities include agenesis or hypoplasia of the corpus callosum, enlarged massa intermedia, deficiency of the falx resulting in interdigitation of cortical gyri across the midline, and enlarged occipital horns (colpocephaly) (Figure 12-14). Chiari III malformations are associated with occipital or high cervical encephaloceles, containing cerebellar tissue, with or without brainstem.

Disorders of histogenesis include the neurocutaneous syndromes, which are a heterogeneous group of disorders with CNS and, for the most part, cutaneous manifestations. Visceral and connective tissue abnormalities may be prominent. Common disorders within this group include neurofibromatosis types I and II, tuberous sclerosis, von Hippel-Lindau disease, and Sturge-Weber syndrome, where the abnormal lesions corresponding to these entities are neurogenic tumors, tubers, hemangioblastomas, and angiomas, respectively.

Neurofibromatosis type 1 is the most common of all the neurocutaneous syndromes, accounting for 90% of all neurofibromatosis cases, and is the only entity discussed here. It is transmitted on the long arm of chromosome 17 and is a disease of childhood. Autosomal dominant transmission occurs in 50%, and the remainder appear sporadically as new mutations in a patient with no known family history of the disease. The diagnosis is established when two or more of the following criteria are present: (1) six or more café-au-lait spots (brown skin pigmentation), (2) two or more Lisch nodules (hamartomas) of the iris, (3) two or more neurofibromas, (4) one or more plexiform neurofibromas, (5) axillary freckling, (6) one or more bone dysplasias (ie, dysplasia of the greater sphenoid wing), (7) optic nerve glioma, or (8) first-degree relative with neurofibromatosis type 1.

The optic pathway gliomas are generally nonaggressive (low-grade) pilocytic astrocytomas, which present in childhood and may not affect vision until greatly increased in size (Figure 12-15 A). Cerebellar, brainstem, and cerebral astrocytomas may additionally be seen. High T2 signal intensity foci may be identified within the peduncles or deep gray matter of the cerebellum, brainstem, basal ganglia (particularly the globus pallidus), and supratentorial white matter (Figure 12-15 B). The nature of these lesions remains unresolved.

EXERCISE 12-2. STROKE

12-3.   In Case 12-3, what is the most likely diagnosis (Figure 12-16 A,B)?
A. Intracranial abscess
B. Arachnoid cyst
C. Metastatic brain tumor
D. Primary brain tumor
E. Cerebral infarction

12-4.   In Case 12-4, what is the likely cause of the patient's problem (Figure 12-17 A,B)?
A. Brainstem infarction
B. Brainstem compression from cerebellar infarction
C. Brainstem tumor
D. Cerebellar astrocytoma
E. Posterior fossa hemorrhage

12-5.   In Case 12-5, what is the most likely diagnosis (Figure 12-18)?
A. Thalamic glioma
B. Subarachnoid hemorrhage
C. Metastatic disease
D. Hypertensive hemorrhage in the basal ganglia
E. Cerebral contusion

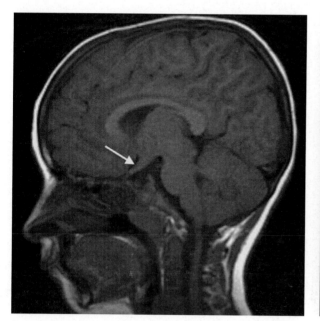

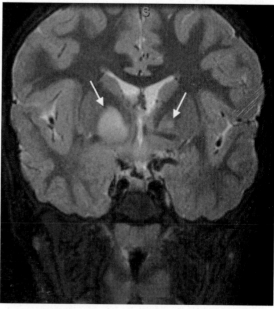

A   B

▲ **Figure 12-15.** Noncontrast parasagittal T1-weighted (**A**) and coronal T2-weighted (**B**) images in a 4-year-old male with neurofibromatosis. (**A**) Bulbous enlargement of the optic chiasm is present (arrow), suggesting an optic glioma. (**B**) Foci of increased T2 signal abnormality are demonstrated within the globus palladi (arrows).

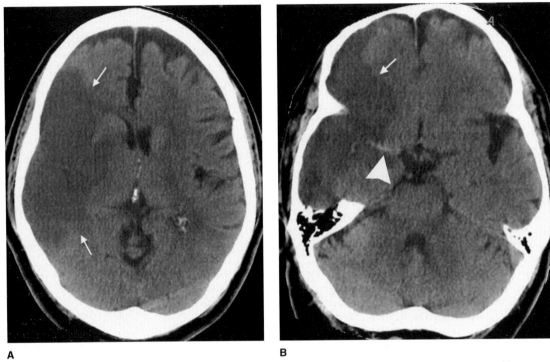

▲ **Figure 12-16.** **(A,B)** Case 12-3. Axial noncontrast head CT images in a 56-year-old male with history of hypertension and diabetes who presents to the emergency department with left hemiparesis.

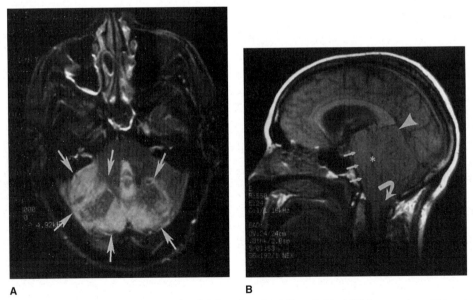

▲ **Figure 12-17.** **(A,B)** Case 12-4. Axial T2-weighted **(A)** and sagittal T1-weighted **(B)** images in a 66-year-old woman who presents with gradual onset of nausea, dizziness, and ataxia. The patient became comatose 24 hours after the onset of symptoms.

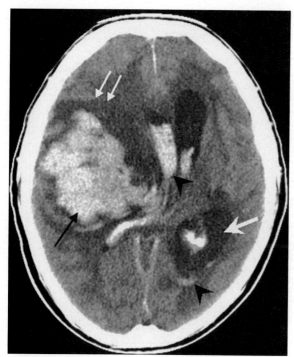

▲ **Figure 12-18.** Case 12-5. A single axial image from a noncontrast head CT in a 68-year-old female patient uncontrolled hypertension who was found unresponsive.

Radiologic Findings

12-3. In this case, the axial CT image (Figure 12-16 A) demonstrates a well-defined area of hypodensity (white arrows) in the right middle cerebral artery (MCA) territory. There is secondary mass effect on the surrounding brain parenchyma with effacement of the cortical sulci. In a more inferior axial image (Figure 12-16 B), note the bright right MCA (arrowhead) corresponding to an acute thrombus in the main trunk of this vessel (E is the correct answer to Question 12-3).

12-4. In this case, the axial T2-weighted MR image (Figure 12-17 A) shows areas of increased T2 signal (arrows) corresponding to edema within the cerebellum. A sagittal T1-weighted image (Figure 12-17 B) shows a swollen cerebellum, as well as upward transtentorial (arrowhead) and downward tonsillar (curved arrow) herniation of cerebellar tissue. Also note compression of the brainstem (small arrows) and fourth ventricle (asterisk). These changes are compatible with a recent cerebellar infarction with brainstem compression caused by the swollen cerebellum (B is the correct answer to Question 12-4).

12-5. In this case, an axial CT scan (Figure 12-18) demonstrates a large, hyperdense intraparenchymal hemorrhage centered in the right basal ganglia (black arrow) with surrounding edema and mass effect (double white arrows). Intraventricular extension of hemorrhage is present (black arrowheads) with entrapment of the left lateral ventricle secondary to midline shift (single white arrow). This is most likely secondary to the patient's known hypertension (D is the correct answer to Question 12-5).

Discussion

Stroke is a lay term for neurologic dysfunction. The usual image of a stroke patient is that of an elderly individual with hemiparesis, often associated with abnormal speech. There are actually many different causes of stroke. These include cerebral infarction, intracerebral hemorrhage, subarachnoid hemorrhage, and miscellaneous causes such as dural sinus occlusion with associated venous infarction. Although these conditions may have similar clinical presentations, they have different treatments and prognoses.

The vast majority of strokes are cerebral infarctions associated with atherosclerosis. The radiologic manifestations of cerebral infarction vary with time. The head CT scan of the patient in Case 12-3 was obtained several days after the onset of symptoms and shows typical findings of a subacute infarct in a major vascular territory, in this case, the right middle cerebral artery region. By this time, the infarct is a very well-defined area of low attenuation compared to normal surrounding brain. There is associated mass effect from the edematous tissue. Acute infarcts (less than 24 hours since onset of symptoms) may be difficult to identify on head CT scans, if at all. However, diffusion-weighted MR imaging often demonstrates brain abnormalities within hours of symptom onset. Subtle changes on head CT scans in acute infarction can sometimes be seen, but may be overlooked if the examination is not closely scrutinized. Sometimes the only apparent change on CT scans is a subtle loss of gray matter/white matter differentiation in the area of infarction. CT scanning is performed in acute cerebral infarction because scans can be quickly obtained, and CT is a very good test for identifying intracranial hemorrhage, an important finding for management considerations. Institutions that are involved in the early management of stroke often have a stroke imaging protocol whereby noncontrast CT is typically obtained along with CT angiography (Figure 12-19 A, B) as well as CT perfusion. If the infarct is not obvious on the initial CT scan, an MR scan is usually obtained to verify high clinical suspicion.

An acute or subacute infarction will exhibit a diffusion signal abnormality that reflects the restricted movement of water molecules and typically persists for 1 to 2 weeks within infarcted tissue (Figure 12-19 C). T2-weighted imaging

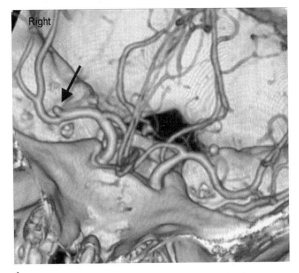

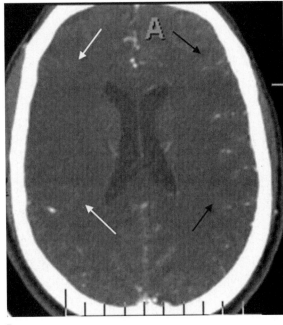

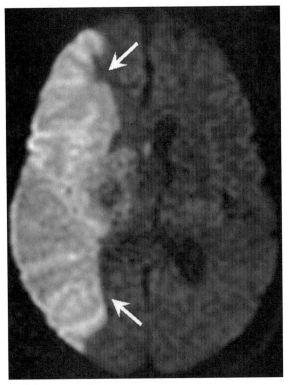

▲ **Figure 12-19.** CT angiographic images corresponding to Case 12-3. (**A**) 3-D vascular rendering demonstrating occluded right superior MCA branch (arrow) and (**B**) axial CT showing generalized poor intravascular contrast opacification of the right MCA territory (white arrows) relative to the left (black arrows). Subsequent diffusion-weighted (**C**) and

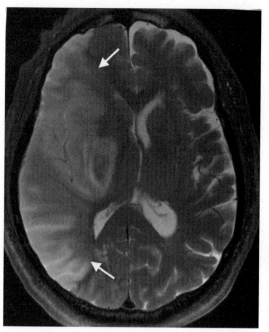

D

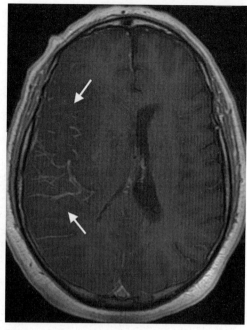

E

▲ **Figure 12-19.** *(Continued)* (**D**) axial T2 MR images demonstrate a large wedge-shaped region of increased signal (arrows) corresponding to right MCA infarct. Postcontrast axial T1-weighted (**E**) MR image reveals intravascular enhancement over the right cerebral cortex (arrows), reflecting slow flow of intravascular contrast.

demonstrates increased signal within the infarcted territory due to the presence of cytotoxic edema (Figure 12-19 D). Intravascular enhancement extending into the cortical sulci may be seen in the acute to early subacute phase of infarct, generally related to prolonged intravascular opacification from slow vascular flow (Figure 12-19 E). Within several days of a cerebral infarction, parenchymal enhancement is commonly identified along the cortex, which usually has a bandlike, tubular, or gyriform appearance and may persist for several weeks. Solid or ring-enhancing areas, as well as more amorphous-appearing patterns of enhancement, can occasionally occur.

Case 12-4 illustrates an important point to consider when deciding which test to order in the setting of acute stroke. In this case, the patient's symptoms were worrisome for a brainstem process. CT scanning of the brainstem and posterior fossa is frequently degraded by streak artifacts emanating from the dense bone of the skull base. Subtle (and sometimes not so subtle) abnormalities may not be apparent. Therefore, for most neurologic conditions that involve the brainstem or posterior fossa, MR scans are much better at depicting an abnormality. Notice that the patient in Case 12-4 did not in fact have a brainstem infarct, as was suspected clinically, but rather had brainstem compression from a large cerebellar infarct.

Case 12-5 illustrates how essential an imaging examination is in managing stroke as the patient initially had signs of

cerebral infarction. The CT scan demonstrated an obvious basal ganglia hemorrhage, probably secondary to the patient's hypertension. Management of these two conditions is considerably different. Hypertension is the main cause of nontraumatic intracranial hemorrhage. In adults, these hemorrhages typically occur in the putamen/external capsule. Other locations for hypertensive hemorrhage include the thalamus, pons, cerebellum, and, rarely, subcortical white matter. Acute parenchymal hematomas, as in this case, are usually hyperdense on CT scans. With time these lesions become darker and eventually appear as round or slitlike cavities. The MR imaging appearance of a parenchymal hematoma is complex and depends largely on the presence of hemoglobin breakdown products within the clot.

EXERCISE 12-3. BRAIN TUMORS

12-6. In Case 12-6, what is the most likely diagnosis (Figure 12-20 A-C)?
   A. Extra-axial brain tumor
   B. Intra-axial brain tumor
   C. Frontal contusion
   D. Subdural hematoma
   E. Encephalocele

12-7. In Case 12-7, what is the most likely cause of the patient's symptoms (Figure 12-21 A, B)?

    A. Multiple sclerosis

    B. Inner ear abnormality

    C. Intraventricular meningioma

    D. Hematoma

    E. Malignant brain tumor

12-8. In Case 12-8, what is the most likely explanation for the patient's mental status changes (Figure 12-22 A, B)?

    A. Metastatic disease

    B. Intracranial hemorrhage

    C. Small infarcts

    D. Sarcoidosis

    E. Arteriovenous malformation

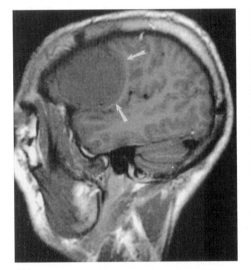

A

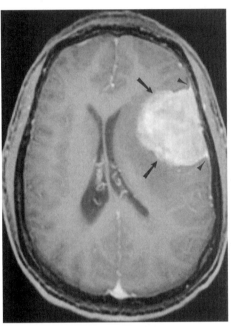

C

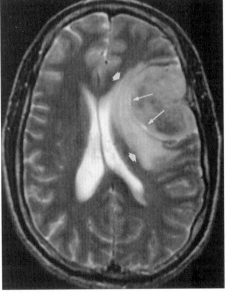

B

▲ **Figure 12-20.** Case 12-6. Noncontrast sagittal T1-weighted (**A**) and axial T2-weighted (**B**) images, as well as postcontrast axial T1-weighted image (**C**) in a 33-year-old Hispanic man who presents with a syncopal episode and involuntary tremors.

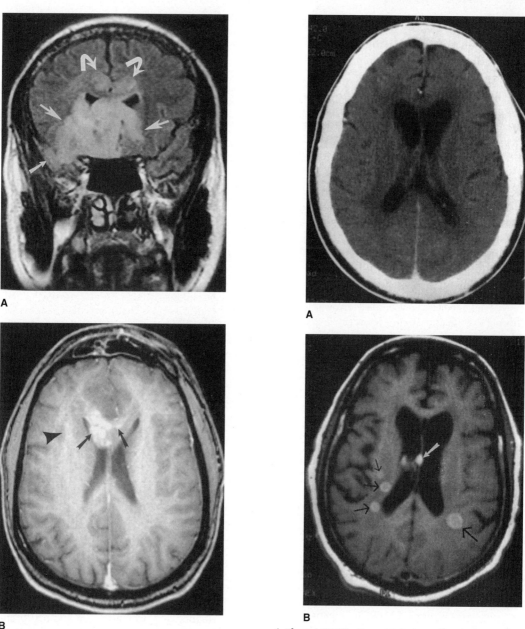

▲ **Figure 12-21.** **A,B.** Case 12-7. Initial coronal T2 FLAIR-weighted (**A**) and axial contrast-enhanced T1-weighted (**B**) images in a 48-year-old woman who presents with a history of headaches and seizures.

▲ **Figure 12-22.** Case 12-8. A contrast-enhanced axial CT scan (**A**) and a gadolinium-enhanced axial T1-weighted MR image (**B**) in a 58-year-old man who presents with a history of lung cancer and mental status changes.

Radiologic Findings

12-6. In this case, the sagittal T1-weighted image before contrast administration shows an extra-axial, left frontal convexity mass (Figure 12-20 A, arrows). This homogenous-appearing, smoothly marginated, mass (arrows) is isointense to the normal gray matter (Figure 12-20 A), and is sometimes difficult to differentiate from normal brain tissue on unenhanced T1 images. On T2-weighted imaging, the mass has a heterogeneous appearance, but is predominantly isointense to gray matter (Figure 12-20 B). The mass is circumscribed by a thin rim (pseudocapsule) of increased T2 signal (long arrows), as well as marginated by a more peripherally located band of T2 signal hyperintensity along its medial and posterior borders (short arrows). There is distortion of the adjacent brain parenchyma, with compression of the left lateral ventricle, and a mild shift of the midline structures to the right. Following intravenous GdDTPA administration, the mass enhances uniformly (arrows), and dural tails are identified (arrowheads), allowing easy identification (Figure 12-20 C). These features are fairly typical of a meningioma (A is the correct answer to Question 12-6).

12-7. In this case, a coronal T2 FLAIR-weighted MR image (Figure 12-21 A) demonstrates a large area of signal hyperintensity involving the inferior frontal regions (large white arrows) and right temporal lobe (small white arrow), with extension into the corpus callosum (curved arrows). On the infused axial view, at the level of the body of the corpus callosum (Figure 12-21 B), subtle, ill-defined enhancement is present within the right cerebral hemisphere (arrowhead) with patchy enhancement (arrows) extending into the body of the corpus callosum. This is one appearance of a malignant brain tumor, in this case, an anaplastic oligodendroglioma (E is the correct answer to Question 12-7).

12-8. In this case, a contrast-enhanced axial CT scan shows no definite abnormality (Figure 12-22 A). A gadolinium-enhanced axial T1-weighted MR image shows multiple enhancing lesions (arrows) within the brain parenchyma (Figure 12-22 B). In a patient with known lung cancer, metastatic disease is the most likely explanation for multiple intracranial enhancing lesions (A is the correct answer to Question 12-8).

Discussion

Brain tumors can be classified in a variety of ways. The traditional classification of intracranial neoplasms is based on histology. In this system, brain tumors are either primary (they arise from the brain and its linings) or secondary (they arise from somewhere outside the CNS, ie, metastases). Primary tumors, which account for approximately two-thirds of all brain neoplasms, can be subdivided into glial and nonglial tumors. Secondary tumors, especially from lung and breast cancer, account for the remaining one-third of brain neoplasms. Metastases are most commonly parenchymal, but can also involve the skull and meninges.

Brain tumors can also be classified according to patient age and general tumor location (ie, adult or child, supratentorial or infratentorial). Finally, brain tumors can be classified according to the specific anatomic region involved. For example, we can generate lists of brain tumors that specifically affect the pineal or the pituitary regions.

Case 12-6 illustrates a useful principle for interpreting studies of patients with suspected brain tumors. It is very important to first decide whether a mass is within the brain parenchyma (intra-axial) or outside the brain (extra-axial). Extra-axial masses usually turn out to be meningiomas, many of which can be removed surgically with a very low incidence of recurrence. Intra-axial masses frequently turn out to be astrocytomas, and the prognosis is less favorable.

The patient in Case 12-6 has an extra-axial, dural-based, frontal convexity mass that markedly enhances with Gd-DTPA. Meningiomas comprise 15% to 20% of intracranial tumors, predominantly occur in females, and exhibit a peak age incidence of 45 years. They are the most common nonglial primary CNS tumors. They can occur anywhere within the head but typically occur along the dural venous sinuses. The parasagittal region and cerebral convexities are the most common locations. Anterior basal or olfactory groove meningiomas account for 5% to 10% of intracranial meningiomas. Anosmia results from involvement of the olfactory tracts by the tumor. These expansile lesions are slow-growing, and the ensuing mass effect on the adjacent brain parenchyma is gradual. The absence of reactive edema in a subset of these lesions can be seen as a result of their slow growth. These masses usually demonstrate intense and uniform enhancement, independent of tumor size. A layer of thickened dural enhancement ("dural tail") is commonly seen extending away from the base of the meningioma. In many cases, this finding represents reactive thickening without tumor involvement.

Case 12-7 demonstrates a large, infiltrating (aggressive or high-grade) glioma involving the majority of the right frontotemporal lobe, with extension into the corpus callosum. Although there is some overlap of the MR imaging features characteristically seen with these invasive neoplasms and their less aggressive (lower-grade) counterparts, the imaging features of higher-grade neoplasms, on the whole, are distinctly different from those seen with lower-grade lesions. High-grade gliomas, namely anaplastic astrocytomas and oligodendrogliomas (as in this case), as well as glioblastoma multiforme (the most highly malignant glioma), demonstrate heterogeneous signal characteristics, generally a reflection of the variable cellularity, in addition

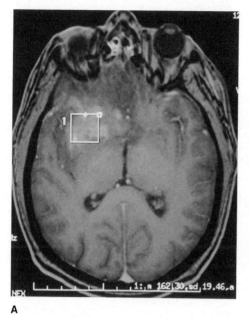
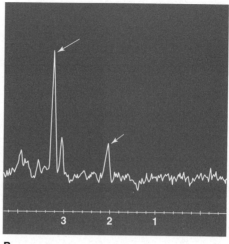

A

B

▲ **Figure 12-23.** The same patient as in Figure 12-21. (**A**) At a more inferior level, the patchy, heterogeneous enhancement of this mass within the right inferior frontal/temporal regions is better appreciated. A region-of-interest or volume element (ie, voxel) was centered within the enhancing tumor volume, and an MR spectrum was obtained. (**B**) MR spectrum. The NAA peak is abnormally decreased (short arrow at 2.0), and the choline signal is elevated (long arrow at 3.2), supporting the diagnosis of a malignant brain tumor.

to the presence of necrosis, hemorrhage, and cystic foci. Calcification and hemorrhage are more common in oligodendrogliomas, often accompanied by cyst formation and necrosis. The spectroscopic findings of decreased NAA and increased choline suggest decreased neuronal/axonal density and increased breakdown of cell membranes (Figure 12-23 A, B).

Oligodendrogliomas account for about 5% of primary gliomas, occurring most frequently within the frontal lobe and often involving the cortex. The majority of patients present with seizures. On the other hand, glioblastoma multiforme is the most common primary malignant brain neoplasm and occurs most frequently in patients over 50 years of age. Patients with glioblastoma multiforme present with neurologic deficits or new-onset seizures. The prognosis in these latter cases is dismal; postoperative survival averages 8 months.

On T2-weighted scans, these high-grade masses usually exhibit heterogeneous signal characteristics, with areas of high T2 signal attributable to tumor tissue, necrosis, cysts, and reactive edema, whereas regions of low signal may reflect hemorrhage or calcification. The corresponding tissue pathology of this region often shows tumor cells residing within and extending beyond the surrounding edema. Enhancement is highly variable within anaplastic oligoden-

drogliomas. Other types of malignant gliomas, such as glioblastoma multiforme, typically demonstrate intense enhancement. The corpus callosum is often involved by a high-grade glial tumor, which may grow medially from an adjacent hemispheric source or may arise independently within this structure. "Wings" may extend symmetrically or asymmetrically into both cerebral hemispheres, exhibiting a butterfly-type appearance (Figure 12-24), appropriately termed butterfly glioma. Perfusion studies on high-grade gliomas generally show increased blood flow and volume, reflecting the increased vascular density and permeability of these tumors. In contrast, low-grade gliomas may appear only as a region of amorphous signal abnormality (most obvious on T2-weighted images), often without associated enhancement or perfusion abnormality.

Case 12-8 illustrates a very important point to remember when working up patients with suspected metastatic disease to the brain: MR imaging is considerably more sensitive than CT in detecting metastases. This is not a trivial point, because surgical resection of single, not multiple, brain lesions is sometimes performed. Conversely, the successful application of radiotherapy protocols relies on sensitively and accurately detecting the entire metastatic tumor burden. Metastatic disease to the brain has a variety of

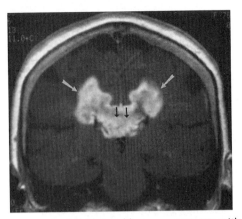

▲ **Figure 12-24.** A 76-year-old woman presents with a 6-month history of progressive gait ataxia and frequent falling. Coronal contrast-enhanced T1-weighted MR image of a glioblastoma multiforme is shown. An enhancing mass (white arrows) extends through the corpus callosum (black arrows) into both hemispheres.

manifestations, the most common being parenchymal involvement. Typical hematogenous brain metastases demonstrate solid or ringlike enhancement on CT or MR scans, occur near gray matter/white matter junctions, and are usually surrounded by a marked amount of edema. They most commonly metastasize from lung or breast primaries.

EXERCISE 12-4. INTRACRANIAL INFECTIONS

12-9. In Case 12-9, what is the most likely diagnosis (Figure 12-25 A, B)?
   A. Frontal contusion
   B. Aneurysm with intraventricular hemorrhage
   C. Parietal lobe abscess
   D. Intracranial lymphoma
   E. Cerebritis

12-10. In Case 12-10, the location of the abnormality is pathognomonic for which type of infection (Figure 12-26 A, B)?
   A. Toxoplasmosis
   B. Tuberculosis
   C. *Cryptococcus*
   D. Herpes
   E. *Staphylococcus*

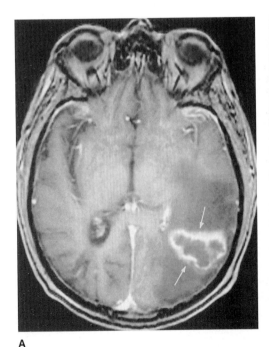

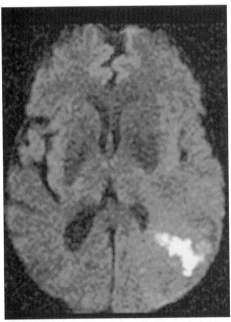

A   B

▲ **Figure 12-25.** Case 12-9. Postcontrast axial T1-weighted (**A**) and diffusion-weighted MR (**B**) images in a 75-year-old man who presents with a history of recurrent lymphoma complicated by multiple infections and new mental status changes.

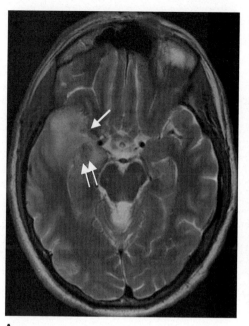

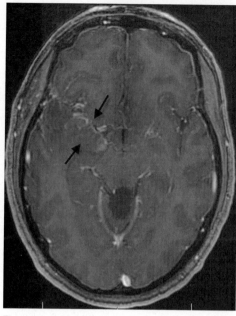

A   **B**

▲ **Figure 12-26.** Case 12-10. Axial T2 (**A**) and axial T1 postcontrast images (**B**) in a 42-year-old female who presents with mental status changes.

12-11. In Case 12-11, the major differential diagnosis for this lesion is toxoplasmosis versus (Figure 12-27)

- **A.** *Cryptococcus*
- **B.** Intracranial lymphoma
- **C.** Sarcoidosis
- **D.** Metastatic disease
- **E.** Cytomegalovirus (CMV)

Radiologic Findings

12-9. In this case, the contrast-enhanced MR scan shows a ring-enhancing lesion (arrows) in the left parietal lobe with decreased surrounding T1 signal (Figure 12-25 A). A diffusion signal abnormality is present on the corresponding diffusion-weighted image (Figure 12-25 B), within the central aspect of the lesion, and is found to be compatible with an area of restricted water motion. The patient's history is compatible with an intracranial infection, and the demonstrated MR imaging findings favor an abscess (C is the correct answer to Question 12-9.)

12-10. In this case, the T2-weighted MR image (Figure 12-26 A) shows increased signal in the medial and anterior aspects of the right temporal lobe (single arrow) with small focus of T2 hypointensity (double arrows) consistent with the presence of blood products. Postcontrast axial T1 (Figure 12-26 B) shows abnormal patchy

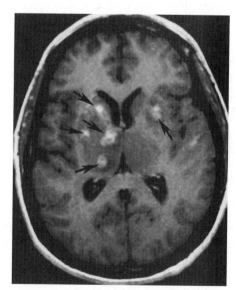

▲ **Figure 12-27.** Case 12-11. An axial contrast-enhanced T1-weighted MR image in a 43-year-old man who presents with headache and weakness.

parenchymal and leptomeningeal enhancement along the medial right temporal lobe. These changes are commonly seen in patients with herpes encephalitis (D is the correct answer to Question 12-10).

12-11. In this case, multiple enhancing lesions are present within the basal ganglia, especially on the right (arrows), on the gadolinium-enhanced T1-weighted MR image (Figure 12-27). The most common lesions with this appearance in an immunocompromised patient, such as a patient with HIV, are toxoplasmosis and intracranial lymphoma (B is the correct answer to Question 12-11). The patient markedly improved after anti-toxoplasmosis therapy, and the lesions shown on the MR image disappeared.

Discussion

A host of infectious diseases can involve the brain and its coverings. Because the CNS has a limited number of ways of responding to an infectious agent, many intracranial infections appear identical on neuroimaging studies. It is, therefore, very important to closely correlate the imaging findings with the clinical presentation and other diagnostic tests, such as lumbar puncture or stereotactic brain aspiration.

For our purposes, it is useful to classify CNS infections according to the intracranial compartment involved, especially because this has treatment implications. Intracranial infections can be either parenchymal or extraparenchymal. Parenchymal manifestations include cerebritis/abscess and encephalitis. Extraparenchymal disease includes epidural abscess, subdural empyema, and leptomeningitis. Bacterial, viral, fungal, and parasitic agents can all affect the CNS. Although a few infectious agents preferentially involve a particular anatomic compartment of the CNS, most are not site specific.

Case 12-9 demonstrates the classic ring-enhancing lesion of an abscess, in this case, due to *Nocardia*. No specific features of this abscess distinguish it from a typical pyogenic abscess. The diffusion signal abnormality has been postulated to arise from restricted water motion in the presence of viscous, purulent material within the abscess cavity and can mimic an area of acute ischemia. Cerebral infection by *Nocardia* usually arises from a pulmonary focus in an immunocompromised host. Similarly, most pyogenic abscesses are the result of hematogenous dissemination from a non-CNS source. Pyogenic brain abscesses can also result from direct extension of an infectious process from an adjacent area (eg, sinusitis or mastoiditis) or from trauma (eg, penetrating wound or surgery).

Abscesses usually occur at gray matter/white matter junctions, although they can occur anywhere in the brain. Patients frequently present with seizures or symptoms related to intracranial mass effect. If abscesses develop near the brain surface, they may rupture into the subarachnoid space, producing meningitis; they may also produce a ventriculitis if they rupture into the ventricular system. Most abscesses are treated surgically.

Herpes encephalitis (Case 12-10) is caused by the herpes simplex virus (HSV). Older children and adults are usually infected by HSV-1, either primarily or as a result of reactivation of a latent virus. The ensuing necrotizing encephalitis in this condition typically involves the temporal and inferior frontal lobes, insular cortex, and cingulate gyrus. Focal abnormalities of attenuation (on CT) or signal (on MR) in these characteristic locations, often with enhancement after contrast administration, are practically pathognomonic of HSV-1 encephalitis. Early diagnosis of this condition is extremely important, because antiviral therapy can significantly affect patient outcome.

Neonatal herpes simplex infection differs from infection in the older child and adult. The offending organism is usually HSV-2, which may be acquired in utero or during birth from mothers with genital herpes. HSV-2 infection can produce severe destructive changes within the developing brain. Unlike HSV-1 infection in older children and adults, neonatal herpes encephalitis can involve any area of the brain, having no predilection for the temporal lobe.

Patients with AIDS (Case 12-11) commonly develop intracranial infections during the course of their disease. Human immunodeficiency virus (HIV) itself can directly infect the CNS, producing encephalopathy in up to 60% of AIDS patients. The most common neuroimaging finding in HIV encephalopathy is cerebral atrophy, often with patchy white matter hypodensity (on CT) or T2 hyperintensity (on MR imaging) from demyelination and gliosis (Figure 12-28). Other common CNS infections in the immunocompromised AIDS patient include toxoplasmosis, cryptococcosis, and progressive multifocal leukoencephalopathy (from a polyomavirus infection).

Toxoplasmosis usually presents as multiple lesions of varying size and demonstrates ring enhancement with surrounding edema on CT or MR imaging. Lesions commonly occur in the basal ganglia or at the gray matter/white matter junction within the cerebral hemispheres. Individual masses may have a solid appearance or demonstrate central necrosis or hemorrhage. The enhancement pattern is variable; both rim-enhancing and more solidly enhancing lesions can be seen. Their appearance is almost identical to that of primary intracranial lymphoma, another common intracranial condition in AIDS. Metabolic studies, such as PET or SPECT scans (no increase in ^{18}F-FDG activity with toxoplasmosis, increased with lymphoma), MR spectroscopy (no choline elevation in toxoplasmosis, elevated in lymphoma), and perfusion-weighted sequences (lower cerebral blood volume in toxoplasmosis) may assist in distinguishing these pathologies.

Meningitis is the most frequent manifestation of cryptococcosis in AIDS, although parenchymal lesions, termed cryptococcomas, are occasionally encountered. In progressive

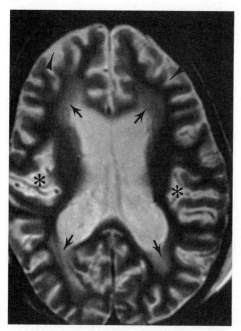

▲ **Figure 12-28.** An 8-year-old girl with AIDS and new onset of seizures. Axial T2-weighted image shows white matter high signal (arrows). Also note the diffuse prominence of gyri and sulci (arrowheads) and sylvian fissures (asterisks), compatible with cerebral atrophy.

multifocal leukoencephalopathy, extensive areas of white matter demyelination are shown on MR imaging. A number of other intracranial infections can occur in AIDS patients, and the reader is referred to the suggested readings at the end of this chapter for sources of further information.

EXERCISE 12-5. HEAD TRAUMA

12-12. In Case 12-12, what is the diagnosis (Figure 12-29 A, B)?
    A. Subdural hematoma
    B. Cerebral contusion
    C. Epidural hematoma
    D. Meningioma
    E. Subdural hygroma

12-13. In Case 12-13, what is the main radiologic finding (Figure 12-30)?
    A. Subdural hematoma
    B. Epidural hematoma
    C. Duret hemorrhage
    D. Cerebral contusions
    E. Shearing injuries

Radiologic Findings

12-12. In this case, a predominantly high-density, extra-axial, hemorrhagic collection (black arrows) is producing mass effect on the right frontal lobe on an

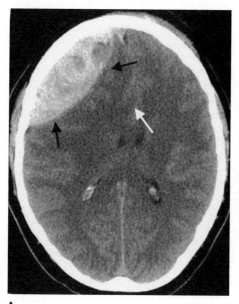
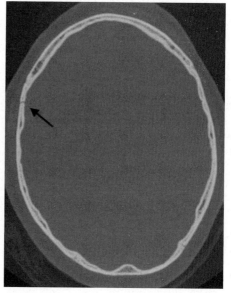

A   B

▲ **Figure 12-29.** Case 12-12. Axial noncontrast head CT with soft tissue (**A**) and bone windows (**B**) in an 18-year-old male who is found unconscious following a motor vehicle collision.

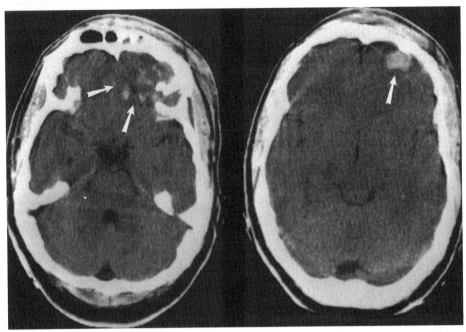

▲ **Figure 12-30.** Case 12-13. Axial noncontrast head CT image in a 24-year-old man who presents with multiple facial fractures and frontal scalp soft-tissue swelling resulting from a motor vehicle accident.

unenhanced head CT scan (Figure 12-29 A). Mass effect results in marked distortion of the underlying cortex and leftward subfalcine herniation (white arrow) (Figure 12-29 A). A linear nondepressed fracture is present along the anterior aspect of the right parietal bone (black arrow) (Figure 12-29 B). The biconvex appearance of this lesion is typical of an epidural hematoma, which is the acute finding in this case (C is the correct answer to Question 12-12).

12-13. In this case, there are multiple areas of increased attenuation within the frontal lobes, especially on the left (arrows) (Figure 12-30). These areas correspond to multiple hemorrhagic contusions involving the brain parenchyma (D is the correct answer to Question 12-13).

Discussion

Intracranial abnormalities in head trauma can be classified as either primary or secondary. Primary lesions occur at the moment of injury and include skull fractures, extracerebral hemorrhage (eg, epidural or subdural hematomas, subarachnoid hemorrhage), and intracerebral hemorrhage (eg, brain contusion, brainstem injury, diffuse axonal injury).

The secondary effects of head trauma are actually complications of the primary intracranial injury. Elevated intracranial pressure and cerebral herniation are responsible for most of the secondary effects of head trauma, which in many cases may be more devastating to the patients than the initial injury.

Epidural hematoma is usually associated with skull fractures that lacerate the middle meningeal artery or a dural sinus. Up to one-half of patients with epidural hematomas have a lucid interval after the head trauma occurs. On CT, epidural hematomas usually appear as biconvex, high-attenuation, extra-axial masses. Most are located in the temporoparietal area. Underlying skull fractures are common. Intracranial brain herniation may also be a prominent feature in this condition. One important imaging feature in epidural hematomas is that they do not cross skull sutures, but may cross the midline.

Subdural hematoma, on the other hand, is usually a crescent-shaped extra-axial collection that may cross suture lines, but is confined by the dural reflections (Figure 12-31). These lesions are more lethal than are epidural hematomas; the subdural hematoma mortality rate is over 50%. CT can usually, but not always, distinguish between epidural hematomas and subdural hematomas. Subdural hematomas are a commonly identified abnormality in the abused child (nonaccidental trauma). CT scans are obtained to detect the

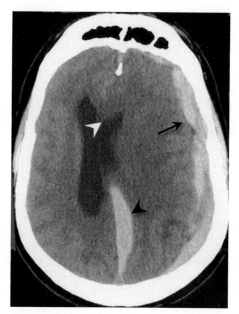

▲ **Figure 12-31.** Axial noncontrast head CT obtained on a 67-year-old male after a fall. A large, crescentic hyperdense extra-axial hemorrhage layers over the left cerebral convexity (black arrow) and extends along the posterior falx (black arrowhead). Secondary mass effect on the adjacent brain parenchyma with effacement of the left lateral ventricle and rightward shift of the midline structures (white arrowhead).

presence of subdural hematomas (Figure 12-32). A brain MRI, however, can more sensitively delineate small extra-axial hematomas, subdural hematomas of varying ages, and coexisting cortical contusions or shearing injuries. A shearing injury (or diffuse axonal injury) is associated with an overall poor prognosis and is recognized as small petechial hemorrhages at the gray-white junction and in the corpus callosum. Interhemispheric (para- and intrafalcial) subdural hematomas may arise from tearing of bridging veins along the falx cerebri in shaking injuries and are nearly pathognomic for nonaccidental trauma. Retinal hemorrhages may be present and are also suspicious, especially if bilateral. In addition, cerebral ischemia/infarction and multiple, complex, unexplained skull fractures may be associated findings.

Cerebral contusions (Case 12-13) are the second most common form of brain parenchymal injury in primary head trauma (diffuse axonal injury is the most common parenchymal injury). Cerebral contusions can be thought of as brain bruises. They result either from the brain striking a bony ridge inside the skull during rapid acceleration/deceleration, as occurs in a motor vehicle accident, or from a depressed

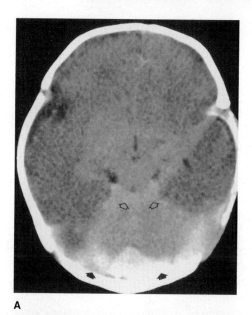

A

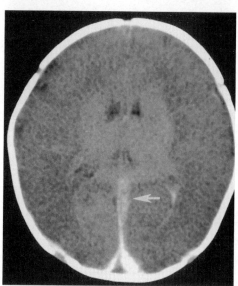

B

▲ **Figure 12-32.** Noncontrast axial CT images (**A, B**) in a 21-day-old male following nonaccidental trauma. Large, bilateral subdural hematomas layer over the tentorium cerebelli in (**A**) (closed arrows) and within the interhemispheric fissure in (**B**) (arrow). In addition, a small amount of subarachnoid hemorrhage is seen within the quadrigeminal plate cistern in (**A**) (open arrows), as well as within the left lateral ventricle (not shown). Loss of the normal cerebral gray-white differentiation is demonstrated. These features are nearly pathognomonic for nonaccidental trauma with diffuse anoxic insult.

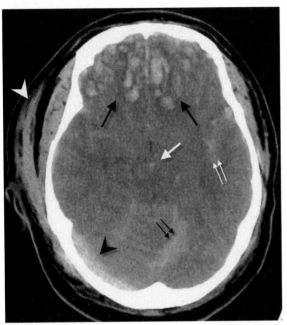

▲ **Figure 12-33.** Axial noncontrast head CT following a high-speed motor vehicle collision. Acute hemorrhage in multiple intracranial compartments is a hallmark of trauma. Hemorrhagic contusions are demonstrated in the inferior bifrontal lobes (large black arrows), subarachnoid hemorrhages in the interpeduncular cistern (white arrow) and Sylvian fissure (double white arrows), subdural hemorrhage along the tentorial incisura (double black arrows), and epidural hemorrhage crossing the right tentorium (black arrowhead), as well as a large scalp hematoma (white arrowhead).

skull fracture. These lesions tend to occur in particular anatomic locations, especially the undersurfaces and poles of the frontal and temporal lobes (Figure 12-33). CT scans show areas of low attenuation (edema) and hemorrhage at the site of injury. Delayed hemorrhage, 1 to 2 days after a head injury, is common with contusions.

EXERCISE 12-6. INTRACRANIAL VASCULAR ABNORMALITIES

12-14. In Case 12-14, what is the reason for the abnormality on the CT scan (Figure 12-34 A–C)?
   A. Cerebral aneurysm
   B. Arteriovenous malformation
   C. Head trauma
   D. Carotid dissection
   E. Vasculitis

12-15. In Case 12-15, what is the reason for the abnormality on the CT scan (Figure 12-35 A-C)?
   A. Cerebral aneurysm
   B. Arteriovenous malformation
   C. Head trauma
   D. Carotid dissection
   E. Vasculitis

Radiologic Findings

12-14. In this case, the CT scan (Figure 12-34 A) shows extensive subarachnoid hemorrhage filling the basal cisterns, more pronounced on the right (black arrows), with extension of hemorrhage into the interhemispheric and Sylvian fissures. Enlargement of the temporal horns (white arrows) is indicative of early hydrocephalus. An oblique craniocaudal view from a CT angiogram (Figure 12-34 B) shows a 4-mm saccular aneurysm arising from the right paraclinoid internal carotid artery (arrow), most likely posterior communicating artery origin. A lateral view taken from a right common carotid catheter angiogram (Figure 12-34 C) confirms a posterior communicating artery origin aneurysm (black arrow) with upward distortion of the normal anterior cerebral artery configuration secondary to hydrocephalus (black arrowheads). (A is the correct answer to Question 12-14.)

12-15. In this case, the noncontrast CT scan (Figure 12-35 A) shows a lobulated, hyperdense mass (black arrows) centered in the medial right occipital lobe with effacement of the right occipital horn. Accompanying axial T2 MRI (Figure 12-35 B) reveals a nidus of low signal vascular "flow-voids" (white arrowheads) in the occipital lobe with a more prominent draining vein extending into the quadrigeminal plate cistern (white arrow). A subsequent catheter angiogram (Figure 12-35 C) of the right vertebral artery (curved arrow) confirms a high-flow vascular lesion with a tangle of vessels (double black arrows) and early venous opacification (arrowhead) characteristic of an arteriovenous malformation. (B is the correct answer to Question 12-15.)

Discussion

Cerebrovascular disorders (strokes) were discussed in Exercise 12-2, which dealt mainly with cerebral infarction secondary to atherosclerosis. For information on other causes of cerebral infarction, the reader is referred to the suggested readings at the end of this chapter. This section addresses two other common vascular conditions affecting the CNS: aneurysms and vascular malformations.

Most cerebral aneurysms, such as Case 12-14, are saccular or "berry" aneurysms. These focal arterial dilatations tend to occur at cerebral arterial branch points. They have traditionally

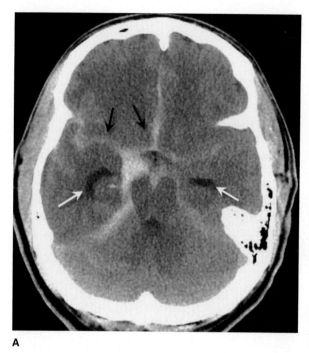

A

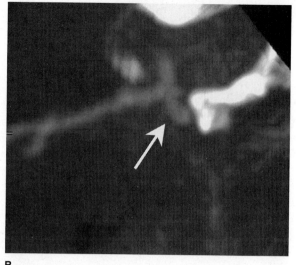

B

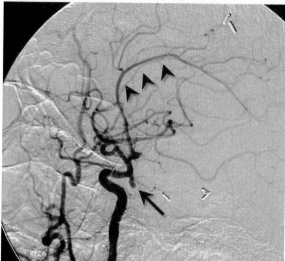

C

▲ **Figure 12-34.** Case 12-14. Axial noncontrast CT (**A**), axial-oblique CT angiographic images (**B**), and catheter angiogram (**C**) in a 41-year-old male who is found unresponsive while at work after complaining of a headache earlier.

been thought to develop at congenitally weak areas of a blood vessel wall. Recent evidence, however, has questioned this view, and many now believe that saccular aneurysms are probably acquired lesions from abnormal hemodynamic stresses that damage the arterial wall.

Intracranial aneurysms are usually asymptomatic until they rupture, at which time the patient typically presents with a severe headache resulting from subarachnoid hemorrhage. The vast majority of nontraumatic SAHs occur as a result of aneurysm rupture. CT is very good at demonstrating SAH. Patients usually undergo CT angiography whenever

nontraumatic SAH is detected, and occasionally cerebral arteriography.

Common locations for intracranial aneurysms include the anterior communicating artery, the internal carotid artery at the origin of the posterior communicating artery, and the middle cerebral artery trifurcation. Posterior fossa aneurysms are less common; they make up only around 10% of all intracranial aneurysms and typically arise from the basilar artery tip.

Vascular malformations can be divided into four major types: true arteriovenous malformations (as demonstrated in

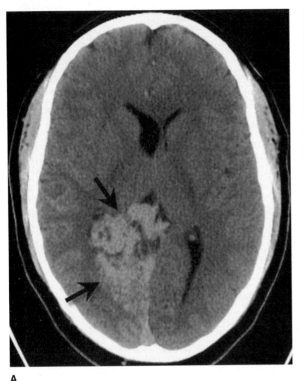

A

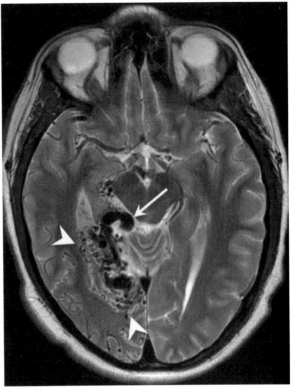

B

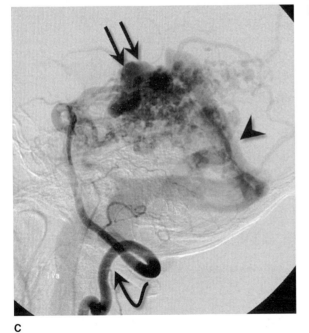

C

▲ Figure 12-35. Case 12-15. Axial noncontrast CT (**A**) and T2-weighted MRI (**B**) and catheter angiogram (**C**) in a 22-year-old male who complains of persistent right-sided headache.

Case 12-15), cavernous hemangiomas, venous angiomas, and capillary telangiectasias. AVMs are congenital lesions consisting of a tangle of abnormal blood vessels, usually within the brain parenchyma, that are fed by enlarged cerebral arteries and drained by dilated, tortuous veins. Because there is no normal intervening brain parenchyma for the blood to flow through, blood is rapidly shunted from the arterial to the venous side. This shunting is dramatically demonstrated on cerebral arteriography. Patients with AVMs usually present with intracranial hemorrhage or seizures. MR imaging or contrast-enhanced CT can demonstrate the tortuous vascular channels of most AVMs, although cerebral arteriography is the definitive study in this condition.

The other intracranial vascular malformations have very characteristic appearances on MR imaging, although they are frequently invisible on cerebral arteriography. Patients with these "low-pressure" malformations can present with headaches, seizures, or, rarely, intracranial hemorrhage. Many of these lesions, however, are incidentally discovered on MR scans performed for other reasons.

EXERCISE 12-7. WHITE MATTER DISEASES

12-16. In Case 12-16, what is the most likely diagnosis (Figure 12-36 A, B)?

    A. Pseudotumor cerebri
    B. Metastatic disease
    C. Septic emboli
    D. Radiation necrosis
    E. Multiple sclerosis

12-17. In Case 12-17, what is most likely responsible for the abnormalities seen on the MR image (Figure 12-37 A, B)?
    A. Cardiac arrhythmia
    B. Chronic hypertension
    C. Remote trauma
    D. Hepatic failure
    E. Carbon monoxide poisoning

Radiologic Findings

12-16. In this case, sagittal T1-weighted and axial FLAIR MR images (Figure 12-36 A, B) show multiple foci of abnormal signal within the periventricular white matter (arrows). These lesions are quite characteristic of multiple sclerosis (E is the correct answer to Question 12-16). The patient's visual difficulties were due to optic neuritis, a common abnormality in multiple sclerosis.

12-17. In this case, there are patchy areas of increased T2 signal (arrows) within the periventricular white matter

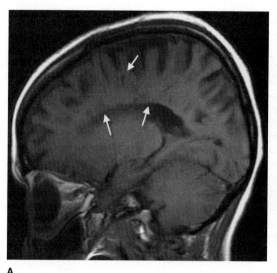

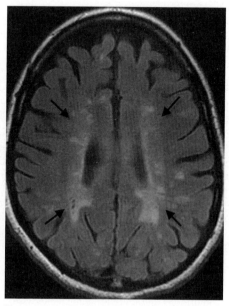

A   **B**

▲ **Figure 12-36. A,B.** Case 12-16. T1-weighted parasagittal (**A**) and axial T2 FLAIR images (**B**) in a 48-year-old female who presents with a history of weakness and visual changes.

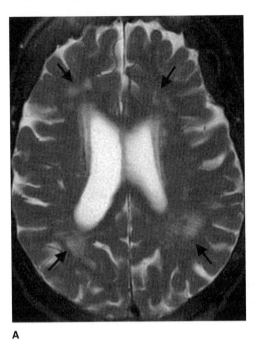
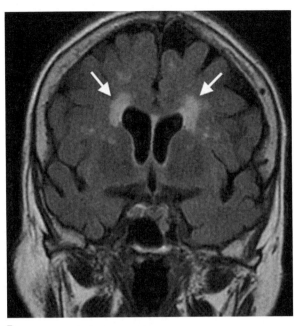

A   **B**

⏶ **Figure 12-37. A, B.** Case 12-17. Axial T2 (**A**) and coronal T2 FLAIR sequences (**B**) in an 83-year-old female who has a history of hypertension, diabetes and worsening dementia.

(Figure 12-37). Usually seen in elderly hypertensive patients, these lesions correspond to focal areas of demyelination secondary to deep white matter ischemia (B is the correct answer to Question 12-17).

Discussion

Diseases that primarily affect the cerebral white matter have a host of causes. Unfortunately, very few of these conditions have specific appearances on CT or MR scans. Neuroimaging is usually performed to determine whether there are changes within the brain that are compatible with one of the white matter diseases and to rule out other conditions that might mimic white matter disease.

White matter diseases include both inherited and acquired conditions. They can be further subdivided into demyelinating conditions (destruction or injury of normally formed myelin) and dysmyelinating conditions (abnormal formation or maintenance of myelin, usually because of an enzyme deficiency). The dysmyelinating conditions are rare and, for the most part, include the leukodystrophies, such as adrenoleukodystrophy and metachromatic leukodystrophy. Although the MR appearance can be striking in some of these diseases, it is often nonspecific. These conditions are not discussed here.

Multiple sclerosis (MS) (Case 12-16) is the most common demyelinating disease. Because there is no generally accepted etiology for MS, it is also referred to as a primary demyelinating disease. Secondary demyelinating conditions are those caused by a known agent or event. MS usually occurs in young adults and more often in women than men (approximately 2:1). The disease is characterized by a relapsing and remitting course and by varying neurologic symptoms, depending on the location of the lesion within the CNS. Although diagnosis of MS is usually based on clinical criteria, MR imaging can be a very helpful confirmatory test. Typical MS plaques appear as ovoid, T2 signal hyperintensities within the periventricular and deep white matter. Lesions are also common within the corpus callosum, brainstem, cerebellar peduncles, spinal cord, and optic nerves. MS plaque enhancement on gadolinium-infused MR images suggests active disease (ie, breakdown of the BBB). Confluent areas of T2 signal abnormality in the periventricular white matter are common in severe cases.

Ischemic demyelination (Case 12-17) is usually seen in patients with small-vessel disease (such as from long-standing hypertension). This condition, also called leukoaraiosis (white matter softening), occurs because of hypertension-induced arteriolar sclerosis of penetrating medullary arteries that supply the deep white matter of the brain. This leads to a

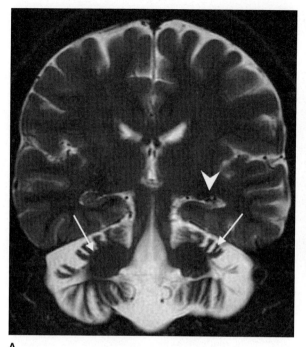

A

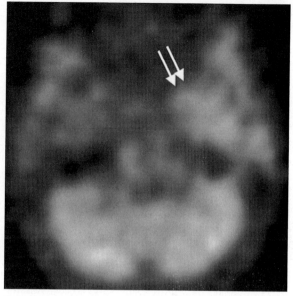

B

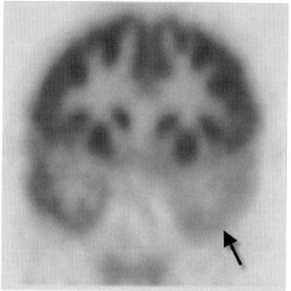

C

▲ **Figure 12-38.** Case 12-18. Coronal fast multiplanar inversion recovery (FMPIR) MRI (**A**), axial ictal SPECT (**B**). and coronal interictal PET images (**C**) in a 34-year-old female with a long-standing history of medical refractory epilepsy who presents with increasing seizure frequency.

reduction in white matter blood flow with accompanying is-chemic demyelination. This condition occurs most commonly in older patients and is associated with small-vessel brain infarcts (lacunar infarcts). MR imaging usually demonstrates patchy areas of increased T2 signal in the deep white matter. The lesions are often bilaterally symmetric and periventricular in distribution.

EXERCISE 12-8. SEIZURE AND EPILEPSY

12-18. In Case 12-18, what is the most likely diagnosis (Figure 12-38 A–C)?

A. Alzheimer's dementia
B. Gray matter heterotopia
C. Hemimegalencephaly
D. Mesial temporal sclerosis
E. Multiple sclerosis

Radiologic Findings

12-18. Coronal FMPIR MRI (Figure 12-38 A) demonstrates marked atrophy of the left hippocampus with loss of normal laminar architecture (white arrowhead). Ictal SPECT (Figure 12-38 B) shows increased radiotracer uptake in the left medial temporal lobe (double arrows), whereas the interictal PET (Figure 12-38 C) demonstrates diminished metabolic activity in the left temporal lobe (black arrow). The constellation of findings is highly suggestive of mesial temporal sclerosis (D is the correct answer to Question 12-18). Pronounced cerebellar atrophy (Figure 12-38 A) in this case is the result of long-standing antiepileptic medication (white arrows).

Discussion

Although a comprehensive review of seizure and epilepsy classification is beyond the scope of this section, it is important to note the central role that imaging serves in the evaluation and management of these patients. The etiology of seizure varies significantly with patient age. In young children (3 months to 5 years), fever is the most common precipitant of seizure. The exact pathophysiology is not fully understood; however, there is likely a relationship to an inflammatory cascade as well as a low seizure threshold in young children. Imaging is generally not performed in the setting of a simple febrile seizure (seizures that last less than 15 minutes, are generalized, and do not recur in a 24-hour period). Febrile seizures that do not meet these criteria are classified as complex and imply a more serious underlying abnormality including meningitis, abscess, or encephalitis, for which imaging may be indicated. Other potential causes of seizure in young children include cerebral anoxia, metabolic abnormalities, cortical malformations (refer to Case 12-2), infection, or inherited neurocutaneous diseases such as tuberous sclerosis.

In older children and adults, common causes of seizure include vascular malformations, cerebral injury due to prior trauma or ischemia, or underlying tumor, among others. Noteworthy tumors associated with intractable seizure include ganglioglioma, dysembryoplastic neuroepithelial tumor (DNET), and pleomorphic xanthoastrocytoma; these generally occur in childhood or in young adulthood.

The most common cause of medically refractory epilepsy is mesial temporal (hippocampal) sclerosis. Although this entity is most commonly seen in adult patients, there is likely a link to febrile seizures earlier in childhood or other remote cerebral insult such as trauma or infection. On MR imaging, there is characteristic atrophy and gliosis of the hippocampus, often with dilation of the ipsilateral temporal horn due to volume loss. There may be atrophy and gliosis of ipsilateral fornix and mammillary body as well. These patients are potential candidates for temporal lobectomy, and additional imaging with ictal SPECT and interictal PET is generally performed as described earlier.

SUGGESTED READING

1. Atlas SW. *Magnetic Resonance Imaging of the Brain and Spine.* 4th ed. Philadelphia: Lippincott Williams & Wilkins; 2009.
2. Grossman RI, Yousem DM. *Neuroradiology: The Requisites.* 2nd ed. St. Louis, Mo: Mosby; 2003.
3. Yock DH. *Magnetic Resonance Imaging of CNS Disease.* St. Louis, Mo: Mosby; 2002.
4. Barkovich AJ. *Pediatric Neuroimaging.* 4th ed. Philadelphia: Lippincott Williams & Wilkins; 2005.
5. Cullen SP, Symons SP, Hunter G, et al. Dynamic contrast-enhanced computed tomography of acute ischemic stroke: CTA and CT perfusion. *Semin Roentgenol.* 2002;37:192-205.
6. Aksoy FG, Lev MH. Dynamic contrast-enhanced brain perfusion imaging: technique and clinical applications. *Semin Ultrasound CT MRI.* 2000;21:462-467.
7. Philips CD, Bubash LA. CTA and MRA in the evaluation of extracranial carotid vascular disease. *Radiol Clin North Am.* 2002;40:783-798.
8. Liu H, Hall WA, Martin AJ, Maxwell RE, Truwit CL. MR-guided and MR-monitored neurosurgical procedures at 1.5T. *J Comput Assist Tomogr.* 2000;24:909-918.
9. McKinney AM, Palmer CS, Truwit CL, Karagulle A, Teksam M. Detection of aneurysms by 64-section multidetector CT angiography in patients acutely suspected of having an intracranial aneurysm and comparison with digital subtraction and 3D rotational angiography. *Am J Neuroradiol.* 2008;29:594-602.

Imaging of the Spine

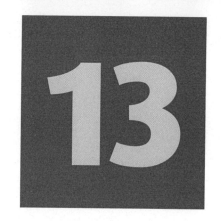

Nandita Guha-Thakurta, MD
Lawrence E. Ginsberg, MD

The spine is critical for normal human function, providing structure, support, and protection of the spinal cord and spinal nerves. Given the wide range of pathologic conditions that can affect the spine, recognition of normal anatomy and variants, differentiation from abnormal anatomy, and diagnosis of different pathologic conditions are the goals of spine imaging.

It is assumed that the reader is already familiar with basic spine anatomy learned early in medical school. With such a foundation, this chapter on the imaging appearance of the spine will serve to solidify and perhaps even enhance this knowledge base.

The purpose of this chapter is to review the different techniques employed in spine imaging, to emphasize normal anatomy as depicted with these techniques, and to highlight the appearance of certain common lesions. Relative advantages and disadvantages of the various imaging modalities are reviewed within the context of an overall imaging strategy. It is not intended that the reader will be an accomplished spine radiologist after reading this chapter. Rather, it is hoped that the reader will gain basic familiarity with normal imaging anatomy and the appearance of certain types of abnormalities, as well as a sense of which test might be the best to order for a given clinical circumstance.

TECHNIQUES

Prior to the advent of computed tomography (CT) in the 1970s, spine imaging consisted primarily of plain-film radiography and an adjunct test, myelography, to be discussed later. Spine imaging was revolutionized by CT, and, subsequently, magnetic resonance (MR) imaging, which for the first time allowed direct acquisition of axial, sagittal, and coronal (multiplanar) images, allowing for better spatial and contrast resolution. Not until the era of CT could the spinal cord be visualized and evaluated. These imaging modalities have so changed the face of diagnosis and treatment of spine pathology that virtually no neurosurgeon today would undertake spine surgery without first obtaining a CT and/or MR imaging study.

This section reviews the major modalities currently employed to image the spine. The highly specialized technique of spinal arteriography, which is used principally to detect vascular malformations, is beyond the scope of this review.

Nuclear medicine scanning also is not discussed, because it is seldom used as a primary diagnostic study in the evaluation of spine disease (though spinal metastases are frequently diagnosed with whole-body isotope bone scanning).

▶ Plain Radiograph

Plain films are conventional radiographs, which are commonly referred to as x-rays. They may be obtained in a frontal projection—anteroposterior (AP) or posteroanterior (PA); the difference is insignificant in the spine—a lateral projection (side view), or an oblique projection (Figures 13-1, 13-2, and 13-3). Plain films are most useful for the visualization of bony structures. Soft-tissue structures (everything but bone) are largely radiolucent and cannot be seen clearly on plain films unless abnormal density such as calcification is present. Although plain films depict bone anatomy quite well, certain structures may be obscured by other structures in front of or behind them. For instance, on a lateral projection, both pedicles would be superimposed on one another (Figures 13-1 B and 13-3 B). For this reason, multiple views are always obtained as part of a routine examination.

On conventional radiographs, bony structures appear white. This appearance is referred to as "radiodense" or simply "dense." Normally, mineralized bones have a recognizable radiodensity, which should always be assessed when viewing

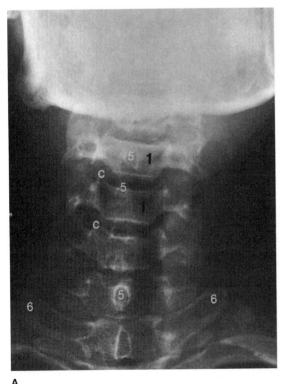

A

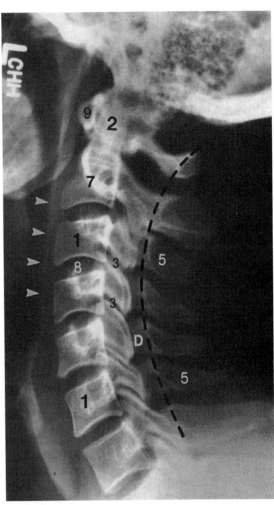

B

▲ **Figure 13-1.** Plain film of normal cervical spine. **(A)** Anteroposterior view. **(B)** Lateral view. Arrowheads indicate pre-vertebral soft-tissue stripe. Note normal lordosis and continuity of spinolaminar line (dashed line).

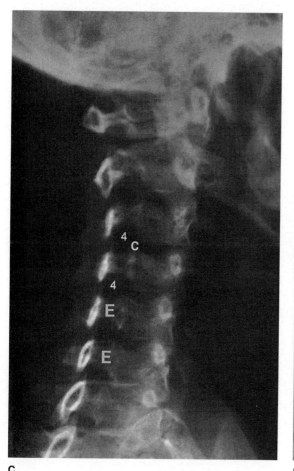

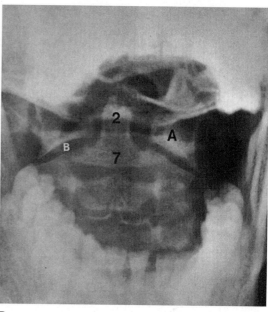

C   D

▲ **Figure 13-1.** *(Continued)* **(C)** Oblique view. **(D)** Open mouth. 1, vertebral body; 2, odontoid process (dens); 3, articular facet joint; 4, intervertebral (neural) foramen; 5, spinous process; 6, transverse process; 7, body of axis (C2); 8, intervertebral disk space; 9, anterior arch of atlas (C1); A, lateral mass of atlas; B, atlantoaxial joint; C, uncinate process; D, lamina; E, pedicle.

x-rays. Certain pathologic conditions (eg, osteopenia and osteolytic metastases) can result in decreased bone density, and other conditions (eg, osteoblastic metastases and some exotic diseases) may result in abnormally increased bone density.

After bone density is assessed, the next evaluation should be the alignment of the spine. A normal spine should show cervical and lumbar lordosis (anterior convexity) (Figures 13-1 and 13-3) and thoracic kyphosis (posterior convexity). Abnormalities in alignment may result from incorrect positioning of the patient or be a reflection of an underlying problem. Such abnormalities may be minor, such as straightening or reversal of normal cervical lordosis in the case of muscle spasm. Abnormal curvature, such as scoliosis, may be idiopathic, congenital, or secondary to an underlying lesion.

Major alterations in alignment, such as subluxation, can result from trauma. In assessing alignment, it is important to determine whether the vertebral bodies, as well as the posterior elements (ie, spinous processes, pedicles, and laminae), are appropriately positioned. The spinal cord rests within the spinal canal formed by the foramen within each vertebra, but the cord is not visible on plain films. Its location is thus defined by identifying the boundaries of the spinal canal. The anterior margin of the spinal canal is the posterior aspect of the vertebral body, and the posterior limit of the spinal canal can be approximated by locating, on a lateral radiograph, the junction of the spinous process and the laminae. Identification of the spinolaminar line also helps in the evaluation of alignment (Figure 13-1 B).

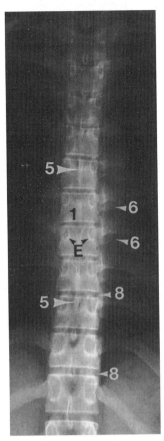

▲ **Figure 13-2.** Plain film of normal thoracic spine, antero-posterior view. 1, vertebral body; 5, spinous process; 6, transverse process; 8, intervertebral disk space; E, pedicle.

cal spinal nerves, 12 pairs of thoracic spinal nerves, and 5 pairs of lumbar spinal nerves. Abnormal bony projections, known as osteophytes, are a common manifestation of degenerative spine disease and, if present within the neural foramen, may be a cause of nerve root compression. Spinal nerves also can be compressed by disk herniations, but this type of neural compression cannot be diagnosed by means of plain films alone.

Small bony structures, such as the cervical transverse foramen (for the vertebral artery) and the small facets for rib articulation in the thoracic spine, are not well visualized on plain radiographs. Because "soft-tissue" structures are also poorly demonstrated on plain radiographs, the intervertebral disk is not well seen with x-rays unless it is calcified (and therefore dense). However, differences in the soft-tissue density can impart additional information. In the cervical spine, for instance, calcification in the region of the carotid artery bifurcation may suggest atherosclerotic vascular narrowing. In the evaluation of cervical trauma, one should always assess the width of the normal soft-tissue stripe that is anterior to

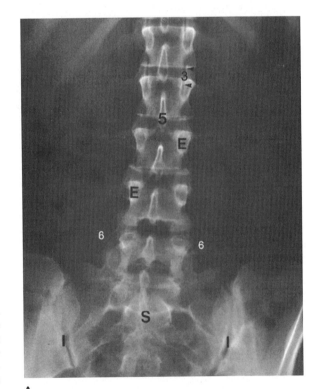

A

▲ **Figure 13-3.** Plain film of normal lumbar spine. **(A)** Anteroposterior view.

Most anatomic features of the spine are readily identifiable on plain radiographs (Figures 13-1, 13-2, and 13-3) such as vertebral bodies, facet joints, disk spaces, pedicles, laminae, transverse and spinous processes, and the neural foramen, whereas certain other areas can be evaluated only on specialized views. For instance, the open-mouth view facilitates visualization of the atlantoaxial (C1-2) articulation and provides an additional view of the dens (Figure 13-1 D). This view is an essential component of a trauma workup. Oblique views allow visualization of the neural foramen in the cervical spine (lateral views are used for this purpose in the thoracolumbar spine) (Figure 13-1 C). The neuroforamina are formed by the pedicles of the vertebrae above and below (Figures 13-1 C and 13-3 B) and allow for the exit of the spinal nerves from the spinal canal. There are 8 pairs of cervi-

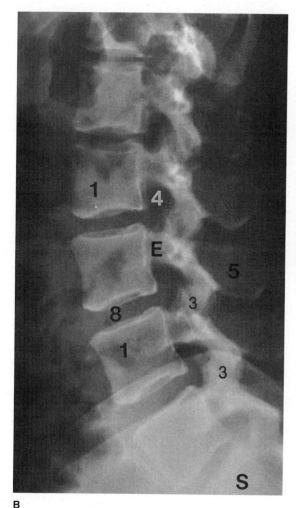

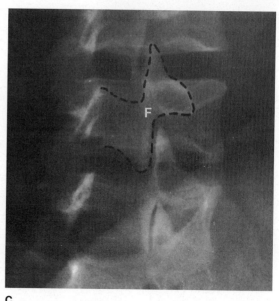

▲ **Figure 13-3.** *(Continued)* **(B)** Lateral view. **(C)** Oblique view. Notice "Scottie dog" configuration formed by facet joints and pedicle in this projection (dashed line). The "neck" of the Scottie dog represents the pars interarticularis. 1, vertebral body; 3, articular facet joint; 4, intervertebral (neural) foramen; 5, spinous process; 6, transverse process; 8, intervertebral disk space; E, pedicle; F, pars interarticularis; S, sacrum; I, sacroiliac joint.

the vertebral bodies (Figure 13-1 B). This prevertebral soft-tissue stripe may become widened in cervical spine trauma (prompting a closer search for fracture) and also in certain inflammatory conditions. When reviewing thoracic or lumbar spine films, attention to the soft tissues may facilitate diagnosis of a host of conditions ranging from pneumonia and lung cancer to retroperitoneal diseases and abdominal aortic aneurysms. Therefore, it is important not to focus only on the spine when interpreting spine radiographs.

▶ Myelography

Contrast myelography has been around since its accidental discovery in 1922, when Sicard and Forestier, intending to administer extradural lipiodol to treat sciatica, inadvertently introduced the material into the subarachnoid space. This radiopaque oil was noted to move freely, and it was immediately recognized that with the use of fluoroscopy (real-time radiography) and conventional radiography, this procedure would be useful for diagnosing intraspinal tumors. Lipiodol quickly replaced air as the medium of choice for myelography (air is lucent and is therefore a "negative" contrast agent; iodinized oils such as lipiodol and, later, the popular Pantopaque (iophendylate) are dense and therefore "positive" contrast agents). Following Mixter and Barr's 1934 report on the syndrome of herniated intervertebral disk, myelography became a widely used test. In the 1980s, the wide availability of less toxic water-soluble agents and, finally, nonionic contrast agents such as iopamidol and iohexol made myelography a readily tolerated procedure.

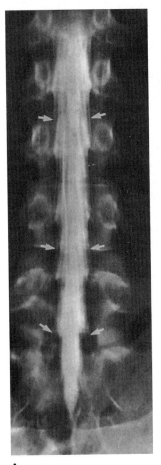

A

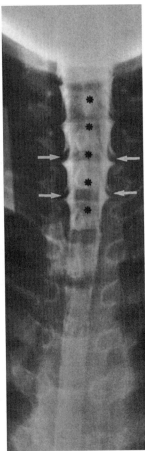

B

▲ **Figure 13-4.** **(A)** Normal lumbar myelogram, antero-posterior view. Note dense white contrast within the thecal sac. The nerve roots are readily identified as a "negative defect" within the dense contrast (arrows). **(B)** Cervical myelogram, anteroposterior view. The spinal cord (asterisks) can be seen as a lower-density "defect" within the contrast column. Exiting nerve roots can also be seen (arrows).

Myelography is employed most commonly to evaluate for disk herniations and to rule out spinal cord compression caused by tumor or trauma. In many parts of the United States, CT and MR imaging have all but replaced myelography. However, in many locations, myelography is still performed. A myelogram is often followed by a postmyelogram CT examination, which is addressed later.

The technique for performing myelography is simple. The patient is placed prone on a fluoroscopy table. Under fluoroscopic guidance, a lumbar puncture (LP) is made with an 18- to 22-gauge spinal needle (a fluoroscopically guided LP is much easier than an LP performed on a sick patient on the ward in the decubitus position). Cerebrospinal fluid (CSF) is then drawn for laboratory tests if needed, and contrast material is placed into the subarachnoid space. Once instillation of the contrast agent is fluoroscopically confirmed, the needle can be withdrawn and the spine studied. Depending on the spinal level to be examined, the patient can be standing, flat, or in Trendelenburg position. Typically, multiple views including lateral, AP, and oblique views are obtained. In the lumbar region, the cauda equina nerve roots are well visualized (Figure 13-4 A). The conus medullaris, usually at L1-2, also can be seen. In the thoracic and cervical levels, the spinal cord can be seen as a "negative" shadow within the dense contrast, and its size and shape can therefore be evaluated (Figure 13-4 B). Cervical spinal nerves are also well seen (Figure 13-4 B). The presence of any lesions and their precise location relative to the dura usually can be determined on the basis of the myelographic appearance. For instance, lesions may be extradural, intradural but extramedullary (not in the spinal cord), or intramedullary (within the spinal cord).

▶ Computed Tomography

CT utilizes x-rays to obtain images by means of multiple sources and detectors surrounding the patient in a radial fashion. This is why the patient appears to be entering a large doughnut-shaped device during the CT examination. The

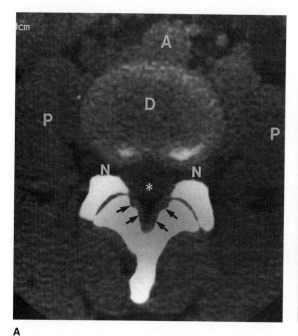

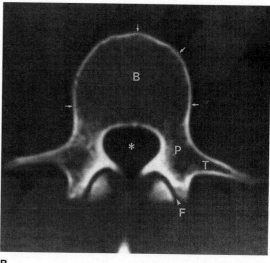

A   **B**

Figure 13-5. CT of normal spine. (**A**) Soft-tissue windows. A, aorta; D, intervertebral disk; N, neural foramen; P, psoas muscles; arrows, ligamentum flavum; asterisk, thecal sac. (**B**) Bone window. Asterisk, spinal canal; P, pedicle; B, vertebral body; T, transverse process; F, facet joint. Notice the excellent bony detail and thin rim of normal dense cortical bone (arrows).

data obtained are processed by a computer, which then generates an image. Nowadays, with multidetector CT, image reconstruction in coronal, sagittal, and oblique planes in addition to the source axial images allows for improved spatial resolution. Once the raw data are obtained, images can be displayed with different "windows" and "level" values that take advantage of density ("attenuation" in CT terminology) differences between tissues. For instance, filming a set of soft-tissue windows allows differentiation of soft-tissue structures that are very similar in attenuation to adjacent structures (eg, muscle and fluid). This is one of the key features of CT, whereas plain films usually cannot distinguish between the different soft tissues as well. In the spine, CT makes it possible to discriminate between CSF, nerve roots, and ligaments, for instance. Therefore, a CT examination can demonstrate the ligamentum flavum, nerve roots, epidural fat, and other structures that cannot be identified discretely on plain films (Figure 13-5 A). Additionally, images can be obtained with a bone algorithm, whose window and level gives detailed information about bony structures (Figure 13-5 B), although on such images, little soft-tissue information is available.

CT is widely used to image the spine in the evaluation of many pathologic conditions. Most common indications include trauma, spine tumors, and degenerative disk disease

(ie, to rule out disk herniation in patients with myelopathy or radiculopathy). Assuming a normal appearance on plain films, CT is often the first study ordered in the evaluation of patients with back pain.

▶ CT Myelography

As mentioned earlier, in patients who have undergone myelography, CT is often obtained immediately afterwards (Figure 13-6). It has been shown that a postmyelogram CT is more sensitive in the detection of pathologic conditions than is either test alone. This is particularly true for lesions within the spinal canal, such as disk herniations or tumors unassociated with a bony component. The presence of subarachnoid contrast allows dramatic visualization of the cauda equina nerve roots and spinal cord in a way that cannot be achieved with regular CT.

▶ MR Imaging

Since the early 1980s, MR imaging has gained widespread acceptance as the most sensitive imaging modality in the study of spine disease. MR imaging undeniably allows visualization of intraspinal anatomy with much higher contrast

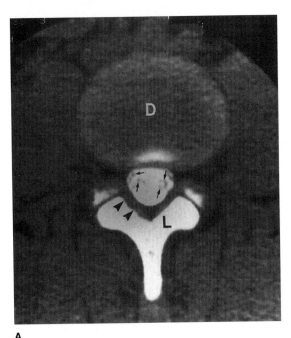

A

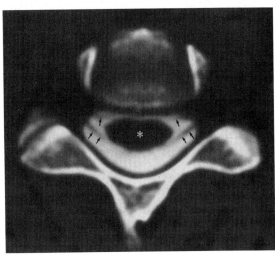

B

Figure 13-6. Postmyelographic CT. (**A**) Lumbar spine, soft-tissue window through L4-5 disk space. Dense contrast can be seen surrounding the small cauda equina nerve roots (arrows). D, disk; L, lamina; arrowheads, ligamentum flavum. (**B**) Cervical spine, bone window, disk space level. Spinal cord is easily seen (∗). Dorsal and ventral nerve roots can be seen as they leave the cord and join to form spinal nerve (arrows).

resolution than does any other modality. The ability to image directly in the sagittal and coronal planes contributes a great deal to the evaluation of the diseased spine. A description of the physics of MR imaging is beyond the scope of this chapter, and the reader is referred elsewhere for this information. Because dense cortical bone has few mobile protons (which are necessary to create an MR signal), MR imaging is sometimes limited in its ability to demonstrate either osteophytes that may be a source of clinical symptoms or calcific components of other lesions. In such cases, CT with its superb depiction of bony detail may be useful as an adjunct examination. On the other hand, MR imaging is very sensitive in its ability to detect abnormalities in bone marrow. The vertebral bodies normally contain a large amount of bone marrow, and an abnormal appearance may be seen in a variety of disorders, such as anemia, infection, and metastatic disease.

MR images can be obtained with a variety of "sequences." The most commonly utilized are called "spin-echo," and these can be "weighted" for either T1 or T2. (A thorough explanation of these parameters can be found elsewhere). On a T1-weighted image, normal adult (yellow/fatty) bone marrow has a "high signal" (ie, it is hyperintense, whitish in color), and CSF has a "low signal" (ie, it is hypointense, or

black in color). Neural tissue, such as the spinal cord or nerve roots, is intermediate in signal intensity (Figure 13-7 A). Cortical bone, lacking mobile protons to produce a signal, is hypointense on all pulse sequences. On T2-weighted images, marrow becomes lower in signal intensity, CSF becomes hyperintense, and neural tissue maintains an intermediate signal intensity. However, the spinal cord appears relatively lower in signal intensity, surrounded as it is by CSF that is hyperintense (Figure 13-7 B). The intervertebral disks in normal individuals are typically of intermediate signal on T1-weighted images and, because of their water content, appear hyperintense on T2-weighted images. Any alterations in the expected normal signal intensity for an anatomic structure should prompt a search for either a technical or a pathologic explanation for the abnormal signal. Postcontrast imaging, scanning after administration of intravenous gadolinium (gadopentetate dimeglumine) or other paramagnetic contrast agents, adds valuable information to either clarify questions raised by the precontrast imaging results or permit detection of lesions that were invisible without contrast. In recent years, the use of fat suppression has increased the utility of contrast-enhanced imaging of the spine, particularly in the evaluation of lesions within the spinal canal (Figure 13-8) and bone.

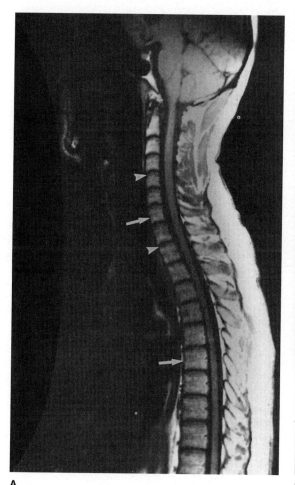
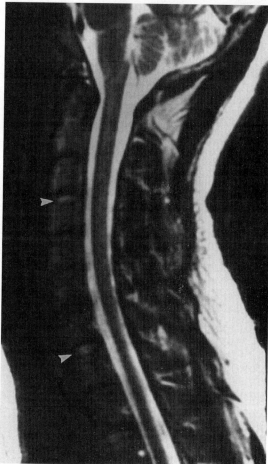

A   B

Figure 13-7. Normal MR images. (**A**) T1-weighted sagittal, cervicothoracic spine. The spinal cord is very easily seen. Note that the CSF anterior and posterior to the cord is hypointense, or low signal intensity. The high signal arising from the vertebral body bone marrow (arrows) is due to the fat content. The disk spaces are readily visualized and are of lower signal intensity (arrowheads). This is the normal relative appearance of bone marrow and disk on T1-weighted images. Any reversal (ie, disk is brighter or higher in signal intensity than marrow) should raise the suspicion of marrow disease. (**B**) T2-weighted sagittal cervical spine. CSF is now very hyperintense, and the spinal cord appears to have relatively low signal intensity. The disks (arrowheads), because of their water content (when normal), appear higher in signal intensity when compared with the T1-weighted image. The bone marrow, on the other hand, is lower in signal intensity (fat fades on T2).

TECHNIQUE SELECTION

A great many clinical circumstances may necessitate spine imaging. The purpose of this section is to convey a sense of which techniques would be most appropriate for the given clinical setting. In some instances, the choice is clear. In others, the test to be performed is determined by the technology available, and often the decision is influenced by the

preferences of the person ordering the test. In some clinical settings, more than one imaging modality is acceptable as a first test. If the clinician consults with the radiologist before deciding on the initial test, unnecessary examinations may be avoided. Perhaps most importantly, however, if the clinician consults with the radiologist and conveys to him or her the clinical information, imaging often can be tailored to hone in on the most likely site or type of abnormality.

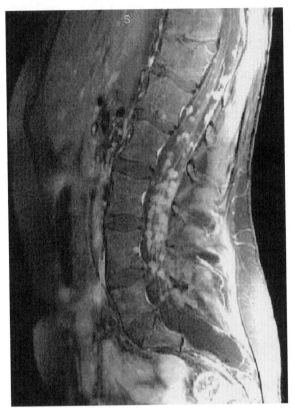

Figure 13-8. Sagittal fat-suppressed, contrast-enhanced T1-weighted MR image. A 22-year-old female with metastatic Ewing's sarcoma presenting with back and leg pain and lower extremity paresthesias. Numerous brightly enhancing nodules indicate subarachnoid tumor deposits. Contrast-enhanced MR imaging may be the only way to confirm this diagnosis, as CSF cytology is often falsely negative.

Still, general guidelines can be established to help decide which imaging test is appropriate. What follows is a brief outline providing general imaging recommendations for common clinical problems related to the spine. Only rarely is a particular test the only useful one for a suspected abnormality. In many cases, any of the modalities would be useful as a baseline examination, with the understanding that additional imaging might be required to answer all clinical questions.

▶ Trauma

Plain films still are used as an initial examination for the evaluation of spine trauma in stable and alert patients. This is followed by CT scan, especially if other parts of the body are being assessed, the patient has altered consciousness, or the clinical examination is positive or equivocal. In the characterization of complex fractures, for conditions in which plain films were inadequate (eg, the cervical thoracic junction), or when additional information is required (eg, to rule out canal compromise by a bone fragment), CT is the best imaging study. In certain circumstances, such as suspected spinal cord injury (contusion or transaction), hemorrhage within the spinal canal, or ligamentous injury, MR imaging is indicated. It is also useful in evaluating the patient with delayed onset of neurological dysfunction after trauma to rule out myelomalacia (softening) of the spinal cord or posttraumatic syrinx.

▶ Back Pain

Back pain is one of the most common medical complaints. Though most cases are caused by muscle strains, new or persistent severe pain, sciatica (a shooting pain down the leg), or neurologic deficits such as weakness, decreased sensation, or abnormal reflexes should prompt a search for an underlying structural abnormality. The most common pathologic conditions are related to bony degenerative disease (osteoarthritis) or intervertebral disk abnormalities. Though disk herniations (protrusion or extrusion of the nucleus pulposus beyond the annulus fibrosus) are not visible on plain films, degenerative changes are generally quite apparent, and any unsuspected lesions such as compression fractures or metastatic disease (both of which are common in older patients) may be detected. For patients with a suspected herniated disk, MR imaging is the most sensitive examination. CT when combined with intrathecal contrast (CT myelography) is still a good examination for the detection of disk herniation, and it can be useful in patients who are unable to obtain an MRI. MRI is most sensitive for detecting disk abnormalities and is especially useful for the identification of other pathologic conditions that might mimic disk herniation, such as lesions of the conus medullaris or metastatic disease. A possible exception to the use of MR imaging as a first-line cross-sectional imaging procedure in degenerative spine disease is for patients suspected of having foraminal nerve impingement by an osteophyte. Osteophytes are small, sharp projections of bone that occur in patients with osteoarthritis, and they may impinge on the spinal cord or nerve roots. Such osteophytes in the cervical spine may be difficult to characterize with MR imaging unless special sequences are employed. However, it is not always possible to differentiate clinically between patients who have disk herniations and those whose nerves are compressed by osteophytes, and MR imaging is the best test to order for these patients.

▶ Myelopathy

In patients who are suspected of having a myelopathy (a true cord syndrome as opposed to radicular symptoms),

MR imaging is unequivocally the first study to be performed. MR imaging is the only imaging procedure that allows direct visualization of the spinal cord, and it is effective for diagnosing or excluding primary spinal cord lesions such as infarct, tumor, hemorrhage, or inflammatory conditions (eg, multiple sclerosis, idiopathic transverse myelitis, or sarcoidosis).

▶ Congenital Spine Lesions

A variety of congenital lesions may affect the spine. Plain films may be useful to initially survey the spine, but ultimately MR imaging is the modality of choice. Multidetector CT with multiplanar reconstruction abilities is gaining usefulness in evaluation of bone lesions and defects.

▶ Metastatic Disease

If metastatic disease in the spine is suspected, plain films are an economical way to carry out a preliminary evaluation for bony lesions. However, plain films do not demonstrate such abnormalities until a significant amount of destruction has taken place. MR imaging, on the other hand, is quite sensitive to replacement of normal bone marrow by tumor and can establish the diagnosis much earlier. Addition of gadolinium-enhanced MR imaging improves detection of bone lesions and of intraspinal spread of tumor to the subarachnoid space (carcinomatous meningitis or leptomeningeal carcinomatosis), if this is suspected clinically.

EXERCISE 13-1. DEGENERATIVE SPINE DISEASE

13-1. What is the abnormality in Case 13-1 (Figure 13-9)?
   A. The bones are too dense.
   B. The bones are not dense enough (osteopenia).
   C. There is a destructive bony lesion.
   D. There is an abnormality of alignment.
   E. There is a soft-tissue abnormality.

13-2. In Case 13-2, the lesion represented by an arrow in Figure 13-10 is most likely to be
   A. a right-sided L4-5 herniated nucleus pulposus.
   B. an extradural tumor.
   C. an epidural abscess.
   D. an intradural mass.
   E. a bony lesion.

13-3. In Case 13-3, the lateral cervical spine plain film in Figure 13-11 suggests that the *most* likely diagnosis is
   A. degenerative disk disease at C2-3 and C3-4.
   B. neoplastic disease at C4.
   C. degenerative disk disease at C5-6 and C6-7.
   D. traumatic injury.
   E. disk space infection at C5-6 and C6-7.

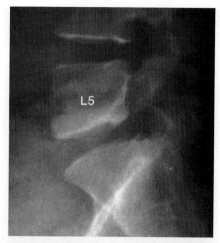

Figure 13-9. Case 13-1. A coned-downed lateral plain film of the lumbar spine in a whiny 45-year-old neuroradiologist who presents with low back pain.

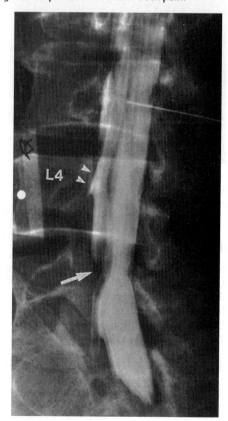

Figure 13-10. Case 13-2. A 58-year-old man with right-sided L5 radiculopathy. A myelogram was performed, and an oblique view demonstrating the right-sided nerve roots is displayed.

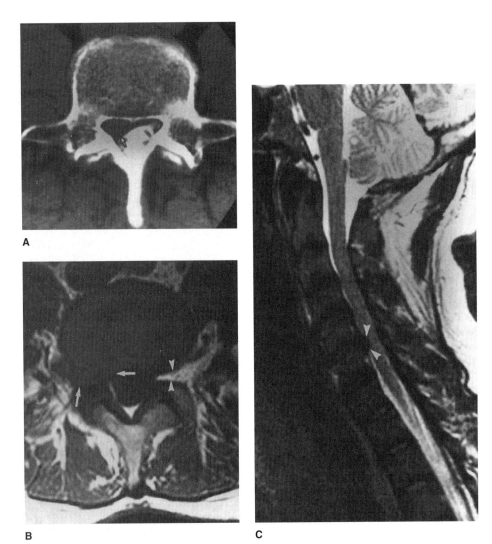

A

B

C

▲ **Figure 13-13.** (**A**) Axial CT (same patient as in Figure 13-10) just below the L4-5 disk space shows compression of the right anterolateral aspect of the thecal sac by the HNP (arrow). The image was obtained below the L4-5 disk space, indicating inferior migration of herniated disk material. (**B**) Axial T1-weighted MR image of a different patient shows a far lateral right-sided HNP (arrows) with replacement of normal foraminal fat by intermediate signal representing the disk. Note normal perineural fat (arrowheads) in the left neural foramen. A far lateral HNP such as this would probably be missed if only myelography were performed. (**C**) Sagittal T2-weighted image shows a midline disk herniation at C5-6 that is compressing the spinal cord (arrowheads).

13-5. In Case 13-5, what is the most likely diagnosis (Figure 13-16)?
  A. Sacroiliitis
  B. A sacral tumor
  C. Constipation
  D. Osteoporosis
  E. Uterine malignancy

13-6. In Case 13-6, on the lateral cervical spine radiograph in Figure 13-17, what is the main radiologic finding?
  A. A lesion of the C7 spinous process
  B. An osteoblastic bony lesion
  C. An abnormality of alignment
  D. A destructive lesion at C2
  E. A fracture

MR imaging is unequivocally the first study to be performed. MR imaging is the only imaging procedure that allows direct visualization of the spinal cord, and it is effective for diagnosing or excluding primary spinal cord lesions such as infarct, tumor, hemorrhage, or inflammatory conditions (eg, multiple sclerosis, idiopathic transverse myelitis, or sarcoidosis).

▶ Congenital Spine Lesions

A variety of congenital lesions may affect the spine. Plain films may be useful to initially survey the spine, but ultimately MR imaging is the modality of choice. Multidetector CT with multiplanar reconstruction abilities is gaining usefulness in evaluation of bone lesions and defects.

▶ Metastatic Disease

If metastatic disease in the spine is suspected, plain films are an economical way to carry out a preliminary evaluation for bony lesions. However, plain films do not demonstrate such abnormalities until a significant amount of destruction has taken place. MR imaging, on the other hand, is quite sensitive to replacement of normal bone marrow by tumor and can establish the diagnosis much earlier. Addition of gadolinium-enhanced MR imaging improves detection of bone lesions and of intraspinal spread of tumor to the subarachnoid space (carcinomatous meningitis or leptomeningeal carcinomatosis), if this is suspected clinically.

EXERCISE 13-1. DEGENERATIVE SPINE DISEASE

13-1. What is the abnormality in Case 13-1 (Figure 13-9)?
 A. The bones are too dense.
 B. The bones are not dense enough (osteopenia).
 C. There is a destructive bony lesion.
 D. There is an abnormality of alignment.
 E. There is a soft-tissue abnormality.

13-2. In Case 13-2, the lesion represented by an arrow in Figure 13-10 is most likely to be
 A. a right-sided L4-5 herniated nucleus pulposus.
 B. an extradural tumor.
 C. an epidural abscess.
 D. an intradural mass.
 E. a bony lesion.

13-3. In Case 13-3, the lateral cervical spine plain film in Figure 13-11 suggests that the *most* likely diagnosis is
 A. degenerative disk disease at C2-3 and C3-4.
 B. neoplastic disease at C4.
 C. degenerative disk disease at C5-6 and C6-7.
 D. traumatic injury.
 E. disk space infection at C5-6 and C6-7.

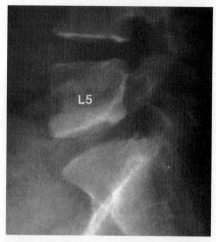

Figure 13-9. Case 13-1. A coned-downed lateral plain film of the lumbar spine in a whiny 45-year-old neuroradiologist who presents with low back pain.

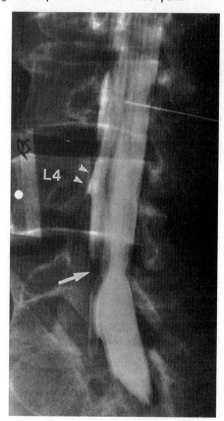

Figure 13-10. Case 13-2. A 58-year-old man with right-sided L5 radiculopathy. A myelogram was performed, and an oblique view demonstrating the right-sided nerve roots is displayed.

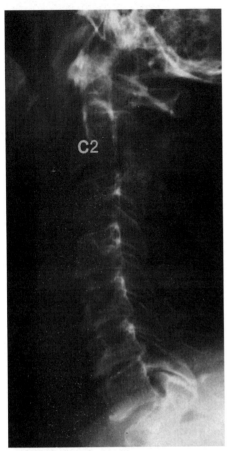

Figure 13-11. Case 13-3. Plain film of the cervical spine (lateral view) of a 53-year-old woman who presents with neck and right arm pain.

Radiologic Findings

13-1. In this case, there is subtle anterior displacement of the L5 vertebral body relative to S1, known as spondylolisthesis (D is the correct answer to Question 13-1).

13-2. In this case, an extradural defect is seen at and below the L4-5 disk space, and the right L5 nerve root does not fill. These changes are most likely caused by a disk herniation (A is the correct answer to Question 13-2). Note the normal filling of the right L4 nerve root (arrowheads).

13-3. In this case, there is disk space narrowing, and osteophytes are seen at the C5-6 and C6-7 disk spaces (C is the correct answer to Question 13-3).

Discussion

Degenerative osteoarthropathy may affect different parts of the spine. When the facet joints are involved, the result is often bony osteophytes, which may project into the neural foramen or spinal canal and compress neural structures. When the disk space is affected, bony changes in the vertebral body endplate can occur. In addition, the intervertebral disk itself may be affected, and disk herniation can occur as a result. Differentiation between disk bulge (generalized extension of the disk, less than 3 mm beyond the edges of the apophyses, with no significant compression of cord or thecal sac) and herniation (protrusion or extrusion, with possible compression of nerves or thecal sac) is not always possible. Treatment decisions must be based on clinical as well as radiologic data.

In Case 13-1 (author's spine), the spondylolisthesis of L5 over S1 is a result of a defect in the pars interarticularis. This is the junction of the superior and inferior articular facet of a given vertebra (Figures 13-3 C and 13-12 A). Spondylolysis, as this defect is known, is usually caused by a chronic stress fracture, though rarely it can be congenital or acute. If, as is commonly the case, the spondylolysis is bilateral, the vertebral body is essentially disconnected from the posterior elements, and this allows the anterior slipping, or spondylolisthesis, shown in Figure 13-9. This entity is included here because it is quite common and predisposes to premature degenerative disease. In older patients, spondylolisthesis can be secondary to degenerative disease in the absence of a pars defect, and this "nonlytic" form is known as pseudospondylolisthesis or degenerative spondylolisthesis. When present, the spondylolysis defect is readily identified on oblique lumbar plain films, as a "broken neck on the Scottie dog" (Figure 13-12 B). The lysis defect is also readily detected on CT (Figure 13-12 C), although it may superficially resemble a facet joint.

Disk herniations are a common medical problem. Though they can usually be diagnosed with noninvasive CT or MR imaging, myelography is still employed in some places to diagnose disk herniations. In Case 13-2, Figure 13-10 shows an extradural defect, seen as an area of low density distorting the lateral aspect of the thecal sac, deviating the nerve roots. This is the typical appearance of a herniated nucleus pulposus (HNP) on myelography. We see the effect of the herniated disk rather than visualizing the actual disk abnormality. On a CT study, the herniated disk can also be visualized (Figure 13-13 A). Most of the myelographic filling defect can be seen to be below the L4-5 disk space, secondary to inferior migration of disk material. This helps explain why the patient had an L5 radiculopathy. The right L4 nerve root (arrowheads in Figure 13-10) had already exited and would be unaffected by an L4-5 HNP unless it was far lateral (Figure 13-13 B). As previously mentioned, MR imaging is excellent in detecting disk herniations (Figures 13-13 B, C) and eliminates the need for painful, invasive procedures such as myelography.

Osteophytic ridging is a common manifestation of degenerative bone disease and in the cervical spine may cause myelopathy (if the cord is compressed) or radiculopathy (if a nerve root is compressed). In Case 13-3, Figure 13-11 shows marked narrowing and osteophyte formation at C5-6 and C6-7. An oblique

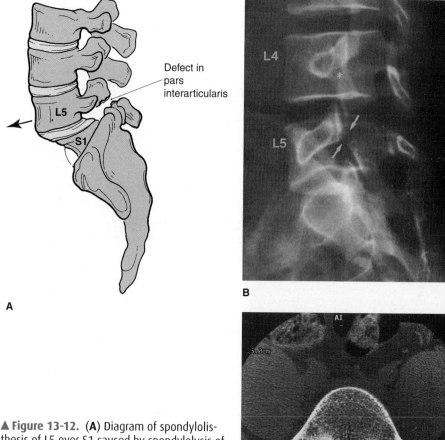

▲ **Figure 13-12.** (**A**) Diagram of spondylolisthesis of L5 over S1 caused by spondylolysis of L5. (**B**) Oblique plain film of lumbar spine (same patient as in Figure 13-9) demonstrates a spondylolysis or pars defect on the right side at L5 (arrows). Note the intact pars at L4 (∗). (**C**) CT bone window of a different patient shows spondylolysis defects (arrows). Though these resemble facet joints, they are more horizontal in orientation and more irregular, lacking a smooth cortical margin.

radiograph is useful in identifying the foraminal compromise that can result if osteophytes occur in that location (Figure 13-14 A). Myelography can demonstrate effacement of nerve roots (Figure 13-14 B). CT, with or without intrathecal contrast material, is excellent in depicting foraminal stenosis caused by osteophytes (Figure 13-14 C). MR imaging may be limited in its ability to depict subtle bony abnormalities, although utilization of newer high-resolution sequences have resulted in improved detection of foraminal stenosis.

EXERCISE 13-2. NEOPLASTIC SPINE DISEASE

13-4. In Case 13-4, what does this the AP view from a thoracic myelogram in Figure 13-15 show?
   A. A bony abnormality
   B. An extradural mass
   C. An intradural-extramedullary mass
   D. An intramedullary mass
   E. A really big disk herniation

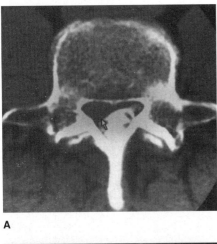

A

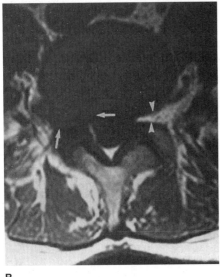

B

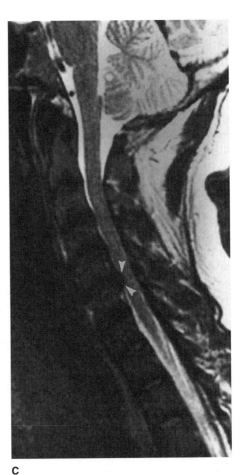

C

▲ **Figure 13-13.** (**A**) Axial CT (same patient as in Figure 13-10) just below the L4-5 disk space shows compression of the right anterolateral aspect of the thecal sac by the HNP (arrow). The image was obtained below the L4-5 disk space, indicating inferior migration of herniated disk material. (**B**) Axial T1-weighted MR image of a different patient shows a far lateral right-sided HNP (arrows) with replacement of normal foraminal fat by intermediate signal representing the disk. Note normal perineural fat (arrowheads) in the left neural foramen. A far lateral HNP such as this would probably be missed if only myelography were performed. (**C**) Sagittal T2-weighted image shows a midline disk herniation at C5-6 that is compressing the spinal cord (arrowheads).

13-5. In Case 13-5, what is the most likely diagnosis (Figure 13-16)?
   A. Sacroiliitis
   B. A sacral tumor
   C. Constipation
   D. Osteoporosis
   E. Uterine malignancy

13-6. In Case 13-6, on the lateral cervical spine radiograph in Figure 13-17, what is the main radiologic finding?
   A. A lesion of the C7 spinous process
   B. An osteoblastic bony lesion
   C. An abnormality of alignment
   D. A destructive lesion at C2
   E. A fracture

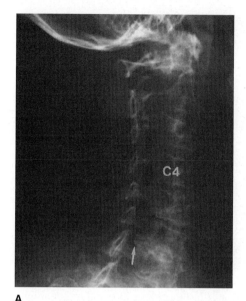

A

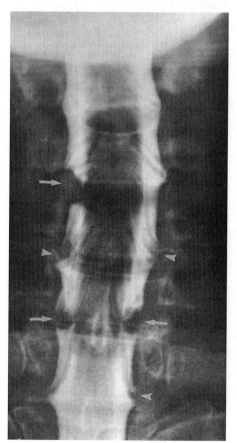

B

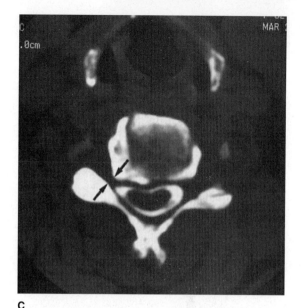

C

▲ **Figure 13-14.** **(A)** Oblique radiograph shows compromise of the right C6-7 neural foramen by osteophytes (arrow). Note that the other foramina are patent. **(B)** AP view, cervical myelogram of a different patient. Effaced nerve roots (arrows) can be seen as defects larger than would be expected for a normal nerve root. Compare with normal nerve roots (arrowheads). **(C)** Axial postmyelographic CT of same patient shows narrowing of the right neural foramen (arrows). The contralateral neural foramen is normal.

13-7. In Case 13-7, Figure 13-18, what diagnostic possibilities should be most seriously considered?
   A. Congenital or traumatic lesions
   B. Metabolic or endocrine disease
   C. Myeloma or metastatic disease
   D. Infectious or inflammatory disease
   E. Degenerative or inflammatory disease

Radiologic Findings

13-4. In this case, the patient has a lower thoracic primary spinal cord astrocytoma (D is the correct answer to Question 13-4). The cord is normal inferiorly but is seen to get wider toward the middle of the image. The contrast column on either side of the lesion is narrowed, most noticeably on the patient's right. This lesion has caused a "block" to the flow of contrast. Subsequent postmyelography CT (Figure 13-19 A) confirmed the spinal cord enlargement. An MR image demonstrated the tumor (Figure 13-19 B) within the spinal cord.

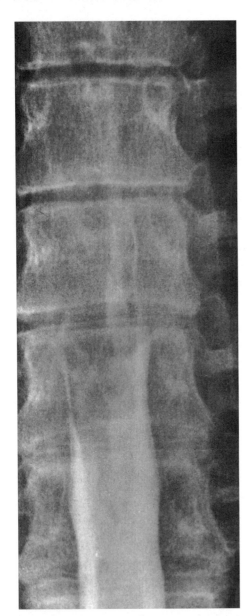

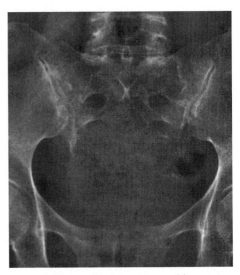

▲ **Figure 13-16.** Case 13-5. A 70-year-old woman presents with a 5-year history of back pain and recent onset of paresthesia in the groin and inner thighs (saddle distribution).

▲ **Figure 13-15.** Case 13-4. A thoracic myelogram in a 39-year-old man who presents with leg pain and weakness. A prior lumbar spine MR examination was normal.

13-5. In this case, the plain film shows a large destructive mass replacing most of the lower sacrum (B is the correct answer to Question 13-5). Notice how normal bone disappears below the midsacrum. A CT showed a large destructive mass with areas of calcification (Figure 13-20).

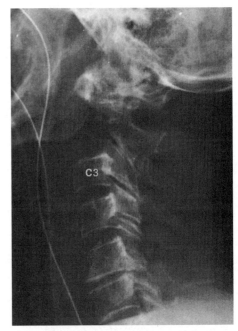

▲ **Figure 13-17.** Case 13-6. A 63-year-old man presents with severe upper neck pain not responding to anti-inflammatory medication.

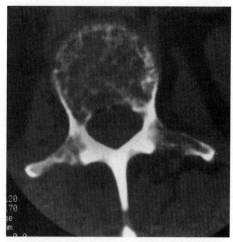

▲ **Figure 13-18.** Case 13-7. A CT bone window in a 65-year-old man who presents with back pain.

13-6. In this case, the plain film shows that the body of C2 has been destroyed (lytic destruction) (D is the correct answer to Question 13-6).

13-7. In this case, the CT image shows multiple small areas of lytic bony destruction. This is characteristic of either multiple myeloma or metastatic disease (C is the correct answer to Question 13-7).

Discussion

Primary tumors of the spine can arise from the bone or the neural elements. In Case 13-4, the diagnosis was primary spinal cord glioma. The two most common spinal cord tumors are astrocytomas and ependymomas. As with this patient, the diagnosis may be elusive for some time while other diseases such as disk herniation are ruled out. This patient even had a normal lumbar MR examination several months prior to the myelogram. Although the thoracolumbar junction is usually visualized on a lumbar MR imaging study, this tumor (at T10) was just missed. A thoracic MR examination would certainly have made the diagnosis, but the patient's doctor ordered a myelogram. Spinal cord tumors are generally very difficult to treat. The more malignant ones, usually astrocytomas, are associated with a poor prognosis. Ependymomas, because they are less infiltrative and more readily resectable, are associated with a much better prognosis.

Primary bone tumors can be benign or malignant. In the sacrum, giant-cell tumor is the most common benign tumor. The most common primary sacral malignancy is chordoma. This is the diagnosis in Case 13-5. Chordomas develop from remnants of the embryonic notochord and represent 2% to 4% of primary malignant bone tumors. The sacrum is the most common site for chordoma, accounting for 50% of these lesions. The skull base accounts for 35% and other vertebrae

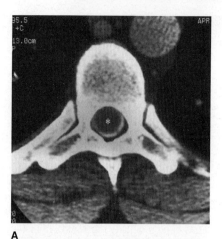

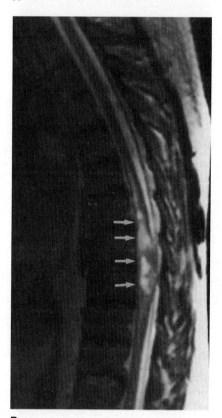

▲ **Figure 13-19. (A)** Axial postmyelographic CT demonstrates enlargement of the spinal cord (asterisk), representing tumor, with narrowing of the subarachnoid/contrast space surrounding the cord. **(B)** Sagittal T2-weighted MR image shows the tumor and resulting enlargement of the thoracic spinal cord, with areas of central hyperintense signal (arrows) probably representing necrosis.

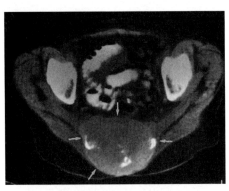

▲ **Figure 13-20.** CT study (without intravenous contrast) shows a large mass replacing the lower sacrum (arrows). Internal areas of high density represent either tumor calcification or remnants of destroyed bone.

account for 15%. Typical presentation of sacral chordoma is low back pain, paresthesias, or rectal dysfunction. Figure 13-16 shows the typical radiographic appearance of expansile, lytic destruction. On CT (see Figure 13-20), a large soft-tissue mass with internal calcifications is characteristic.

A common type of malignant spine tumor is metastatic disease, with lung and breast being the most frequent primary sites. Virtually any tumor may metastasize to the spine. In general, certain tumors tend to result in osteoblastic or dense metastases, and prostate adenocarcinoma falls in this category. Other primary malignancies, such as those in the lung and breast, tend to have osteolytic, destructive spine metastases. The patient in Case 13-6 had lung carcinoma, and Figure 13-17 represents a hematogenous spread of tumor to the C2 vertebral body. Metastatic disease may affect the spine by other mechanisms. Tumors adjacent to the spine may grow directly into it (Figures 13-21 A, B). This may occur in lung carcinoma and lesions such as neuroblastoma or lymphoma (with retroperitoneal/paraspinal lymphadenopathy). Finally, the spinal canal may be affected by spread of malignant neoplasm. Rarely, a metastatic lesion may occur in the spinal cord itself, usually as a terminal event. Metastatic disease may occur in the subarachnoid space by two methods. First, an intracranial malignancy (ie, glioma, medulloblastoma) can seed the subarachnoid space. These are known as "drop" metastases. Hematogenous spread to the subarachnoid space may occur in non-CNS primary tumors. Such involvement is known as leptomeningeal carcinomatosis or carcinomatous meningitis (see Figure 13-8) and is associated with a very poor prognosis.

Multiple myeloma is a disseminated malignancy caused by a proliferation of plasmacytes, typically occurring in the middle-aged and elderly, with a slight male predominance. The

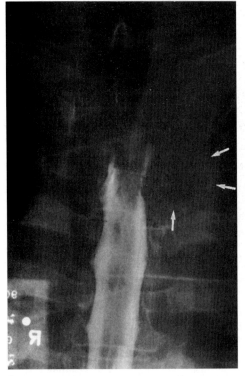

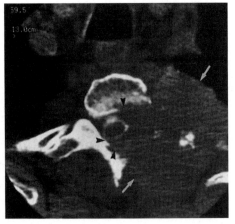

B

▲ **Figure 13-21. (A)** A 49-year-old man with lung carcinoma and direct contiguous spread into the spine. AP view, thoracic myelogram shows a mass in the left upper lung with bone destruction (arrows). The contrast column was blocked, and there was no flow cephalad to the lesion despite steep Trendelenburg positioning. The appearance of this block is typical for an extradural process. **(B)** Postmyelographic CT of same patient at the level of the block demonstrates the large lung mass (arrows) extending into the spine, destroying bone and involving the epidural space (arrowheads).

A

spine may be affected primarily or secondarily, and bone pain caused by pathologic compression fracture is the most common symptom. Plain films may be normal early in the course of the disease or show only mild osteopenia. Later, multiple, small, lytic, "punched out" lesions may be seen. CT is very sensitive, and Figure 13-18 shows the typical CT appearance of multiple myeloma. The findings, however, would be indistinguishable from those of small lytic metastases of other origin, and for this reason, metastases and myeloma are often mentioned together in the context of multiple small lytic bony lesions. MR imaging of multiple myeloma may have different appearances, but the typical pattern would be multiple, small foci of decreased signal intensity replacing the normal hyperintense bone marrow on T1-weighted images (Figure 13-22).

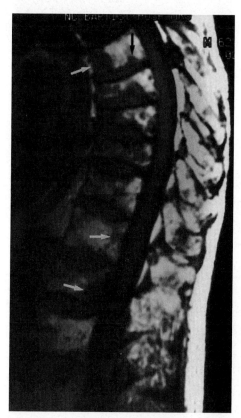

▲ **Figure 13-22.** Sagittal T1-weighted MR image of the thoracic spine shows multiple small hypointense foci of myeloma (arrows) replacing normal bone marrow. Compression fractures are also seen, indicated by loss of height of several upper thoracic vertebral bodies. The spinal cord is intact, but spread of tumor or retropulsion of fractured bone could result in cord compression. Note that metastatic tumor other than myeloma could have an identical appearance.

EXERCISE 13-3. SPINE TRAUMA

13-8. What is the most likely diagnosis in Case 13-8 (Figure 13-23)?
A. Spinal tumor, aggravated by trauma
B. Abnormality of bone density
C. Disruption of facet joints at multiple levels
D. Subluxation of L4 over L5
E. L2 compression fracture with kyphotic angulation

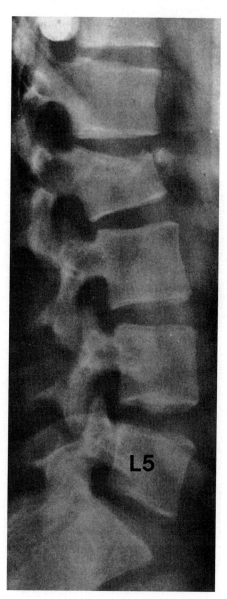

▲ **Figure 13-23.** Case 13-8. A 23-year-old woman was involved in a motor vehicle accident.

13-9. Regarding the patient in Case 13-9 shown in Figure 13-24, which of the following is true?
- A. The condition probably predated the trauma.
- B. The prospects for a full recovery are good.
- C. Surgical repair will likely be successful.
- D. The patient will probably never have normal neurologic function below C6.
- E. The spinal cord is intact.

13-10. In Case 13-10, the MRI in Figure 13-25 most likely demonstrates
- A. delayed posttraumatic syrinx.
- B. subluxation.
- C. spinal cord tumor.
- D. abnormal bone marrow.
- E. disk abnormality.

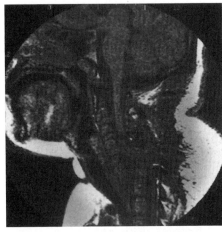

▲ Figure 13-24. Case 13-9. A 21-year-old quadriplegic woman had a motor vehicle accident 4 weeks ago.

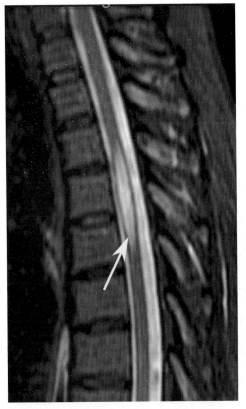

A

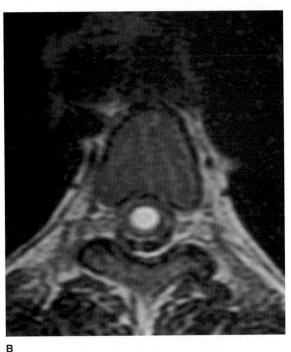

B

▲ Figure 13-25. (A,B) Case 13-10. A 38-year-old woman presents slowly with progressive upper extremity and upper trunk sensory deficits 3 years after a motor vehicle accident.

Radiologic Findings

13-8. In this case, there is a compression fracture of the L2 vertebral body with kyphotic angulation (E is the correct answer to Question 13-8).

13-9. In this case, the sagittal T1-weighted MR image shows a complete subluxation of C6 on C7 and a complete transection of the cervical spinal cord at that level. In all likelihood this patient will never regain use of her legs or have any normal neurologic function below C6 (D is the correct answer to Question 13-9).

13-10. In this case, the sagittal T2-weighted MR image shows a high signal abnormality (arrow) within the upper thoracic spinal cord, and on the axial T2-weighted image, an epicenter in the central canal region is confirmed. This is a typical appearance of syringomyelia or syrinx (A is the correct answer to Question 13-10).

Discussion

Spinal trauma is a major medical problem, usually caused by motor vehicle and occupational accidents. Accurate and complete diagnosis is essential to maintain spine stability and ensure preservation of neurologic function. As mentioned previously, plain films are commonly obtained initially. However, additional imaging tests are often necessary to fully evaluate a case of spine trauma, especially in high-risk injury cases, patients with clinical signs and symptoms, or those with altered cognition. In Case 13-8, there was clinical concern that the spinal canal was compromised. Small bony fragments within the spinal canal may not be visible with plain film alone. For this reason, CT was performed (Figures 13-26 A, B). This allowed a better appreciation of the extent of the fractures and ruled out neural compression. An example of spinal canal compromise is shown in Figure 13-26 C.

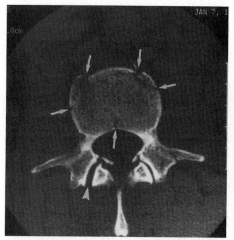

A

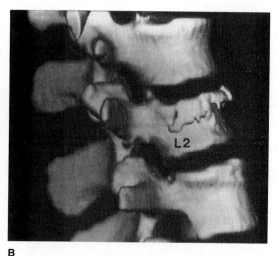

B

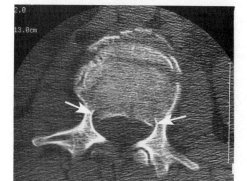

C

▲ **Figure 13-26. (A)** Axial CT bone window shows different components of the fracture (arrows). The spinal canal was intact. Note the separation of the facet joint on the right (arrowhead). **(B)** Three-dimensional reconstruction shows compression of L2 and fracture sites. Such reconstructions are sometimes useful in cases of spine trauma. **(C)** Axial CT bone window of a different patient demonstrates multiple fractures and retropulsion of a bone fragment, causing narrowing of the spinal canal (arrows).

In severe trauma, the spinal cord may be affected. Contusions may occur with or without fracture/subluxation, and MR imaging would be required for diagnosis. In a severe fracture/subluxation, the spinal cord can be completely transected. In Case 13-9, the patient was known to have a severe C6-7 subluxation, but because of obesity, plain film and CT imaging were very limited. In this case, only MR imaging was able to demonstrate the full extent of her spinal cord injury.

Rarely, patients who have recovered from an acute spinal injury experience a delayed onset of neurologic symptoms, occurring 1 to 15 years after the trauma. This suggests the possibility of delayed posttraumatic syrinx (Case 13-10). Symptoms include pain on coughing or exertion, sensory disturbances, or motor deficits. MR imaging is essential for diagnosis. The condition is sometimes amenable to surgical shunting. Syringomyelia can also be idiopathic or can be secondary to certain congenital or inflammatory conditions. Imaging often cannot distinguish among different possible etiologies, and history is important.

EXERCISE 13-4. SPINE INFECTION AND INFLAMMATION

13-11. What is the most likely diagnosis in Case 13-11 (Figure 13-27)?
   A. Spine metastases
   B. Posttraumatic changes
   C. Discitis and osteomyelitis
   D. Epidural abscess
   E. Degenerative changes

13-12. Regarding Case 13-12, what is the main abnormality visualized in Figure 13-28?
   A. None
   B. Artifact
   C. Subarachnoid lesion
   D. Intramedullary lesion
   E. Syrinx

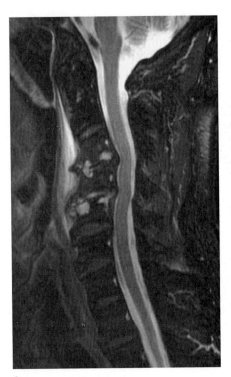
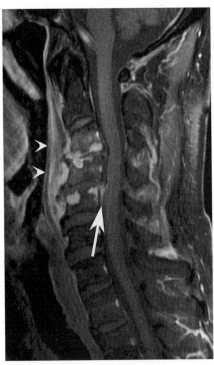

A   B

▲ **Figure 13-27.** **(A,B)** Case 13-11. A 44-year-old male with history of intravenous drug use presents to the emergency department with neck pain.

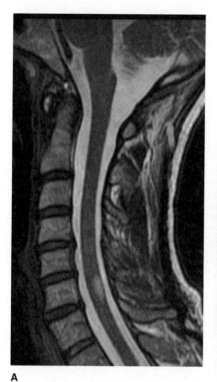

A

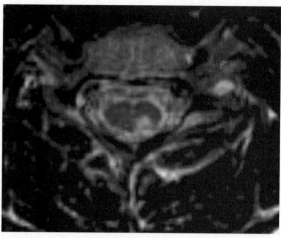

B

▲ **Figure 13-28. (A,B)** Case 13-12. A 35-year-old female with recent onset of paresthesias in her extremities.

Radiologic Findings

13-11. In this case, there is discitis and osteomyelitis (C is the correct answer to Question 13-11). Enhancement is identified within the C3-4 and C4-5 intervertebral disks with involvement of the adjacent vertebral bodies on the sagittal T1-weighted postcontrast images (Figure 13-27 A) and an increase in the T2 hyperintensity in Figure 13-27 B. Additionally, enhancement, T2 hyperintensity, and increased thickness within the prevertebral soft tissues from C2-C5 levels (arrowhead) is present. There is linear epidural enhancement seen at the C5 level (arrow).

13-12. In this case, the sagittal T2-weighted image demonstrates an intramedullary T2 hyperintense lesion at the C6 level that on the axial image is localized to the left posterior cord (D is the correct answer to Question 13-12).

Discussion

Spine infections include vertebral osteomyelitis and discitis, which occur most commonly as a result of hematogenous spread. Penetrating trauma, contiguous spread from adjacent

infection, or iatrogenic causes are additional routes of dissemination. The presenting feature is usually pain. A majority of the lesions occur in the lumbar spine, followed by the thoracic spine, with peak incidences between 60 and 80 years of age. *Staphylococcus aureus* is the most common organism in adults. Epidural abscess can result as a complication of osteomyelitis and is commonly associated with diabetics, patients with chronic renal failure, alcoholics, and intravenous drug users. Ventral location of the epidural abscess is usually seen in cases secondary to osteomyelitis. MR imaging has a specificity, sensitivity, and accuracy of 92%, 96%, and 94%, respectively, for detection of vertebral osteomyelitis. Imaging characteristics include increase in T1 hypointensity and T2 hyperintensity, along with variable enhancement in the intervertebral disk and adjacent vertebral body as seen in Case 13-11, Figure 13-27. Although T2 hyperintensity and contrast enhancement can be seen in degenerative changes, infection of the spine is commonly associated with paraspinal and epidural inflammatory changes.

Inflammatory diseases of the spinal cord can result from both infectious and noninfectious causes. The noninfective etiologies are more common and include disorders such as multiple sclerosis, acute disseminated encephalomyelitis

(ADEM), idiopathic transverse myelitis, Devic's disease, and sarcoidosis. Multiple sclerosis (MS) is diagnosed with temporal and spatially varied clinical signs and symptoms of white matter involvement supplemented by CSF analysis and MRI findings that are seen in more than 90% of cases. The cervical cord is more likely to be affected. Abnormality in the cord ranges from one to multiple lesions, although diffuse involvement of the cord can also be seen. Typically, lesions occupy a segment less than two vertebral bodies in length (Figure 13-28 A), are peripherally located within the posterior or lateral white matter, and involve less than half the cross-sectional area of the cord as seen in Figure 13-28 B. Presence of enhancement is thought to be reflective of active disease. ADEM is histopathologically inseparable from MS and can be differentiated from MS on account of its monophasic nature. Idiopathic acute transverse myelitis lesions, on the other hand, are frequently greater than two vertebral segments in length and clinically present with bilateral signs or symptoms as well as a clearly defined sensory level.

Acknowledgments *Special thanks to Stanley P. Bohrer, MD, for providing Figures 13-1 D and 13-3 C for use in this chapter. Thanks also to William Copen, MD, for providing Figures 13-28 A and 13-28 B for use in this chapter.*

SUGGESTED READING

1. Atlas SW. *Magnetic Resonance Imaging of the Brain and Spine.* 4th ed. Baltimore: Lippincott Williams & Wilkins; 2008.
2. Ross JS, Brant-Zawadzki M, Chen MZ, Moore KR. *Diagnostic Imaging: Spine.* Philadelphia: Elsevier; 2004.
3. Harris JH. *The Radiology of Emergency Medicine.* 4th ed. Baltimore: Lippincott Williams & Wilkins; 1999.

Index

Note: Page numbers in italics refer to figures; page numbers followed by *t* indicate tables.